TROPICAL ANEMIA

TROPICAL ANEMIA

VIROJ WIWANITKIT

Nova Science Publishers, Inc.
New York

NOTICE TO THE READER
The Publisher has taken reasonable care in the preparation of this book, but makes no expressed or implied warranty of any kind and assumes no responsibility for any errors or omissions. No liability is assumed for incidental or consequential damages in connection with or arising out of information contained in this book. The Publisher shall not be liable for any special, consequential, or exemplary damages resulting, in whole or in part, from the readers' use of, or reliance upon, this material.

This publication is designed to provide accurate and authoritative information with regard to the subject matter covered herein. It is sold with the clear understanding that the Publisher is not engaged in rendering legal or any other professional services. If legal or any other expert assistance is required, the services of a competent person should be sought. FROM A DECLARATION OF PARTICIPANTS JOINTLY ADOPTED BY A COMMITTEE OF THE AMERICAN BAR ASSOCIATION AND A COMMITTEE OF PUBLISHERS.

Library of Congress Cataloging-in-Publication Data
Viroj Wiwanitkit.
　Tropical anemia / Viroj Wiwanitkit.
　　p. ; cm.
　Includes bibliographical references and index.
　ISBN 1-59454-586-3
　1. Anemia.　2. Tropical medicine.　　I. Title.
　[DNLM: 1. Anemia--classification.　2. Anemia--etiology.
　3. Hematologic Tests.　4. Tropical Medicine--methods.　　WH 155
　V819t 2006]
　RC641.V57 2006
　616.1'52--dc22
　　　　　　　　　　　　2005034979

Published by Nova Science Publishers, Inc. ✤ New York

Contents

Preface

Anemia is a common health problem all over the world. The term "tropical anemia" means anemic disorders, predominant in the tropical regions of the world. The purpose of this book is to summarize and present the topics specifically relating to anemia in the forms that are unique in tropical countries. Due to globalization in the present day, a change in the epidemiology of diseases from one site to others all around the world can be expected. The summative on the common anemic problems in the tropical countries can be and should be performed. This book can make them at least realize and become familiarized with the problems. The details of this book focus on anemia in the aspects relating to tropical medicine. This book will cover specifically the clinical aspect, the scientific laboratory aspect, and the public health aspects as well as the social sciences relating to anemia in important tropical diseases. The common tropical diseases, including inherited disorders and infectious diseases, which relate to anemia will be summarized, presented and discussed. Mainly the book will present summative data from molecular to population scales, as well as additional meta-analysis for important topics. In addition, the diagnostic guidelines and clinical practice guidelines of the mentioned conditions will be presented. This work can be a useful reference for practitioners who are not familiar with the unique problems of the developing world and who might face those problems due to the possible migration of diseases. The academic level of this book is aimed at a wide range from the medical student, resident, general practitioner, specialist in hematology and tropical medicine to researchers in medical sciences. It can also be useful for medical personnel in allied health sciences.

Viroj Wiwanitkit, M.D.

Chapter 1

Introduction to Tropical Anemia

Some Basic Knowledge on Anemia

In laboratory medicine, anemia (uh-NEE-mee-uh) means the condition in which the level of hemoglobin is lower than the lower normal limit (-2 standard deviation: - 2 S.D.) [1 – 2]. In some cases, it can be easily referred to as a deficiency of red blood cells. However, sometimes the word "anemia" is used as a term for the condition called "pale". Indeed, "pale" is not equal to "anemia" but "pale" is an important manifestation of anemia. Recently, Kent *et al.* performed a study to assess the correlation of the bulbar conjunctival blood column (BCBC) with anemia [3]. In this study, observations of the palpebral conjunctival hue (PCH) and BCBC by two observers masked to the patient's diagnosis and laboratory test results were assessed [3]. The PCH and BCBC were correlated by slit-lamp examination with serum hemoglobin values, and different threshold levels for anemia were defined as hemoglobin <10, <11, and <12 mg/dl [3]. According to this study, the sensitivity of the BCBC and PCH for anemia was 83%-94% and 38%, respectively, regardless of the definition of anemia, but the specificity of BCBC improved with increasing hemoglobin threshold levels for anemia [3]. Kent *et al.* concluded that the BCBC is significantly associated with anemia, with higher sensitivity and only slightly less specificity than PCH [3].

According to the definition of anemia, it is necessary to perform a laboratory investigation to document an anemic case. The hematological investigation that is necessary for detection of anemia is hemoglobin determination or hemoglobinometry.

Naturally, hemoglobin is a red blood cell pigment, consisting of globin and heme. This red blood cell pigment's main function is to carry oxygen from the lung to the tissue. At present, there are many methods for hemoglobin determination. Those methods for hemoglobinometry can be grouped into 5 main classes depending on the basic technique as colorimetric methods, gasometric methods, specific gravity methods, chemical methods and mathematical model methods (Table 1.1). Of those several methods, cyanmethemoglobin method, a colorimetric method, is the standard reference method [1]. The principle of this method is that when blood is mixed with a solution containing potassium ferricyanide and potassium cyanide (Drabkin's solution), the potassium ferricyanide oxidizes iron to form methemoglobin. The potassium cyanide then combines with methemoglobin to form cyanmethemoglobin, which is a stable color pigment read photometrically at a wave length of 540nm [1,4 - 5] (Figure 1.1). The advantages of this method are a) the measurement covers all forms of hemoglobin except sulfhemoglobin, b) standardization is not difficult and c) the reagent, Drabkin's solution, is very stable [1, 4 - 5]. The reference value of hemoglobin by this method depends on age and sex. For male and female adults, the reference values are equal to 15 gm/dL and 14 gm/dL, respectively. Concerning the WHO criteria for anemia, the cutoff hemoglobin value is equal to 11 gm/dL [1 – 2].

Table 1.1. Comparison between the main hemoglobin determination methods [1, 4 – 5]

Aspects	Colorimetric	Gasometric	Specific gravity	Chemical	Mathematical model
Basic principle	Measurement of color change	Measurement of gas change	Measurement of specific gravity	Measurement of chemical reaction	Measurement by calculation
Disadvantage	Require specific reagent	Require specific analyzer	Poor coverage	Poor coverage	Lack of accuracy
Advantage	Easy to perform, stable	Hard to perform	Easy to perform	Easy to perform	Low cost

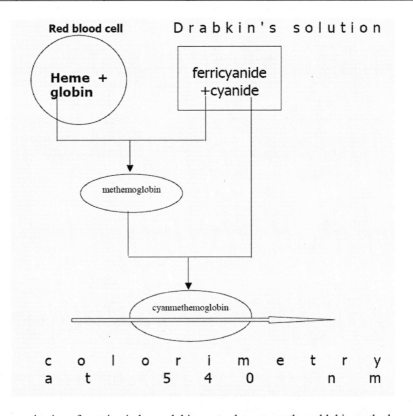

Figure 1.1. Summarization of reaction in hemoglobinometry by cyanmethemoblobin method

The other hematological investigation widely used for detection of anemia is hematocrit determination. Indeed, hematocrit determination cannot replace the hemoglobin determination, especially in abnormal cases. In 1982, Bhokaisawan and Chinayon proposed the correlation between hemoglobin and hematocrit as " $Y = 2.62X + 3.67$ " when Y means hematocrit and X means hemoglobin [6]. In addition, according to this study, the good correlation between hematocrit and hemoglobin, as shown by coefficient of correlation (r) equal to 0.98 and p value less than 0.001, can be seen [6]. The validity of the equation had also been verified, since the actually measured hematocrit values of 30 patients were not statistically different from the calculated ones [6]. It can be estimated that the hemoglobin was equal to hematocrit divided by 3 [6]. In 1995, Chung *et al.* performed a rheological study to assess the relations among hemoglobin contents, hematocrit and viscosity of hemosome and found that the hemoglobin content correlated with viscosity of hemosome but not with hematocrit [7]. The rheological equation as "viscosity = 0.315 ln (hemoglobin contents) + 0.435" was proposed [7].

However, before diagnosis of anemia by the hematological laboratory investigation, the patient must be suspected for this disorder. The symptomatology of the anemia is therefore the necessary basic knowledge for the general practitioners. In medicine, the anemia is a disorder with a wide spectrum of clinical manifestation, ranging from asymptomatic to arrest, however, the common manifestation is paleness. The complete history taking and physical examination to formulate the hypothesis of the existence of anemia in the patients before laboratory determination is rational (Figure 1.2).

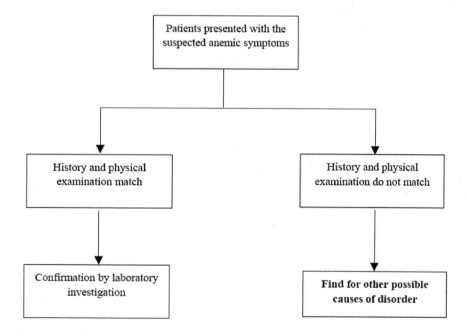

Figure 1.2. Conceptual framework in diagnosis of anemia

After confirming the existence of anemia by laboratory determination, the next step in coping with anemia is classification of the anemic disorder. There are several methods for the classification of anemia, however, the two frequently used methods are pathophysiological and morphological classification. Using pathophysiological classification, two main groups of anemia, decreased red blood cell production and increased red blood cell destruction can be derived. The first group, decreased red blood production, might result from the nutritional deficiency (such as iron deficiency anemia, folate deficiency anemia and vitamin B12 deficiency anemia) or bone marrow disorder (such as aplastic anemia, leukemic infiltration of bone marrow). The later group, increased red blood cell destruction, might result from blood loss (both acute and chronic form) or red blood destruction due to defect (such as autoimmune hemolytic anemia, G-6-PD deficiency, thalassemia) [8] (Figure 1.3)

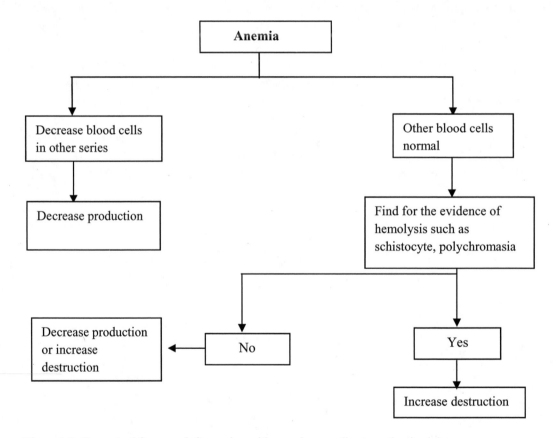

Figure 1.3. Conceptual framework for coping with anemia according to pathophysiology

The necessary laboratory investigations for morphological classification of anemia include blood smear interpretation and red blood cell index determination, especially for mean corpuscular volume (MCV) and mean corpuscular hemoglobin (MCH), by automated hematology analyzer. Using the morphological classification, three groups of anemia can be derived. The first group is hypochromic microcytic anemia, low MCV and MCH. This type of anemia is based on the protocol for patients who have an automated MCV of less than 80 fl [8]. The three most common causes of microcytic anemias are iron deficiency, thalassemia, and anemia of chronic disease [8]. The second group is normochromic normocytic anemia, normal MCV and MCH. This type is the largest, most frequently encountered anemia.

If acute blood loss can be ruled out, the diagnosis remains to be intrinsic or extrinsic [8]. Hereditary spherocytosis, drug induced anemia, and anemia secondary to other malignancies are a few of the anemias in this classification [8]. The last group is macrocytic anemia, high MCV. This type is less common than the previous two types. These anemias may be caused by marrow failure such as aplastic anemia and myelodysplasis, or caused by deficiencies of vitamin B12 or folic acid or caused by autoimmune hemolysis [8]. The MCV is usually greater than 100 fl. in macrocytic anemia [8].

Risch *et al.* proposed that the combined use of morphologic and pathophysiologic classification allowed for understanding and correct classification of anemia [9]. They also proposed that the determination of reticulocyte counts was of special importance, and further targeted biochemical, morphological and immunological analysis lead to the definitive diagnosis of anemia [9]. Although a large proportion of the anemias can be diagnosed and treated by the general practitioner, involvement of a haematologist is recommended in several clinical situations, such as newly diagnosed haemolytic anemia, as well as in patients with complex, equivocal or therapy-refractory anemia or certain normocytic hyporegenerative anemias [9 - 10]. In addition, Beris and Tobler proposed that no anemic patient should be treated by trial and error [10] (Table 1.2). The treatment of anemia can be easily planned by general practitioners. The best way for management is treatment based on the underlying pathophysiology. The anemias that resulted from decreased production required promotion of production. The methods for promotion of production are according to the types of anemia such as nutritional supplement for nutritional deficiency cases. Concerning the anemias that resulting from increased destruction, required a limitation of this destruction.

Table 1.2. Summary for the diagnosis and management of anemia

Type		Example	Diagnosis	Treatment
Decrease production	microcytic	Iron deficiency	• Iron study • Stool examination	• Iron supplement • Antiparasitic drug
	normocytic	Aplastic anemia	• Bone marrow study	• Bone marrow transplantation (BMT)
	macrocytic	Folate deficiency, vitamin B12 deficiency	• Vitamin B12 folate	• folate supplement • vitamin B12 supplement
Increase destruction	microcytic	Thalassemia	• Hemoglobin typing • OF test	• Blood transfusion (supportive) • BMT
	normocytic	Blood loss	• Occult blood • Reticulocyte count	• Blood transfusion
	macrocytic	Autoimmune hemolysis	• Antiglobulin test • Autoimmune profile	• Immunosuppressive therapy

Blood replacement should be considered in anemias of any origin if there are any overt anemic symptoms, such as fainting, and there is no contraindication for blood transfusion [11 – 12]. Hardy proposed that numerous theoretical arguments had been put forward either to support or to condone the classic transfusion threshold of 10 g/dL in the absence of definitive outcome studies and the limited data available from random control trials suggested that a restrictive transfusion strategy (transfusion threshold between 7 and 8 g/dL) was associated with decreased transfusion requirements, that overall morbidity (including cardiac morbidity) and mortality, hemodynamic, pulmonary and oxygen transport variables were not different between restrictive and liberal transfusion strategies [11]. Hardy concluded that the majority of existing guidelines were rarely indicated when the hemoglobin concentration was greater than 10 g/dL and was almost always indicated when it fell below a threshold of 6 g/dL in healthy, stable patients or more in older, sicker patients [11]. Last but not least, the follow up of the patients who have anemia is necessary. The follow up for the success of the treatment as well as the recurrent of anemia is indicated.

Tropical Anemia, What – How?

The term "tropical anemia" means those anemic disorders that are predominant in the tropical regions of the world. Several anemias are members of the tropical anemic group. Some important examples of tropical anemia are parasitic infestation – induced anemias, anemias due to nutritional disorders, anemia due to the tropical endemic genetic disorders. In other words, many common tropical diseases, including inherited disorders and infectious diseases, relate to the anemia.

Due to globalization in the present day, the change in the epidemiology of these anemic diseases from one site to others around the world can be expected [13]. The summative on the common anemic problems in tropical countries is therefore not limited to doctors in the tropics at present.

1. Factors Contributing to Tropical Anemia

Similar to general disorders in medicine, two main factors contributing to tropical anemia are inherited and non-inherited factors.

1.1. Inherited Factor

Pathogenesis of Disease

Several genetic disorders presented with anemia are unique to the tropics. Recently, Weatherall indicated that molecular and cellular biology had a great deal to offer tropical medicine [14]. Understanding the population genetics and dynamics of both infectious and non-infectious diseases, provides a new generation of diagnostic and therapeutic agents, and plays a major role in the development of management and approach to the control of disease in tropical communities [14]. The examples of those inherited diseases, which usually cause tropical anemia, are hemoglobinopathies and thalassemic disorders hemoglobinopathies found in tropical countries contribute to severe anemic disease cell anemia is a well-known tropical anemia caused by hemoglobinopathy. Fleming that about 120,000 infants are born each year with sickle cell disease in Africa, especia West Africa, and the majority had Hb SS, but Hb SC and Hb S/beta+ thalassaemia [15]. Another well-known hemoglobinopathy, usually mentioned for its high endemicity in the Indochina region, hemoglobin E is also the problematic tropics anemia at present [16]. The tropical splenomegaly syndrome subsequently from this hemoglobinopathy is a major tropical disease as well [17]. Principles of control of these hemoglobinopathies disoders are (1) early diagnosis through appropriate laboratory techniques and selective screening, (2) education of parents, patients, health professionals and the public, and (3) the maintenance of health at specific clinics [15].

The other common group of inherited tropical anemia is anemia due to inherited red blood cell enzyme defects. The Glucose-6-phosphate dehydrogenase (G-6-PD) deficiency is the widely mentioned defect leading to hereditary hemolytic anemia. G6PD deficiency is the most common enzymopathy in the world with the highest frequency values in tropical Africa, in the Middle East, in some areas of the Mediterranean, in tropical and sub-tropical Asia and in Oceania [18]. This genetic defect shows sex-linked inheritance and a marked heterogeneity and at least 400 abnormal variants with different biochemical characteristics and about 100 diverse mutations have been identified [18]. The most common clinical consequences are neonatal jaundice and sporadic haemolytic crises caused by a number of drugs, by infections or by ingestion of fava beans [18]. Salvati *et al.* Noted that since early diagnosis, education and epidemiologic surveillance had been proved to be cornerstones in the prevention of the haemolytic disease, therefore they should be taken into account in the national health programmes, especially in the tropical countries with high prevalence rates [18].

Response to Disease

Not only the effect of the inherited factor on the pathogenesis of tropical anemia, but also the response to disease are mentioned in tropical medicine. The inherited factor has been widely studied for its role in response to many diseases, especially for the response to tropical infectious diseases. Of those infectious diseases, malaria has been the most widely investigated. Lell *et al.* noted that red cell polymorphisms that confer resistance to severe disease are widespread in regions highly endemic for Plasmodium falciparum malaria [19]. They found that the severity of malaria is partly determined by the presence of blood group A and the sickle cell trait [19]. Lell *et al.*proposed that the different presentations of reinfections in severe versus mild cases probably reflected different susceptibility to malaria [19]. In 1999, Stirnadel *et al.* performed a study to investigate the effects of host polymorphisms on malaria morbidity and infection in Tanzania [20]. In this study, there were no differences in malariametric indices between infants with normal TNF alpha promoter gene and those who were heterozygous for this trait. The heterozygous cases for the sickle cell trait had significantly lower parasite densities, but similar prevalence, and MSP-2 infections compared to those with normal haemoglobin [20]. Stirnadel *et al.* found that the TNF alpha promotor polymorphism appeared not to have any protective effect on malaria in contrast to the sickle cell trait [20].

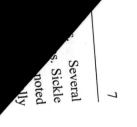

eptibility to the parasite, parasite susceptibility to the antimalarial gated. Le Bras and Durand mentioned that an established and low antiparasitic immunity probably explained the multidrug- rests of Southeast Asia and South America and frequent genetic um originate from a high level of malaria transmission, and stant prevalence brought to stabilise at an equal level as in Africa [21]. They also noted that resistance levels might place and time [21]. Finally Le Bras and Durand pointed out that in vivo and in vitro tests were insufficient in giving an accurate map of resistance, and that biochemical tools at a low cost were urgently needed for a prospective monitoring of resistance [21].

1.2. Non-Inhertied Factor

Sima Zue *et al.* proposed that despite enormous progress in medical science, health care coverage in poor underdeveloped tropical countries remains incomplete, uncertain and minimal and the probability of death is high in these countries [22].

Several inherited factors including malnutrition, poverty, poor hygiene, infections and pollution can bring trauma and illness; straightforward and consequently vital or functional prognosis is poor [22]. In addition, due to difficult field conditions and limited medical facilities in tropical countries, care is often delayed [22]. As a result, most patients are admitted with an advanced, complicated disease to facilities that are often poorly equipped, undersupplied and lacking in qualified personnel, and basic medication [22]. These situations are also the main problematic concerns for tropical anemia as well.

Nutritional Problem

Monte pointed out that despite recent world prevalence reduction, malnutrition is a major public health problem in developing tropical countries [23]. Monte noted that malnutrition, in any of its forms, contributed for more than 50% of deaths among children under 5 years in those countries and the mortality rates of severely malnourished children treated as inpatients had been unchanged for the last five decades [23]. In addition to children, nutrition in developing countries has also focused upon maternal nutrition with regard to the effect of maternal nutritional status on birth weight and lactational performance [24]. The current challenge is the proper use of the available scientific knowledge on nutrition to further reduce the figures for all the types of malnutrition in developing countries [23].

At present, tropical anemia is a common and worldwide problem that deserves more attention. The relationship between anemia and mortality and morbidity is widely studied. Micronutrient deficiency and especially iron deficiency is believed to be the main underlying cause for tropical anemia due to nutritional disorder [25]. However, some specific nutritional disorders are related to the local life styles of the populations in the tropics. A good example is vegetarianism, which can bring folate and vitamin B12 deficiency and subsequently megaloblastic anemia [26].

Kasili noted that anemia is the most common disorder in hospital patients in tropical Africa, and it is demonstrated in up to 70% of inpatients and nutritional disorder was the most common etiology [27]. Kasili also noted that although the anemia is multifactorial in etiology, the interplay between malnutrition and infection was still the most important element in causing the morbidity and mortality attributed to childhood anemia in Africa and that although iron deficiency is the most common cause of nutritional anemia, *Plasmodium falciparum* malaria is the leading cause among the anemias of infectious origin [27]. Therefore, the co-effect of several factors in anemic cases can be demonstrated and this should be realized by the general practitioners.

The effectiveness of interventions against malnutrition must be based on any approaches which reassure the confidence of health professionals about achieving positive results with the proper treatment of malnourished cases, establishment of an effective relationship between health professionals and the patients, as well as practical support to the patients and their families in recognizing them as valuable active agents for their nutrition rehabilitation at the household level [23].

Poverty

Poverty can bring several poor outcomes including low education, poor hygiene, infections and malnutrition, which can lead to anemia as a final result.

In other words, poverty leads to the lack of opportunity to get good health and brings many health disorders including tropical anemia. Recently Gomber *et al.*. performed a study to find out the prevalence and etiology of nutritional anemia among corporation school children from urban slums in India [28]. They found that childhood anemia continued to be a significant public health problem in those school children and iron deficiency, either alone or in combination, was the most common nutritional cause of anemia [28]. Gomber *et al.* also reported another similar study in India. In that study, prevalence of anemia, as judged by WHO recommended 'cut-off' value of haemoglobin < 11 g/dl, was 76 per cent while a comparable value of 74.8 per cent was derived by response to haematinic supplementation [29]. In addition, pure iron deficiency anemia (IDA) was detected in 41.4 % of anaemic children, and vitamin B12 deficiency alone or in combination with iron was diagnosed in 14.4 % and 22.2 % of anaemic children respectively.

childhood anemia continues to be a sig
by far the most common nutritional ca
is an important factor leading to anemi

Therefore, development based on
countries is necessary and become
Development stands for an improved q
standards, and higher income [30]. How
development: GDP per capita, average
been rising in almost all countries, i
decades, economic growth did not lead
[30]. Brinkmann also noted that the
economic growth were often different fi
urbanization could be described as one
affecting human health today, and po
countries where rapid urban growth has

One of the adverse effects of development, pollution has also been proposed as an important factor leading to tropical anemia at present.

Poor Hygiene

As already mentioned, poor hygiene can result from poverty. The population, especially the underprivileged group, in the tropics usually poses poor hygienic behaviors. Mata proposed that the physical environment in tropical areas and the socioeconomic characteristics of the population inhabiting such regions, favor maintenance and transmission of a variety of viruses, bacteria, and parasites that make agricultural progress and social development difficult, and they contribute to poor fetal growth, nutrient wastage, and deficient postnatal physical growth, accounting for most of the morbidity and mortality [32]. Several poor hygienic behaviors result in the nutritional disorder. Awated *et al.* performed an interesting study in India and reported the high prevalence of various nutritional disorders, anemia and vitamin A deficiency were the most common among them [33]. Wiwanitkit and Sodsri also reported similar findings; high rate of nutritional disorder and high corresponding poor hygienic behaviors among the children near the Thai-Cambodia border, where a high endemic area of anemia was located [34]. Awated *et al.* recommended dietary modification: improvement of school sanitation and personal hygiene, strengthening school health services and building awareness are the key strategies to cope with the problems [33].

Those poor hygienic behaviors can also bring several infections that can induce anemia, especially a round the world, geohelminth infestations. Control measures through improved sanitation, hygiene and de-worming are needed to prevent infection and re-infection and it can subsequently reduce the anemia [34]. UNICEF has supported many governments in the tropical regions to assist in the provision of water supply and sanitary facilities and intensive hygiene education in many schools through the Water, Environment and Sanitation (WES) program aiming at enhancing behaviour change in the population to break the routes of worm transmission and other waterborne diseases [34].

Infections

Many infections are prevalent in the tropics. Some of these infections can bring anemia. Examples of those tropical infections are anemia and hookworm infestation. Malaria is a well-known tropical infection caused by protozoa, *Plasmodium* spp. The vector of this se, mosquito, is common in the tropical countries, therefore, this disease is endemic in ics. Spielman *et al.* proposed that present public health entomology should focus on tion biology of vector-borne infections especially malaria, seeking to understand ogens perpetuate over time and attempting to devise methods for reducing the impose on human health [35].

station is another infestation that usually leads to tropical anemia. This harboring hookworm parasites in the intestinal lumen [36 – 37]. The well in the monsoon type climate, the nature of the tropics, and larvae, which can penetrate into human bodies [36 – 37]. In l countries pose poor hygienic behavior such as not wearing hus, the transmission of disease is easy. Iron depletion and ks of hookworm disease [37]. The course and outcome of pregnancy and development during childhood and the extent of worker productivity are diminished during hookworm disease [37].

Pollution

Exposure to environmental pollution remains a major source of health risk throughout the world, though risks are generally higher in developing countries, where poverty, lack of investment in modern technology and weak environmental legislation combine to cause high pollution levels [38]. Briggs noted that associations between environmental pollution and health outcome were, however, complex and often poorly characterized [38]. Briggs also mentioned that about 8-9% of the total disease burden might be attributed to pollution, but considerably more in developing countries [38]. To summarize, unsafe water, poor sanitation and poor hygiene are seen to be the major sources of exposure, along with indoor air pollution [38].

Some toxic pollutants such as benzene and other volatile hydrocarbons can induce anemia as well as malignant hematologic disorders. In addition, lead intoxication as a possible cause of anemia should also be a concern of physicians [39]. Kakosy mentioned that besides the classical, professional, and alimentary sources, the environmental pollution caused first of all by leaded petrol plays a more and more important role in the lead exposure of the people [39]. Both volatile hydrocarbons and lead become important pollutants in many big cities all over the world at present.

Arsine is another important pollutant mentioned for its possibility to damage the erythrocytes' membranes, resulting in anemia [40]. Badman and Jaffe also said that the extensive use of pesticides and herbicides might be associated with the development of Hodgkin's disease, non-Hodgkin's lymphoma, and aplastic anemia as well [40].

2. Magnitude of Tropical Anemia

Anemia is considered to be a common public health problem worldwide. Tropical anemia shows similar high prevalence in each region of the world, however, there might be differences in types of anemic disorders. Here, the summary of reports concerning the magnitude and patterns of tropical anemia in many tropical regions is presented.

South Asia

Khor said that prevalence of stunting and underweight were high especially in South Asia where one in every two preschool children is stunted [41]. Khor mentioned that iron deficiency anemia affects 40.0-50.0% of preschool and primary school children and nearly half of all vitamin A deficiency and xeropthalmia in the world occurs in South Asia, with large numbers of cases in India (35.3 million) [41].

While significant progress has been achieved over the past 30 years in reducing the proportion of malnourished children in these developing countries, nonetheless, malnutrition persists affecting large numbers of children and subsequently has resulted in a high prevalence of anemia [41].

In India, Awasthi *et al.* conducted a study to assess the prevalence of anemia among preschool children and its association with malnutrition in the rural Barabanki district of Uttar Pradesh, India [42]. They found that among the 67.3% underweight children the mean hemoglobin level was 9.85 as compared to 10.39 in those without malnutrition, and stunted children (87.6%) had statistically significantly lower mean hemoglobin levels than those not stunted [42]. In this study, the odds ratio of an underweight and stunted child having moderate to severe anemia was 1.66 [42].

Rao et al. also noted a high prevalence of intestinal parasitic infections and anemia that could be due to indiscriminate defecation, low socio-economic status, ignorance and low standard of personal hygiene in Madhya Pradesh [43]. In this study, a high prevalence of anemia, 86.7%, was observed [43]. Not only the non-inherited anemic disease, the inherited anemic disease especially the hemoglobinopathies are also prevalent in India. According to the study of Chhotray *et al.* Hb E was found mainly in higher castes like Khandayat and Karan, residing in the coastal region of Orissa [44].

West Asia

There are some interesting reports concerning the prevalence of anemia in West Asia. Kardiva *et al.* reported that the prevalence of iron deficiency anemia in South Iran was about 19.7%, less than the prevalence reported in other developing countries, however, higher compared to industrialized countries [45]. They mentioned that the nutritional status had improved, which was probably because of obligatory iron supplements given to the pregnant mothers and their under two year old infants, by the Health Care Centers [45]. Concerning the hemoglobinopathies, Beta-thalassemia is the most common hereditary disease in Iran. Yavarian *et al.* reported that IVS-I-5 (G-->C) was the most frequent mutant in the province of Hormozgan (69%), followed by the IVS-II-1 (G-->A) (9.6%) [46]. Najmabadi *et al.* performed a similar study in Tehran (34 %) and reported that IVS-II-I (G --> A) was the most common mutation while IVS-I-5 (7.55%), codons 8/9 (+ G) (4.76%), and IVS-I-110 (G --> A) (4.76%) were the other most common mutations. The difference in the prevalence of mutations according to the geographical sites of the two studies can be demonstrated [46 – 47]. Concerning the G-6-PD deficiencies, Gandapur *et al.* indicated that these disorders are common in the central region of Saudi Arabia and a lot of patients present with haemolytic episodes. They mentioned that the haemolytic crisis, however, was not related to the intake of fava beans [48].

Southeast Asia

Anemia is still an important public health problem in Southeast Asia.

This area, especially Laos and the northeastern part of Thailand, has been mentioned as a highly prevalent area for inherited hemoglobin diseases, especially for hemoglobin E disorders. Piyapromdee performed a study to determine the prevalence rate of anemia in pregnant women attending an antenatal care (ANC) unit at a tertiary hospital in Thailand by retrospective study and found that the prevalence rates of anemia in these studied groups was 2.95 [49]. The importance of those inherited hemoglobin disorders can be repeatedly confirmed. At present, several screening methods, including a new combination between osmotic fragility test [50], have been launched for screening in the ANC unit and added in national strategy.

Concerning iron deficiency anemia, the high prevalence can still be observed in some underprivileged groups of the populations such as the refugee. According to a recent study of Kemmer *et al.*, the prevalence of anemia in refugee children was 85.4% [51]. Also, another tropical anemic disease that should be mentioned for this area is malarial anemia. According to a recent study of Suyaphan and Wiwanitkit, a high prevalence of anemia among hilltribers in Mae Jam district, Chiangmai Province Thailand, could be seen [52].

Latin America

Iron deficiency anemia is still one of the major micronutrient deficiencies in Latin America [53]. Recently Cohen and Haas proposed a high prevalence of iron deficiency anemia (24%) in Costa Rica [54]. Many national strategies are suggested by the Pan American Health Organization of the World Health Organization (PAHO/WHO) for adoption by individual countries [53].

Similar to Southeast Asia, the chloroquine-resistant strains *P. falciparum* are widely spread in the countries of Latin America and can lead to a severe hemolytic anemia [55]. The importance of malarial anemia in Latin America should be mentioned as well.

Africa

Africa can be mentioned as the area with the highest poverty in the world.

Several tropical diseases are endemic to Africa. Van den Broek said that anemia was responsible for an estimated 20% of maternal deaths in West Africa and contributed to still more deaths through obstetric hemorrhage [56]. Van den Broek noted that those anemic disorders have been linked to iron and folate dietary deficiencies, the secondary effects of malaria and hookworm infestations, infections such as human immunodeficiency virus, and hemoglobinopathies [56]. Concerning iron deficiency anemia, Khosrof-Ben Jaafar et al. performed a study in Tunisia and found that the anemic children who suffer from an iron deficiency had shown an average supply of iron inferior to the required needs of 86% [57]. They also detected that 22.7% of these children had an available iron supply below the recommended average, which represents the limit of a severe deficiency risk [57]. Therefore, a nutritional supplement is recommended. However, Oppenheimer noted that several subsequent studies in Africa using oral iron showed many deleterious effects [58].

Concerning the folate deficiency, Allain *et al.* performed a study in Zimbabwe and revealed a large amount of occult haematological abnormality and interesting differences between rural and urban subjects [59]. They proposed that more attention be given to low levels of folate, an extensive problem in the community [59], which should be preventable by simple nutritional education. The nutritional supplementation for folate is another program corresponding with iron supplementation. Concerning parasitic –related anemia, malarial anemia is still the extremely problematic public health issue in Africa. In 1995, Guyatt and Snow performed a metanalysis for eighteen studies from areas with stable malaria transmission in sub-Saharan Africa and found that the median prevalence of severe anemia in all-parity pregnant women was approximately 8.2% [60]. If it is assumed that 26% of these cases were due to malaria, as many as 400,000 pregnant women might have developed severe anemia as a result of infection with malaria in sub-Saharan Africa [60]. In addition to malaria, the high prevalence of anemia relating to hookworm infestation is reported as well. Brooker *et al.* performed a study in Kenya and found that almost one-third (28.7%) were infected with hookworm and 76.3% of all subjects were anemic, with the prevalence decreasing with age [61]. Anemia was significantly worse in children with heavy hookworm infection (> 200 eggs per gram) and this relationship held for all ages, both sexes, and was independent of socioeconomic factors [61].

Concerning the inherited hemoglobin disease, a well-known hemoglobin disorder, sickle cell anemia is widely described in Africa. It can be said that Africa is the main birthplace of sickle mutations; the number of newborns affected by sickle cell disease is estimated at 200,000 per year [62]. Diallo and Tchernia mentioned that because of low family income and public health funding and, to a lesser extent, because of local beliefs about sickle cell disease, overall treatment of patients was still poor and, in some places, inadequate [62].

References

[1]   Lee GR, Foerster J, Lukens J, Paraskevas F, Greer JP, Rodgers GM. *Wintrobe's Clinical Hematology.* 10th ed. Baltimore:Williams and Wilkins, 1999.

[2]   CDC. CDC criteria for anemia in children and childbearing-aged women. *MMWR* 1989;38:400-4.

[3]   Kent AR, Elsing SH, Hebert RL. Conjunctival vasculature in the assessment of anemia. *Ophthalmology* 2000;107:274-7.

[4]   *Hemoglobin.* Available at *http://cls.umc.edu/COURSES/CLS312/hgbproc.doc*

[5]   Alison FS. An historical review of quality control in hematology. *Am J Med Technol* 1983;49:625-32.

[6]   Bhokaisawan N, Chinayon S. The correlation between hematocrit and hemoglobin. *Chula Med J* 1982 ; 26: 15-21.

[7]   Chung TW, Chu SN, Chen WK, Lee CJ. A rheological equation to express the relations among hemoglobin contents, hematocrits, and viscosity of hemosome. *Artif Cells Blood Substit Immobil Biotechnol* 1995;23:153-61.

[8]   *Thai Hematology Society. Anemia.* Available at Thaihemato.org/public/anemia.htm

[9]   Risch L, Herklotz R, Huber AR. Differential diagnosis of anemia. *Ther Umsch* 2004;61:103-15.

[10] Beris P, Tobler A. Differential anemia diagnosis. *Schweiz Rundsch Med Prax* 1997;86:1684-6.

[11] Hardy JF. Should we reconsider triggers for red blood cell transfusion? *Acta Anaesthesiol Belg* 2003;54:287-95.

[12] Goodnough LT. Indications for red cell transfusion. *Vox Sang* 2002;83 Suppl 1:7-9.

[13] Wiwanitkit V. Amazing Thailand Year 1998-1999 Tourist's health concepts. *Chula Med J* 1998; 42: 975 – 84.

[14] Weatherall D. The future role of molecular and cell biology in medical practice in the tropical countries. *Br Med Bull* 1998;54:489-501.

[15] Fleming AF. The presentation, management and prevention of crisis in sickle cell disease in Africa. *Blood Rev* 1989;3:18-28.

[16] Nusse GT. Haematological genetics. Part 2: Oceania. *Clin Haematol* 1981;10:1051-67.

[17] Crane GG. The pathogenesis of tropical splenomegaly syndrome--the role of immune complexes. *P N G Med J* 1977;20:6-13.

[18] Salvati AM, Maffi D, Caprari P, Pasquino MT, Caforio MP, Tarzia A. Glucose-6-phosphate dehydrogenase deficiency and hereditary hemolytic anemia. *Ann Ist Super Sanita* 1999;35:193-203.

[19] Lell B, May J, Schmidt-Ott RJ, Lehman LG, Luckner D, Greve B, Matousek P, Schmid D, Herbich K, Mockenhaupt FP, Meyer CG, Bienzle U, Kremsner PG. The role of red blood cell polymorphisms in resistance and susceptibility to malaria. *Clin Infect Dis* 1999;28:794-9.

[20] Stirnadel HA, Stockle M, Felger I, Smith T, Tanner M, Beck HP. Malaria infection and morbidity in infants in relation to genetic polymorphisms in Tanzania. *Trop Med Int Health* 1999;4:187-93.

[21] Le Bras J, Durand R. Molecular aspects of chloroquine and antifols resistance in P. falciparum. *Ann Pharm Fr* 2001;59:85-92.

[22] Sima Zue A, Chani M, Ngaka Nsafu D, Carpentier JP. Does tropical environment influence morbidity and mortality? *Med Trop* (Mars) 2002;62:256-9.

[23] Monte C. Malnutrition: a secular challenge to child nutrition. *J Pediatr* (Rio J). 2000;76 Suppl 3:S285-97.

[24] Walker SP. Nutritional issues for women in developing countries. *Proc Nutr Soc.* 1997;56:345-56.

[25] Van den Broek N. Anemia and micronutrient deficiencies. *Br Med Bull* 2003;67:149-60.

[26] Craig WJ. Iron status of vegetarians. *Am J Clin Nutr* 1994;59(5 Suppl):1233S-1237S.

[27] Kasili EG. Malnutrition and infections as causes of childhood anemia in tropical Africa. *Am J Pediatr Hematol Oncol* 1990;12:375-7.

[28] Gomber S, Bhawna, Madan N, Lal A, Kela K. Prevalence and etiology of nutritional anemia among school children of urban slums. *Indian J Med Res* 2003;118:167-71.

[29] Brinkmann UK. Economic development and tropical disease. *Ann N Y Acad Sci* 1994;740:303-11.

[30] Stephens C. The urban environment, poverty and health in developing countries. *Health Policy Plan.* 1995;10:109-21.

[31] Mata LJ. The environment of the malnourished child. *Basic Life Sci* 1976;7:45-66.

[32] Awate RV, Ketkar YA, Somaiya PA. Prevalence of nutritional deficiency disorders among rural primary school children (5-15 years). *J Indian Med Assoc* 1997;95:410-1.

[33] Wiwanitkit V, Sodsri P. Underweight schoolchildren in a rural school near the Thai-Cambodian border. *Southeast Asian J Trop Med Public Health* 2003;34:458-61.

[34] Luong TV. De-worming school children and hygiene intervention. *Int J Environ Health Res* 2003;13 Suppl 1:S153-9.

[35] Spielman A, Pollack RJ, Kiszewski AE, Telford SR 3rd. Issues in public health entomology. *Vector Borne Zoonotic Dis* 2001;1:3-19.

[36] Kucik CJ, Martin GL, Sortor BV. Common intestinal parasites. *Am Fam Physician* 2004;69:1161-8.

[37] Crompton DW, Nesheim MC. Nutritional impact of intestinal helminthiasis during the human life cycle. *Annu Rev Nutr* 2002;22:35-59.

[38] Briggs D. Environmental pollution and the global burden of disease. *Br Med Bull* 2003;68:1-24.

[39] Kakosy T, Soos G. An undying civilization damage: lead poisoning. *Orv Hetil* 1995;136:1091-7.

[40] Badman DG, Jaffe ER. Blood and air pollution: state of knowledge and research needs. *Otolaryngol Head Neck Surg* 1996;114:205-8.

[41] Khor GL. Update on the prevalence of malnutrition among children in Asia. *Nepal Med Coll J* 2003; 5:113-22.

[42] Awasthi S, Das R, Verma T, Vir S. Anemia and undernutrition among preschool children in Uttar Pradesh, India. *Indian Pediatr* 2003;40:985-90.

[43] Rao VG, Yadav R, Bhondeley MK, Das S, Agrawal MC, Tiwary RS. Worm infestation and anemia: a public health problem among tribal pre-school children of Madhya Pradesh. *J Commun Dis* 2002; 34:100-5.

[44] Chhotray GP, Dash BP, Ranjit M. Spectrum of hemoglobinopathies in Orissa, India. *Hemoglobin* 2004;28:117-22.

[45] Kadivar MR, Yarmohammadi H, Mirahmadizadeh AR, Vakili M, Karimi M. Prevalence of iron deficiency anemia in 6 months to 5 years old children in Fars, Southern Iran. *Med Sci Monit*. 2003; 9:CR100-4.

[46] Yavarian M, Harteveld CL, Batelaan D, Bernini LF, Giordano PC. Molecular spectrum of beta-thalassemia in the Iranian Province of Hormozgan. *Hemoglobin* 2001;25:35-43.

[47] Najmabadi H, Karimi-Nejad R, Sahebjam S, Pourfarzad F, Teimourian S, Sahebjam F, Amirizadeh N, Karimi-Nejad MH. The beta-thalassemia mutation spectrum in the Iranian population. *Hemoglobin* 2001;25:285-96.

[48] Gandapur AS, Qureshi F, Mustafa G, Baksh S, Ramzan M, Khan MA. Frequency of glucose 6 phosphate dehydrogenase deficiency and related hemolytic anemia in Riyadh, Saudi Arabia. *J Ayub Med Coll Abbottabad* 2002;14:24-6.

[49] Piyapromdee S. Prevalence of Anemia, Syphilitic, HBV and HIV infections in pregnant women attending ANC unit at Maharat Nakhon Ratchasima Hospital Maharat Nakhon *Ratchasima Hosp Med Bull* 1994; 18: 153-165.

[50] Wiwanitkit V, Suwansaksri J, Wiwanitkit V. Combined one-tube osmotic fragility (OF) test and dichlorophenol-indolphenol (DCIP) test screening for hemoglobin disorders, an experience in 213 Thai pregnant women. *Clin Lab* 2002;48:525-8.

[51] Kemmer TM, Bovill ME, Kongsomboon W, Hansch SJ, Geisler KL, Cheney C, Shell-Duncan BK, Drewnowski A. Iron deficiency is unacceptably high in refugee children from Burma. *J Nutr* 2003;133:4143-9.

[52] Suyaphan A, Wiwanitkit V. The prevalence of anemia among the hilltriber in Mae Jam District, Northern Thailand. *Haema* 2003; 6: 260 – 1.

[53] Cohen JH, Haas JD. The comparison of mixed distribution analysis with a three-criteria model as a method for estimating the prevalence of iron deficiency anemia in Costa Rican children aged 12-23 months. *Int J Epidemiol* 1999;28:82-9.

[54] Freire WB. Strategies of the Pan American Health Organization/World Health Organization for the control of iron deficiency in Latin America. *Nutr Rev* 1997 ;55:183-8.

[55] Loban KM, Polozok ES, Efimov LS, Khorin AT. Treatment of imported tropical malaria caused by chloroquine-resistant strains of P. falciparum. *Ter Arkh* 1987;59:69-72.

[56] Van den Broek N. The aetiology of anemia in pregnancy in West Africa. *Trop Doct* 1996;26:5-7.

[57] Khosrof-Ben Jaafar S, el Fazaa S, Kamoun A, Beji C, Farhat A, Cherif S, Haddad S, Gharbi N. Iron-deficiency anemia and protein-energy status in children aged 6 to 59 months in Tunisia. *Tunis Med* 2003;81:540-7.

[58] Oppenheimer SJ. Iron and infection in the tropicss: paediatric clinical correlates. *Ann Trop Paediatr* 1998;18 Suppl:S81-7.

[59] Allain TJ, Gomo Z, Wilson AO, Ndemera B, Adamchak DJ, Matenga JA. Anemia, macrocytosis, vitamin B12 and folate levels in elderly Zimbabweans. *Cent Afr J Med* 1997;43:325-8.

[60] Guyatt HL, Snow RW. The epidemiology and burden of Plasmodium falciparum-related anemia among pregnant women in sub-Saharan Africa. *Am J Trop Med Hyg* 2001;64(1-2 Suppl):36-44.

[61] Brooker S, Peshu N, Warn PA, Mosobo M, Guyatt HL, Marsh K, Snow RW. The epidemiology of hookworm infection and its contribution to anemia among pre-school children on the Kenyan coast. *Trans R Soc Trop Med Hyg* 1999;93:240-6.

[62] Diallo D, Tchernia G. Sickle cell disease in Africa. *Curr Opin Hematol* 2002;9:111-6.

Chapter 2

Malarial Anemia

Introduction to Malarial Anemia

Malaria is an important potentially deadly mosquito-borne disease characterized by cyclical bouts of fever with muscle stiffness, shaking and sweating , highly endemic in tropical countries, especially those in Africa, Southeast Asia and Latin America [1]. Malaria is the most important parasitic disease of people, affecting over 200 million people and causing more than one million deaths each year. Members of 3 anopheline species complexes, *Anopheles dirus*, *Anopheles minimus*, and *Anopheles manculatus*, considered to be primary malaria vectors, are also common in tropical countries [1]. Because of its dependence on human/vector (mosquito) contact, malaria is considered to be a disease of poverty. Underprivileged people in the rural endemic area become infected with malaria. Also it causes economic loss and impacts social functions. Despite decades of control success and a competent network of country-wide health infrastructure, malaria remains an important health threat in rural areas in the tropics [2].

Indeed, malaria is an old disease with a long history. First, this disease was believed to be due to breathing bad air, however, the protozoa in *Plasmodium* spp is identified as its true etiology. This disease can manifest a wide clinical spectrum from silent carrier to fatal shock. According to a recent report of Suyaphan *et al.*, the commonest clinical manifestation of malaria was fever (96.8%), followed by chills (in 60.6%) [3]. Interestingly, some unusual presentations such as petechiae [4] and jaundice [5] were also found. Concerning anemia in malarial infection, Rogerson *et al.* screened 4,764 Malawian women at first antenatal visits for malaria and anemia [6]. According to this study, a total of 42.7% had a malaria infection, which was more common and of higher density in primigravidae (prevalence = 47.3%) and teenagers (49.8%) than in multigravidae (40.4%) or older women (40.6%) [6]. In addition, prevalences of malaria and anemia were highest in the rainy season and the women with moderate/severe anemia had higher parasite prevalence and densities than women with mild/no anemia [6]. In 2000, Murthy *et al.* studied 158 consecutive cases of falciparum malaria with respect to the clinical presentation, complications, and response to treatment in Hyderabad and found that the frequently encountered complications were anemia (74.68%), jaundice (40.50%), cerebral malaria (45.56%), thrombocytopenia (40.50%) and renal failure

(24.68%) [7]. In 1998, Richards *et al.* conducted a retrospective analysis of hematologic changes in 89 patients with imported Plasmodium falciparum malaria and found that thirteen (15%) were anemic at presentation, 67% had thrombocytopenia, and 63% had lymphopenia [8]. According to those reports, malarial anemia is still an important presentation of malarial infection. General practitioners should know about this abnormality and manage it properly.

Genetic Basis of Malarial Anemia

At present, there are several investigations on the genetic basis of malarial anemia. Many genes have been shown to be involved in host susceptibility to the severe forms of malaria including malarial anemia, but it is likely that there are undetected malaria-susceptibility genes. However, the genetic molecular basis of this event has been unclear. Weatherall *et al.* mentioned that the pathophysiology of the disease, its protean hematological manifestations, and how carrier frequencies for the common hemoglobin disorders had been maintained by relative resistance to the malarial parasite has been of interest [9]. McGuire *et al.* found that severe malarial anemia was associated with the TNF-238 A allele, with an odds ratio of 2.5 after stratification for the HLA type. They suggested that severe malarial anemia and cerebral malaria were influenced by separate genetic factors situated near the TNF gene [10]. In 1994, Taverne *et al.* performed a study in transgenic mice and found that a factor in the anemia of human malaria might be macrophage activation caused by the secretion of TNF [11].

According to recent experimental animal studies, more than 400 genes in the brain and 600 genes in the spleen displayed transcriptional changes and dominant patterns revealed strongly suppressed erythropoiesis, starting early during infection [12]. Sexton *et al.* proposed that interferon-regulated gene transcripts dominated the inflammatory response to cytokines and these results demonstrated previously unknown transcriptional changes in the host that might underlie the development of malarial syndromes, such as anemia and metabolic dysregulation, and increase the utility of murine models in investigation of basic malarial pathogenesis [12].

Recently, Praba-Egge *et al.* performed an experimental study in animal model and found that the repeated malarial infection stimulated a wide variety of responses; most included expression of tumor necrosis factor-alpha, a cytokine that had been associated with inflammatory and host-destructive effects, which included weight loss, fever, and anemia [13]. In 2002, Gourley *et al.* performed a cohort investigation in Kenya and concluded that Interferon (IFN)-gamma and Interleukin (IL)-6 genotypes might play roles in the development of severe malaria and could contribute to the relative frequency of severe malarial anemia in exposed populations [14]. Bellamy *et al.* studied 1200 children in Gambia for polymorphisms of the intercellular adhesion molecule 1 (ICAM-1), complement receptor 1 (CR-1) and interleukin 1 receptor antagonist (IL-IRA) genes. They found that none of the polymorphisms typed were significantly associated with a severe disease, including malarial anemia [15].

The genes relating to the susceptibility to malarial anemia and the genes relating to malarial anemia resistance are also mentioned. In 2002, Hobbs *et al.* studied the NOS2 promoter polymorphisms with the primary hypothesis that it would affect resistance to severe

malaria [16]. In this study, they found that a novel single nucleotide polymorphism, -1173 C-
->T, in the NOS2 promoter was significantly associated with protection from symptomatic
malaria (odds ratio 0.12), and significantly associated with protection from severe malarial
anemia (adjusted relative risk 0.25) [16]. In 2001, May *et al.* performed a four-year
longitudinal study and proposed that associations were found between the HLA class II allele
DQB1*0501 and protection from malaria anemia and malarial reinfections in Gabonese
children. They also found that children carrying DQB1*0501 had a higher frequency of
interferon-gamma responses to plasmodium liver stage antigen (LSA)-1 T cell epitopes,
compared with noncarriers [17].

In addition to the general genes, the specific genes for common inherited diseases found
in the tropics are mentioned for their role in malarial anemia resistance. The effects of those
genes are believed to be good examples in natural selection process in the tropical area. The
first widely referred gene is the gene found in sickle cell anemia. The high frequencies of the
Hb S genes in the tropics are explained by their relative resistance against malarial infection,
and they may confer an advantage through lower infection rates or through lower
parasitaemia. Bienzle and Guggenmoos-Holzmann said that there is evidence that
heterozygote carriers of these genes are partially protected [18]. In 2002, Aidoo *et al.*
reported a study that HbAS provides significant protection against all-cause mortality, severe
malarial anemia, and high-density parasitaemia [19]. In their study, this significant reduction
in mortality was detected between the ages of 2 and 16 months, the highest risk period for
severe malarial anemia area [19]. Finally, Feng *et al.* proposed the increased frequency of
resistance in a population might be expected to decrease the frequency of malaria and reduce
selection for resistance over longer time scales [20]. However, they noted that possession of
the sickle-cell gene led to longer-lasting parasitaemia in heterozygote individuals, and
therefore the presence of resistance might actually increase infection prevalence [20].

Another hemoglobinopathy gene that is mentioned for its role in malarial resistance is the
hemoglobin E gene. Lachant and Tanaka performed a study in individuals with hemoglobin E
and found that those subjects had increased incubated Heinz body formation compared to
normal RBC [21]. In addition, The 2,3-diphosphoglycerate (DPG) content of the EE RBC
was increased to 5.59 +/- 0.69 mumol/ml RBC as compared to normal (4.51 +/- 0.77) and
there was a direct correlation between Heinz body formation and DPG content in the EE
RBC [21]. They proposed that impaired antioxidant defense might account for the persistence
of the hemoglobin E gene in areas where malaria is endemic, especially in Southeast Asia
[21]. In 1999, Hutagalung *et al.* performed a retrospective study in 42 patients and 175
controls to determine if hemoglobin E trait influences the course of acute malaria, adults
hospitalized for the treatment of symptomatic infection with Plasmodium falciparum [22].
They found that one patient (2.4%) with hemoglobin E trait had a severe complication of
malaria, while 32 subjects in the control group (18.3%) had one or more severe complications
including severe anemia [22].

Concerning thalassemia, there are several studies concerning the inhibition effect of ther
thalassemic gene on malarial anemia. Haldane's attractive hypothesis that the high gene
frequencies for thalassaemia in the tropical population may have resulted from heterozygote
advantage in regions where Plasmodium falciparum malaria was common in the past but has
been extremely difficult to verify at the population or experimental level [23]. Weatherall

mentioned that alpha thalassaemia provided protection against severe malaria [23]. In 2004, Cockburn *et al.* showed that RBC complement receptor (CR) 1 deficiency occurs in up to 80% of healthy individuals from the malaria-endemic regions [24]. They noted that this RBC CR1 deficiency was associated with polymorphisms in the CR1 gene and with alpha-thalassemia, a common genetic disorder in tropical populations [24]. They mentioned that analysis of a case-control study demonstrated that the CR1 polymorphisms and alpha-thalassemia independently conferred protection against severe malaria [24].

Concerning another commonly inherited hematologic disorder, Glucose-6-phosphate dehydrogenase (G6PD) deficiency, Ruwende *et al.* reported the natural selection of hemi- and heterozygotes for G6PD deficiency in Africa by resistance to severe malaria [25]. Saunder *et al.* said that deficiency alleles for this X-linked disorder were geographically correlated with historical patterns of malaria, and the most common deficiency allele in Africa (G6PD A-) had been shown to confer some resistance to malaria in both hemizygous males and heterozygous females [27]. Tishkoff *et al.* proposed that the deficiency alleles are thought to provide reduced risk from infection by the *Plasmodium* spp parasite and were maintained at high frequency despite the hemopathologies that they caused [27]. Another enzyme deficiency disorder that is reported for its resistant effect on malaria infection is pyruvate kinase deficiency. In 2003, Min-Oo *et al.* identified a loss-of-function mutation (269T-->A, resulting in the amino acid substitution I90N) in the pyruvate kinase gene (Pklr) that underlies the malaria resistance [28].

Finally, the abnormal genes in hereditary elliptocytosis (HE), a common disorder of erythrocyte shape, occurring especially in individuals of African and Mediterranean ancestry, probably confers some resistance to malaria [29]. Pathophysiologically, HE is mechanical weakness or fragility of the erythrocyte membrane skeleton due to defects in alpha-spectrin, beta-spectrin, or protein 4.1 [29].

O'Donnell *et al.* found that the degree of ovalocytosis was lower in children with Southeast-Asian ovalocytosis band 3 during acute malaria, suggesting that a selective loss of ovalocytes may contribute to malaria anemia in Southeast-Asian ovalocytosis [30].

Table 2.1. Summary on some genes that affect malarial anemia

gene	Description
1. TNF	macrophage activation promoting malarial anemia
2. IL-6	immune response induction promoting malarial anemia
3. NOS2 promoter	Increased NO production supporting to a protective role for NO
4. S	against malarial anemia
5. E	deformity of red cell increase resistance to malarial anemia

Pathophysiology of Malarial Anemia

The primary pathophysiological events contributing to fatal malaria are cerebral syndrome, anemia, and lactic acidosis [12]. Severe and refractory anemia leads to hypoxia and cardiac decompensation in malarial patients [31]. Those fatal malaria symptoms are common for falciparum malaria. Several mechanisms have been proposed to play a role in the pathogenesis of malarial anemia, such as erythrocyte lysis and phagocytosis, and sequestration of parasitized red blood cells [31]. Concerning erythrocyte lysis, it is believed to be due to several cytokine productions especially TNF [10]. Waitumbi *et al.* looked for changes in the red cell surfaces of children with severe malarial anemia that could explain this accelerated destruction and they found that red cells from patients with severe anemia were more susceptible to phagocytosis and also showed increased surface IgG and deficiencies in CR1 and CD55 compared with controls [32]. In addition, red cell surface CD59 was elevated in cases of severe anemia compared with asymptomatic controls but not as compared with symptomatic controls [32]. Waitumbi *et al.* concluded that the surface of red cells of children with severe P falciparum anemia was modified by the deposition of IgG and alterations in the levels of complement regulatory proteins and these changes could contribute to the accelerated destruction of red cells in these patients by mechanisms such as phagocytosis or complement-mediated lysis [32].

In 1995, Mohan *et al.* found that uninfected erythrocytes within the parasite culture revealed a significant increase in the lipid peroxide formation and susceptibility to lysis [33]. Furthermore, there was a direct correlation between membrane lipid peroxidation and peroxide hemolysis, both before and after monocyte exposure, suggesting a primary role of membrane peroxidation in red cell lysis [33]. Mohan *et al.* proposed the contribution of intraerythrocytic parasites and nonspecific activation of blood monocytes in the pathophysiology of erythrocyte damage and anemia of *Plasmodium falciparum* infection [33].

Concerning microvascular sequestration of parasitized red blood cells, Weatherall *et al.* said that after an acute malarial infection there was a steady fall in the haemoglobin level with an inappropriate reticulocyte response [34]. They proposed that this form of anemia might result from a combination of acute sequestration of iron in the reticuloendothelial system associated with a shortened red cell survival [34]. In addition, Davis *et al.* studied the mathmetical model of the microvascular sequestation phenomenon and found the mean fall in hematocrit over 84 hours in the patients conformed to a three-term equation [35]. Concerning the autoimmune hemolytic anemia, this phenomenon is very rare in malaria and not proposed as a common mechanism for malarial anemia [31].

Although those evidences support the nature of the normocytic normochromic anemia with hemolytic evidence of malarial anemia, recent data indicate that these mechanisms (singly or in combination) do not adequately explain the severity of this anemia [31]. Westherall *et al.* indicated that there may be a dyserythropietic component as well [34]. Westherall *et al.* proposed that although malarial anemia might be due in part to sequestration of parasitized cells, the haemoglobin level continued to fall for several weeks after the acute episode, and other factors should be involved [34]. It is apparent that severe dyserythropoiesis with minimal haemolysis plays a major role in the anemias of Plasmodium falciparum infection, particularly in immune individuals [34]. Hematologic studies have shown that bone marrow suppression and ineffective erythropoiesis contribute importantly to the severe anemia of malaria infection [31]. McDevitt *et al.* said that the host mechanisms were responsible for suppression of erythropoiesis might involve an excessive or sustained innate immune response or a pathologic skewing of the T-cell differentiation response with the attendant production of certain proinflammatory cytokines [31]. In 1998, Mohan and Stevenson performed a study in an animal model and found that dyserythropoiesis and severe anemia associated with malaria correlate with deficient interleukin-12 production [36].

McDevitt *et al.* also indicate that severe malarial anemia is associated with the immunologic expression of a circulating inhibitor of erythropoiesis that functionally antagonizes the action of erythropoietin (EPO) [31]. This phenomenon has been studied by both light and electron microscopy and by assessing the in vitro kinetics of erythroid precursor proliferation [34]. Chang *et al.* suggested that during malaria, EPO-induced proliferation of early EPOR-positive erythroid progenitors was suppressed, which might lead to a suboptimal generation of TER119(+) erythroblasts [37]. They concluded that the shift in CD71 expression may result in impaired terminal maturation of these erythroblasts, thus, inadequate reticulocytosis during malaria was associated with suppressed proliferation, differentiation, and maturation of erythroid precursors [37]. However, Verhoef *et al.* indicated that in asymptomatic malaria, the erythropoietic response is adequate for the degree of anemia, and that inflammation probably plays no or only a minor role in the pathogenesis of the resulting anemia [38]. The difference in the results from those studies might be due to the difference of the time-course of malarial infection since the data from the experimental infection is limited. Recently, Paritpokee *et al.* proposed the corresponding elevation of serum transferrin receptor to the hemoglobin change and parasitemia in time sequence in an animal model study [39].

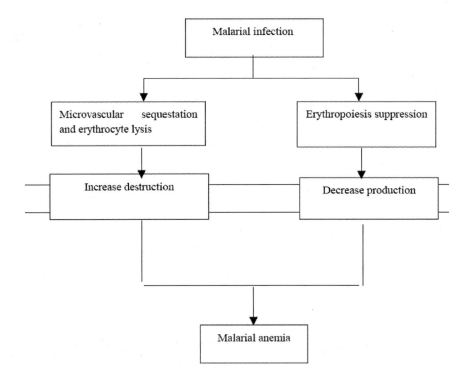

Figure 2.1. Summary on the pathophysiology of malarial anemia

In conclusion, the malarial anemia seems to have a very complex pathogenesis. Westherall *et al.* indicated a major defect in erythroid maturation with a significant degree of erythrophagocytosis [31]. However, further research is needed to answer the clear pathophysiology of malarial anemia.

Concerning non-falciparum malaria, the anemia is not common. However, anemia can be seen in the non-falciparum malarial patients, especially in cases with G-6-PD deficiency and those receiving some drug inducing hemolysis. The most common problematic drug in those cases is primaquine, an effective antimalarial drug recommended for vivax malaria. In 1997, Menendez *et al.* performed a study to investigate the usage of primaquine in the vivax malarial patients with G-6-PD deficiency. In that study, it was determined that 87.5% of the patients presented hemolysis but its relation with the enzymatic activity was not significant, and 50% of the patients could not finish their treatment because of the appearance of important hemolysis [40]. Menendez *et al.* concluded that primaquine should not be used indiscriminately among those patients with deficit G-6-PD.

Clinical Manifestation of Malarial Anemia

As already mentioned, malarial anemia is common for falciparum malaria [8].

In 1992, Rojanasthien *et al.* studied 126 patients with malaria (30 cases of vivax and 96 cases of falciparum malaria) for evidence of hematological abnormalities. In this study, anemia associated with malaria was observed only in *Plasmodium falciparum* infections and there was no correlation between the degree of anemia and the percentage of parasitemia, however, decreased hematocrit levels were found to be statistically significant in *Plasmodium vivax* infected patients [41]. In 2002, Verhoef *et al.* performed a community-based cluster survey among Kenyan children aged 2 to 36 months asymptomatic for malaria or anemia [42]. They concluded that nutritional inadequacies causing stunting also impaired host immunity, thus increasing the degree to which malaria was associated with decreased concentrations of hemoglobin, with increased inflammation, and with increased iron demand in developing erythroblasts [42]. Verhoef *et al.* proposed that increased intake of micronutrients might not only reduce stunting and nutritional anemia, but also reduce malaria-associated anemia [42]. Conclusively, Verhoef *et al.* mentioned that stunting may determine the severity of malaria-associated anemia [42].

Muhe *et al.* said that anemia from malaria was a common problem in development and children who were severely anaemic and who may require urgent blood transfusion usually go to peripheral first-level health facilities from where they should be referred to hospitals [43]. Paleness is the most common presentation of malarial anemia which can be confirmed by simple hemoglobinometry, however, hemoglobin cannot be easily detected in rural settings where the laboratory instruments are unavailable [43]. Muhe *et al.* performed a study to compare clinically detected pallor with measured blood hemoglobin concentrations [43]. They concluded that moderate and severe anemia could be identified clinically in most cases for treatment and referral purposes [43]. In addition, a systolic ejection murmur, altered sensorium, the presence of splenomegaly or malarial parasitaemia may be used as additional tools in considering urgent referral for blood transfusion [43]. Concerning the severe presentation of malarial anemia, Charles and Bertrand proposed that cardiac symptoms could be caused by a myocardiopathy resulting from malarial chronic anemia [44]. English et al. found that in children with severe malaria anemia (SMA), severe symptoms and severe lactic acidosis could be detected [45]. They suggested that some children with SMA and respiratory distress accumulated an oxygen debt when a relatively high oxygen demand outstrips supply, this debt being repaid when supply was increased during transfusion [45].

Concerning vivax malaria, parasite density significantly influences the fragility of the erythrocytes, Heinz body formation, MCV, MCH and MCHC levels, thus, the erythrocytes of the patients repeatedly infected with *Plasmodium vivax* parasite are subjected to structural and functional impairment, ultimately culminating in anemia [46]. However, the anemia is not a common presentation in the patients with vivax malaria. But the anemia becomes very important in some cases of vivax malaria, the drug-induced hemolytic anemia. This situation is common in the antimalarial treatment in G-6-PD deficient cases. Similar to other drug-induced hemolytic anemia, drug-induced hemolytic anemia in vivax malaria requires prompt diagnosis and early management [40]. Luckily the G-6-PD deficient cases who did get the antimalarial drugs did not manifest very severe symptoms [40]. Another type of hemolytic anemia in malarial patients presented with such classical signs as hemoglobinuria, the well-known Blackwater fever has been mentioned [47]. This fever is a clinical entity characterized by acute intravascular hemolysis classically occurring after the re-introduction of quinine in long-term residents in malaria endemic areas and repeatedly using the product. Acute intravascular haemolysis, haemoglobinurea and renal failure are common triads [48 - 49]. This complication is totally unwanted and usually severe.

Management of Malarial Anemia

The principles of management of malarial anemia is based on both principles of management for anemia "promotion of red blood cell production in cases that have decrease red blood cell production as basic pathophysiology accompanied with red blood cell replacement and decrease red blood cell destruction in cases that have increase red blood cell destruction as basic pathophysiology" and principles of management for infection "getting rid of source of infection and control of complications from pathogen virulence, host responses and treatment".

Promotion of Red Blood Cell Production

Decreased erythropoiesis is an important underlying pathophysiology for malarial anemia [31]. The bone marrow suppression in the malarial infected patients can be demonstrated [31]. The EPO for management of malarial anemia has been mentioned for a few years. In 2004, Chang et al. investigated the roles of erythropoietin (Epo) and erythropoiesis during blood-stage malaria in an animal model [50]. By treating *Plasmodium chabaudi* AS-infected mice, which are resistant to malaria, with polyclonal anti-human Epo neutralizing antibody, Change et al. demonstrated that Epo-induced reticulocytosis was important for alleviating malarial anemia and for host survival [50]

Red Blood Cell Replacement

The blood transfusion for malarial anemia has been practiced for a long time. Hall mentioned that fresh blood transfusion might be helpful in small doses for severe anemia and to replace clotting factors [51]. In 2002, Meremikwu and Smith performed a metanalysis on this topic and proposed that there was insufficient data to be sure whether routinely giving blood to clinically stable children with severe anemia in endemic malarious areas reduced death, or resulted in higher haematocrit measured during one month [52]. However, the blood transfusion for treatment of malarial anemia posed a high risk for blood-borne infections, especially in the setting where screening in the blood bank process is not effective. Greenberg *et al.* proposed that the treatment of malaria with blood transfusions is an important factor in the exposure of Kinshasa children to HIV infection [53].

Decrease Red Blood Cell Destruction

Since the autoimmune hemolytic anemia is rare in malarial infection, the role of immunosuppressive drugs in treatment of malarial anemia is limited.

Getting Rid of Source of Infection

The prompt getting rid of the source of infection in malaria is the blood exchange. In severe malarial patients, cell exchange transfusion results in a marked decrease in the parasitaemia, before a response to quinine therapy would have been anticipated, leading to a successful outcome thereafter [54]. This practice is widely indicated for those cases with cerebral malaria, acute respiratory distress syndrome, acute renal failure, and disseminated intravascular coagulation [55]. The usage of this technique in malarial anemia is very limited.

Concerning the slower method for getting rid of the source of infection, antimalarial drug therapy, it is no doubt needed to manage malarial anemia. If the practitioners do not get rid of the infection, the malarial anemia which is its subsequent complication cannot be gotten rid off. Beales noted that the asymptomatic parasitaemia remaining after poor response to full antimalarial treatment might lead to life-threatening anemia; as drug-resistant strains of the malarial parasite proliferate this was becoming increasingly important [56]. Nevertheless, the usage of antimalarial drug in the tropics should be considered for the other important inherited hematologic disorder, G-6-PD deficiency, which is common in the tropics as well.

Control of Complications

As already mentioned, estimation of anemia should become an additional parameter in the traditional malariometric survey [56]. Hemoglobin concentrations should also be taken into consideration in the management of malaria patients at the primary-care level, particularly in deciding whether a patient should be referred to an appropriate treatment center [56]. Follow up for the patients to determine the response to treatment is necessary. Control of complications of malarial anemia are necessary. Close monitoring for the possible complications of malarial anemia especially for cardiac and respiratory complications is recommended. In addition, the corresponding monitoring for selected treatment methods such as monitoring for adverse transfusion reaction in transfusion management and monitoring for adverse drug reaction in antimalarial therapy is needed.

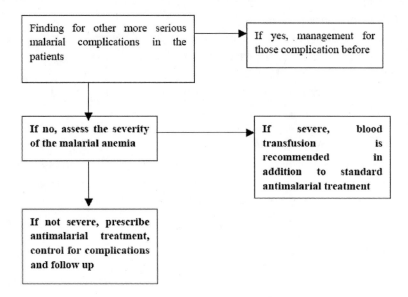

Figure 2.2. Brief recommended guideline for management of malarial anemia

References

[1]   Chareonviriyaphap T, Bangs MJ, Ratanatham S. Status of malaria in Thailand. *Southeast Asian J Trop Med Public Health* 2000;31:225-37.

[2]   Thimasarn K, Jatapadma S, Vijaykadga S, Sirichaisinthop J, Wongsrichanalai C. Epidemiology of Malaria in Thailand. *J Travel Med* 1995;2:59-65.

[3]   Suyaphun A, Wiwanitkit V, Suwansaksri J, Nithiuthai S, Sritar S, Suksirisampant W, Fongsungnern A. Malaria among hilltribe communities in northern Thailand: a review of clinical manifestations. *Southeast Asian J Trop Med Public Health* 2002;33 Suppl 3:14-5.

[4]   Wiwanitkit V, Suyaphan A. Prevalence of thrombocytopenia in vivax malarial patients: an observation. *Platelets* 2003;14:395.

[5]   Wiwanitkit V, Suyaphan A Jaundice as co-presentation in Thai malarial patients. *J Indian Med Assoc* 2004;102:107.

[6]   Rogerson SJ, van den Broek NR, Chaluluka E, Qongwane C, Mhango CG, Molyneux ME. Malaria and anemia in antenatal women in Blantyre, Malawi: a twelve-month survey. *Am J Trop Med Hyg* 2000;62:335-40.

[7]   Murthy GL, Sahay RK, Srinivasan VR, Upadhaya AC, Shantaram V, Gayatri K. Clinical profile of falciparum malaria in a tertiary care hospital. *J Indian Med Assoc* 2000;98:160-2, 169.

[8]   Richards MW, Behrens RH, Doherty JF. Short report: hematologic changes in acute, imported Plasmodium falciparum malaria. *Am J Trop Med Hyg* 1998;59:859.

[9]   Weatherall DJ, Miller LH, Baruch DI, Marsh K, Doumbo OK, Casals-Pascual C, Roberts DJ. Malaria and the red cell. *Hematology* (Am Soc Hematol Educ Program) 2002;1:35-57.

[10] McGuire W, Knight JC, Hill AV, Allsopp CE, Greenwood BM, Kwiatkowski D. Severe malarial anemia and cerebral malaria are associated with different tumor necrosis factor promoter alleles. *J Infect Dis* 1999;179:287-90.

[11] Taverne J, Sheikh N, de Souza JB, Playfair JH, Probert L, Kollias G. Anemia and resistance to malaria in transgenic mice expressing human tumour necrosis factor. *Immunology* 1994;82:397-403.

[12] Sexton AC, Good RT, Hansen DS, D'Ombrain MC, Buckingham L, Simpson K, Schofield L. Transcriptional profiling reveals suppressed erythropoiesis, up-regulated glycolysis, and interferon-associated responses in murine malaria. *J Infect Dis* 2004;189:1245-56.

[13] Praba-Egge AD, Montenegro S, Cogswell FB, Hopper T, James MA. Cytokine responses during acute simian Plasmodium cynomolgi and Plasmodium knowlesi infections. *Am J Trop Med Hyg* 2002;67:586-96.

[14] Gourley IS, Kurtis JD, Kamoun M, Amon JJ, Duffy PE. Profound bias in interferon-gamma and interleukin-6 allele frequencies in western Kenya, where severe malarial anemia is common in children. *J Infect Dis* 2002;186:1007-12.

[15] Bellamy R, Kwiatkowski D, Hill AV. Absence of an association between intercellular adhesion molecule 1, complement receptor 1 and interleukin 1 receptor antagonist gene polymorphisms and severe malaria in a West African population. *Trans R Soc Trop Med Hyg* 1998;92:312-6.

[16] Hobbs MR, Udhayakumar V, Levesque MC, Booth J, Roberts JM, Tkachuk AN, Pole A, Coon H, Kariuki S, Nahlen BL, Mwaikambo ED, Lal AL, Granger DL, Anstey NM, Weinberg JB. A new NOS2 promoter polymorphism associated with increased nitric oxide production and protection from severe malaria in Tanzanian and Kenyan children. *Lancet* 2002;360:1468-75.

[17] May J, Lell B, Luty AJ, Meyer CG, Kremsner PG. HLA-DQB1*0501-restricted Th1 type immune responses to Plasmodium falciparum liver stage antigen 1 protect against malaria anemia and reinfections. *J Infect Dis* 2001;183:168-72.

[18] Bienzle U, Guggenmoos-Holzmann I. Malaria hypothesis--the significance of the hereditary red cell traits Hb S and glucose-6-phosphate dehydrogenase deficiency in malaria. *Immun Infekt* 1979;7:196-201.

[19] Aidoo M, Terlouw DJ, Kolczak MS, McElroy PD, ter Kuile FO, Kariuki S, Nahlen BL, Lal AA, Udhayakumar V. Protective effects of the sickle cell gene against malaria morbidity and mortality. *Lancet* 2002;359:1311-2.

[20] Feng Z, Smith DL, McKenzie FE, Levin SA. Coupling ecology and evolution: malaria and the S-gene across time scales. *Math Biosci* 2004;189:1-19.

[21] Lachant NA, Tanaka KR. Impaired antioxidant defense in hemoglobin E-containing erythrocytes: a mechanism protective against malaria? *Am J Hematol* 1987;26:211-9.

[22] Hutagalung R, Wilairatana P, Looareesuwan S, Brittenham GM, Aikawa M, Gordeuk VR. Influence of hemoglobin E trait on the severity of Falciparum malaria. *J Infect Dis* 1999;179:283-6.

[23] Weatherall DJ. Thalassaemia and malaria, revisited. *Ann Trop Med Parasitol* 1997; 91:885-90.

[24] Cockburn IA, Mackinnon MJ, O'Donnell A, Allen SJ, Moulds JM, Baisor M, Bockarie M, Reeder JC, Rowe JA. A human complement receptor 1 polymorphism that reduces Plasmodium falciparum rosetting confers protection against severe malaria. *Proc Natl Acad Sci U S A* 2004;101:272-7.

[25] Ruwende C, Khoo SC, Snow RW, Yates SN, Kwiatkowski D, Gupta S, Warn P, Allsopp CE, Gilbert SC, Peschu N, et al. Natural selection of hemi- and heterozygotes for G6PD deficiency in Africa by resistance to severe malaria. *Nature* 1995;376:246-9.

[26] Saunders MA, Hammer MF, Nachman MW. Nucleotide variability at G6pd and the signature of malarial selection in humans. *Genetics* 2002;162:1849-61.

[27] Tishkoff SA, Varkonyi R, Cahinhinan N, Abbes S, Argyropoulos G, Destro-Bisol G, Drousiotou A, Dangerfield B, Lefranc G, Loiselet J, Piro A, Stoneking M, Tagarelli A, Tagarelli G, Touma EH, Williams SM, Clark AG. Haplotype diversity and linkage disequilibrium at human G6PD: recent origin of alleles that confer malarial resistance. *Science* 2001;293:455-62.

[28] Min-Oo G, Fortin A, Tam MF, Nantel A, Stevenson MM, Gros P. Pyruvate kinase deficiency in mice protects against malaria. *Nat Genet* 2003;35:357-62.

[29] Gallagher PG. Hereditary elliptocytosis: spectrin and protein 4.1R. *Semin Hematol* 2004;41:142-64.

[30] O'Donnell A, Allen SJ, Mgone CS, Martinson JJ, Clegg JB, Weatherall DJ. Red cell morphology and malaria anemia in children with Southeast-Asian ovalocytosis band 3 in Papua New Guinea. *Br J Haematol* 1998;101:407-12.

[31] McDevitt MA, Xie J, Gordeuk V, Bucala R. The anemia of malaria infection: role of inflammatory cytokines. *Curr Hematol Rep* 2004;3:97-106.

[32] Waitumbi JN, Opollo MO, Muga RO, Misore AO, Stoute JA. Red cell surface changes and erythrophagocytosis in children with severe plasmodium falciparum anemia. *Blood* 2000;95:1481-6.

[33] Mohan K, Dubey ML, Ganguly NK, Mahajan RC. Plasmodium falciparum: role of activated blood monocytes in erythrocyte membrane damage and red cell loss during malaria. *Exp Parasitol* 1995 ;80:54-63.

[34] Weatherall DJ, Abdalla S, Pippard MJ. The anemia of Plasmodium falciparum malaria. *Ciba Found Symp* 1983;94:74-97.

[35] Davis TM, Krishna S, Looareesuwan S, Supanaranond W, Pukrittayakamee S, Attatamsoonthorn K, White NJ. Erythrocyte sequestration and anemia in severe falciparum malaria. Analysis of acute changes in venous hematocrit using a simple mathematical model. *J Clin Invest* 1990;86:793-800.

[36] Mohan K, Stevenson MM. Dyserythropoiesis and severe anemia associated with malaria correlate with deficient interleukin-12 production. *Br J Haematol* 1998;103:942-9.

[37] Chang KH, Tam M, Stevenson MM. Inappropriately low reticulocytosis in severe malarial anemia correlates with suppression in the development of late erythroid precursors. *Blood* 2004;103:3727-35.

[38] Verhoef H, West CE, Kraaijenhagen R, Nzyuko SM, King R, Mbandi MM, van Laatum S, Hogervorst R, Schep C, Kok FJ. Malarial anemia leads to adequately increased erythropoiesis in asymptomatic Kenyan children. *Blood* 2002;100:3489-94.

[39] Paritpokee N, Wiwanitkit V, Nithiuthai S, Boonchaermvichian C, Bhokaisawan N. Change of serum transferrin receptor in *Plasmodium gallinaceum* infected chicken model. *Presented at the Joint International Tropical Medicine Meeting 2002.* Bangkok Thailand, 2002.

[40] Menendez Capote R, Diaz Perez L, Luzardo Suarez C. Hemolysis and primaquine treatment. Preliminary report. *Rev Cubana Med Trop* 1997;49:136-8.

[41] Rojanasthien S, Surakamolleart V, Boonpucknavig S, Isarangkura P. Hematological and coagulation studies in malaria. *J Med Assoc Thai* 1992;75 Suppl 1:190-4.

[42] Verhoef H, West CE, Veenemans J, Beguin Y, Kok FJ. Stunting may determine the severity of malaria-associated anemia in African children. *Pediatrics* 2002;110:e48.

[43] Muhe L, Oljira B, Degefu H, Jaffar S, Weber MW. Evaluation of clinical pallor in the identification and treatment of children with moderate and severe anemia. *Trop Med Int Health* 2000;5:805-10.

[44] Charles D, Bertrand E. The heart and malaria. *Med Trop* (Mars) 1982;42:405-9.

[45] English M, Muambi B, Mithwani S, Marsh K. Lactic acidosis and oxygen debt in African children with severe anemia. *QJM* 1997;90:563-9.

[46] Selvam R, Baskaran G. Hematological impairments in recurrent Plasmodium vivax infected patients. *Jpn J Med Sci Biol* 1996;49:151-65.

[47] George CR, Parbtani A, Cameron JS. Mouse malaria nephropathy. *J Pathol* 1976;120:235-49.

[48] Bruneel F, Gachot B, Wolff M, Bedos JP, Regnier B, Danis M, Vachon F. Blackwater fever. *Presse Med* 2002;31:1329-34.

[49] Pe Than Myint, Tin Shwe. A case of black water fever treated with peritoneal dialysis and artemether (quinghaosu derivative). *Southeast Asian J Trop Med Public Health* 1987;18:97-100.

[50] Chang KH, Tam M, Stevenson MM. Modulation of the course and outcome of blood-stage malaria by erythropoietin-induced reticulocytosis. *J Infect Dis* 2004;189:735-43.

[51] Hall AP. The treatment of malaria. *Br Med J* 1976;1:323-8.

[52] Meremikwu M, Smith HJ. Blood transfusion for treating malarial anemia. *Cochrane Database Syst Rev* 2000;2:CD001475.

[53] Greenberg AE, Nguyen-Dinh P, Mann JM, Kabote N, Colebunders RL, Francis H, Quinn TC, Baudoux P, Lyamba B, Davachi F, et al. The association between malaria, blood transfusions, and HIV seropositivity in a pediatric population in Kinshasa, Zaire. *JAMA* 1988;259:545-9.

[54] Mainwaring CJ, Leach MJ, Nayak N, Green ST, Jones DA, Winfield DA. Automated exchange transfusion for life-threatening plasmodium falciparum malaria--lessons relating to prophylaxis and treatment. *J Infect* 1999;39:231-3.

[55] Lercari G, Paganini G, Malfanti L, Rolla D, Machi AM, Rizzo F, Cannella G, Valbonesi M. Apheresis for severe malaria complicated by cerebral malaria, acute respiratory distress syndrome, acute renal failure, and disseminated intravascular coagulation. *J Clin Apheresis* 1992;7:93-6.

[56] Beales PF. Anemia in malaria control: a practical approach. *Ann Trop Med Parasitol.* 1997;91:713-8.

Chapter 3

Non-Malarial Protozoa
Induced Anemia

Introduction to Non-Malarial Protozoa
Induced Anemia

Protozoa infestation is common in the tropics. Several protozoa infestations, especially blood and intestinal protozoa, are the public health problems for many tropical countries. Of those protozoa infestations, malaria is the most mentioned disease associated with anemia. However, other protozoa infestations can cause anemia as well. The two main types of non-malarial protozoa induced anemia are anemia due to non-malarial blood protozoa and anemia due to intestinal protozoa.

First, human protozoa, which spend a part of their life-cycle within erythrocytes or extracellularly in human blood or in monocyte-derived macrophages, are considered as blood protozoas [1]. These blood protozoas elicit a common hematological syndrome essentially consisting in hemolytic anemia and splenomegaly [1]. Rosenmund said that some basic factors of host/parasite interaction in these protozoa infestations were very similar: (1) Specific cell attachment through receptor/ligand mechanisms such as the integrin/RGD-oligopeptide system, (2) competition for essential nutrients such as iron, which might be influenced therapeutically to the disadvantage of the parasite by the use of iron chelators, and (3) provocation of host defense through T-cell dependent, cytokine-mediated macrophage activation [1]. As already mentioned, the well-known blood parasites causing anemia is *Plasmodium* spp, which is the etiology for anemia. The other blood parasites mentioned for leading to anemia are babesia, leishmania and trypanosoma.

Secondly, human protozoa, which spend a part of their life-cycle within intestinal lumen, are considered as intestinal protozoa. Recently there has been considerable progress in understanding the physiopathologic aspects of the direct parasitic action of the products that they release, that affect the digestive function [2]. Note that the pathogenetic effects of intestinal parasites were important, not only for the adult forms that occupied the lumen or the intestinal mucosa, but for the migratory forms, and the most important clinical manifestations were in direct relation with the host response to the aggression or trauma caused by the migratory protozoas, the signs and symptoms depend on the infestation phase and on the severity or in the agent "virulence" [2]. However, the intestinal protozoas do not directly lead to anemia but indirectly via the digestion disturbance.

Anemia Due to Non-Malarial Blood Protozoa

A. Anemia and Babesia

Introduction to Babesia

Babesia is a group of malarial-like blood protozoa causing an infectious disease namely babesiosis. At present, babesiosis is considered as an important infection caused by protozoal parasites and transmitted by the same tick, *Ixodes ricinus*, that transmits Lyme disease [3]. Babesiosis is found throughout the world as a disease in animal especially in cattle. Human babesiosis is now considered as an important emerging disease [4]. *Babesia divergens*, and *Babesia microti* are the two agents of zoonotic infections from deer, sheep, cattle, dogs, and horses. This human zoonotic is endemic in Latin America [5], however, this infection is spreading to non-tropical regions including the northeastern and northern midwestern United States [3] and Europe [4]. Gray *et al.* noted that the vast majority of European cases had been caused by *Babesia divergens* in splenectomised patients, and although rare, this disease was very dangerous, requiring aggressive treatment [4]. They also noted that most human babesiosis caused by *Babesia microti* have occurred in the northeastern states of the USA and can affect spleen-intact as well as asplenic patients [6].

Concerning the symptomatology of babesiosis, the infected patients usually experience a flu-like illness that usually lasts for 1 or 2 weeks but may require hospital admission [3]. Similar to malaria, the clinical manifestations of babesiosis range from subclinical illness to fulminant disease resulting in death [7]. At present this tick-borne illness is being recognized with increased frequency [8]. Coinfection with ehrlichiosis and Lyme disease is also being recognized as an important feature of these tick-borne illnesses [8].

Krause notes that those at greatest risk of fatal disease include individuals older than age 50 years; asplenic individuals; and immunocompromised individuals as a result of immunosuppressive drugs, malignancy, or HIV infection [3].

Prompt and accurate diagnosis is difficult because the signs and symptoms are non-specific [4]. Specific diagnosis is made through examination of a Giemsa-stained thin blood smear, DNA amplification using polymerase chain reaction (PCR), or detection of specific antibody [3].

Gray *et al.* noted that a CBC was a useful screening test since anemia and thrombocytopenia are commonly observed and parasites might be visualized on blood smear and conclusive diagnosis of this disease generally depended upon microscopic examination of thin blood smears [8]. However, Gray *et al.* noted that babesia frequently were underdiagnosed because parasitemia tended to be sparse, often infecting fewer than 1% of erythrocytes early in the course of the illness, hence, identification of amplifiable babesial DNA by PCR should be used to increase diagnostic sensitivity and specificity while serologic testing provides useful supplementary evidence of infection because a robust antibody response characterizes human babesial infection, even at the time that parasitemia first becomes detectable [4]. Due to the increased importance of this disease, screening for babesia is recommended as a part of blood bank screening in many countries [9].

Anemia in Babesiosis

As already mentioned, anemia is common in babesiosis. Hatchers *et al.* reported their experience in 34 human babesiosis cases that complicated babesiosis was more commonly associated with the presence of severe anemia and higher parasitemia levels [10]. Rosner *et al.* studied 22 cases of human babesiosis and found that most of the 22 patients had moderate to severe clinical disease including hemolytic anemia, yet all but six recovered [11]. Clark and Jacobson said that anemia with dyserythropoiesis can be seen in babesiosis similar to malaria. They proposed that humans require very much smaller loads of *Plasmodium* or *Babesia* spp. before becoming ill, and likewise were very sensitive to endotoxin, the harmful effects of which were mediated by the pro-inflammatory cytokines, hence, the diseases caused by these two genera of intra-erythrocytic protozoan parasites would probably prove to be conceptually identical [12]. Slovut *et al.* mentioned that the symptoms consisting of fever, anemia, elevated liver function tests, and hemoglobinuria-might be especially severe in asplenic orimmunocompromised patients and bone marrow biopsy might reveal hemophagocytosis and marrow histiocytosis [13].

Management of Anemia Due to Babesiosis

The management of anemia due to babesiosis must follow the principles of management for anemia and infection similar to malaria. In severe cases, the red blood cell exchange can be considered [14 – 15]. In 1981, Cahill *et al.* reported the first use of pentamidine and red blood cell exchange transfusion in human babesiosis, one of the most severe clinical case to survive [14]. Gray *et al.* concluded that exchange transfusion was a potentially life-saving therapy for patients suffering from severe disease with high parasitemia (>5%), significant hemolysis, or renal or pulmonary compromise [4]. In non-severe cases, an antiprotozoan drug such as clindamycin and quinine is recommended for getting rid of the source of infection. The currently recommended therapy for babesiosis is a 7-10-day course of clindamycin (600 mg every 6 h) and quinine (650 mg every 8 h) [4,6]. Weiss said that despite the superficial resemblance of babesia to malaria, these piroplasms do not respond to chloroquine or other similar drugs and noted that the treatment of babesiosis using a clindamycin-quinine combination had been successful [8]. The other recommended antiprotozoan drugs are atovaquone, a recently developed anti-protozoan agent for human treatment and azithromycin [6]. Recently, azithromycin (500-600 mg on day 1, and 250-600 mg on subsequent days) and atovaquone (750 mg every 12 h) was found to be equally effective in babesiosis treatment with fewer adverse reactions than clindamycin and quinine [4,6].

B. Anemia and Leishmania

Introduction to Lesihmania

Leishmania is a group of haemoflagellate protozoa causing an infectious disease namely leihmaniasis. Leishmaniases are widespread in most tropical countries in the Mediterranean basin [16]. Two main groups of leishminaisis are described: *Leishmania infantum*, *Leishmania chagasi* and *Leishmania donovani* responsible from visceral leishmaniasis (VL), and *Leishmania tropica* causes cutaneous leishmaniasis (CL) and mucocutaneous leishmaniasis (MCL) [16 - 17]. *Phlebotomus sergenti*, *P. papatasi*, *P. major* and *P. syriacus* are considered to be the probable vectors, and dogs are the main reservoir of *L. infantum*, *L. chagasi* and *L. donovani* while *P. sergenti* is the main suspected vector of *L. tropica* [16]. The leishmaniasis was first reported by Leishman and Donovan in splenic tissue from patients in India with the life-threatening disease, now called visceral leishmaniasis, in 1903 [18]. At present, leishmanioses are widespread in 88 countries of the tropical and subtropical zone, including regions of the Mediterranean Sea basin of Southern Europe [17]. Stefaniak *et al.* said that approximately 350 million people live in Leishmania endemic areas and about 12 million individuals were infected [17].At present, there are more than 21 species causing human infection and the infection is transmitted to humans through the bites of female sandflies belonging to 30 species [17, 19]. The worldwide spread of human immunodeficiency virus (HIV) infection is also another underlying factor that modifies the endemicity of leishmaniasis at present [19].

At present, diagnosis of leishmaniasis still typically relies on classic microbiological methods, but molecular-based approaches are being tested [17, 19]. The diagnosis of visceral form is conventionally made by the demonstration of amastigotes of the parasite in the aspirated fluid from the bone marrow, the spleen, and rarely from the lymph nodes, or the liver [17, 19]. The protozoa demonstration and isolation rates are rather poor from cutaneous and mucocutaneous lesions due to low parasite load and high rate of culture contamination [17, 19]. Singh and Sivakumar proposed that recombinant kinesin protein of 39 kDa called rK 39 was useful in the diagnosis of HIV-Leishmania co-infection and as a prognostic marker [19].

Anemia in Leishmaniasis

Anemia is a common manifestation of VL. Elnour *et al.* performed a study aiming to study the epidemiological and clinical characteristics of VL in 33 children in Oman and found that all subjects presented with fever, anemia and splenomegaly [20]. Kafetzis said that the children with leishmaniasis usually present with intermittent fever, paleness, refusal to eat or anorexia, weight loss, and abdominal distension [21]. In addition, splenomegaly, hepatomegaly, lymph node enlargement, thrombocytopaenia, anemia, leukopaenia and hypergammaglobulinemia are the most common findings in those cases [21]. According to a recent study of Collin *et al.* in Sudan, anemia was an important risk factor for mortality in the patients with leishmaniasis (OR = 4.0) [22]. Similar findings were reported by Werneck *et al.* In that study [23], variables significantly associated with death in VL patients were severe anemia, fever for more than 60 days, diarrhea and jaundice [23].

Management of Anemia Due to Leishmaniasis

The management of anemia due to leishmaniasis must follow the principles of management for anemia and infection. Since anemia is an important prognostic factor implying bad outcome [22 – 23], blood transfusion for correction of anemia is recommended in severe cases. Due to the study of Grech *et al.* in Malta, blood transfusions for anemia were required in 93% of the patients [24]. Similar high rate of blood transfusion requirement, 73 %, was reported in a previous study, Yemen [25]. In non-severe cases, the antiprotozoan drug is recommended for getting rid of sources of infection. Pentavalent antimony compounds have been the mainstay of antileishmanial therapy for half a century, but lipid formulations of amphotericin B represent a major advance for treating visceral leishmaniasis [17, 19]. Sundar and Rai said that generic stibogluconate enabled the cost effective treatment of all forms of leishmaniasis as it remained the most important antileishmanial drug in most parts of the world [26]. They also noted that a single dose AmBisome for VL made therapy simple and enables mass treatment. They also noted that the two new oral drugs, fluconazole and miltefosine, provided wider options to the clinician for CL and MCL [26].

C. Anemia and Trypanosoma

Introduction to Trypanosoma

Trypanosoma is a group of protozoa causing an infectious disease namely trypanosomiasis. Trypanosomiasis is endemic in the tropics. In sub-Saharan Africa, the final decade of the 20th century witnessed an alarming resurgence in sleeping sickness, human African trypanosomiasis [27]. In South and Central America, Chagas' disease, American trypanosomiasis remains one of the most prevalent infectious diseases [27]. Similar to other blood protozoa, trypanosomiais is an arthropod vector transmitable disease [27]. Tsetse flies (Diptera: Glossinidae) are vectors of several species of pathogenic trypanosomes in tropical countries [28]. Aksoy *et al.* said that Central to the control of these diseases was control of the tsetse vector, which should be very effective since trypanosomes rely on this single insect for transmission [28].

At present, diagnosis of leishmaniasis still typically relies on classic microbiological methods, but molecular-based approaches are being proposed [29]. Similar to leishmaniasis, blood smear interpretation is still an important and easily available tool for diagnosis of leishmaniasis in the tropical developing countries [29]. In order to select a correct treatment after primary diagnosis of trypanosomiasis infection, accurate assessment of the disease stage, haemo-lymphatic or meningo-encephalitic, is essential [30].

Anemia in Trypanosomiasis

Anemia is an abnormal hematologic manifestation described in leishmaniasis. In 1979, Rickman and Cox studied the rats experimentally infected with *Trypanosoma brucei rhodesiense* which developed a syndrome characterized by anemia, splenomegaly, and glomerulonephritis [31]. They noted that serologic evaluation revealed that the syndrome was accompanied by the presence of 3 autoantibodies--cold-active hemagglutinin, immunoconglutinin, and antibody to fibrinogen/fibrin products [31]. In this study, fluorescein isothiocyanate conjugated antibody tests showed the presence of fixed complement and fibrinogen on both trypanosomes and erythrocytes [31].

Rickman and Cox said that anemia, thrombocytopenia, and sharp reductions in parasitemia were associated with elevated titers of cold-active hemagglutinin, antibody to fibrinogen/fibrin-related products, and immunoconglutinin [32]. They noted that depletion of lytic complement, prolonged partial thromboplastin times, and presence of fibrin monomers in the blood occurred at the time anemia and significant elevations in precipitable immune complexes were observed [32]. It was also suggested that microthrombiosis might have resulted from the immunologic interaction of complex-coated blood cells with immunoconglutinin and contributed to the terminal disease signs [32]. Conclusively, the anemia in trypanosomiasis is believed to be due to the immunological reactions. Luckily, anemia in human trypanosomiasis is not common and usually mild.

Management of Anemia Due to Trypanosomiasis

The management of anemia due to trypanosomiasis must follow the principles of management for anemia and infection. Since most anemic cases in human trypanosomiasis are mild the blood transfusion is rarely indicated. In general cases, chemotherapy is available for both American and African trypanosomioses, but existing drugs are far from ideal due to differences in the ways that trypanosome species interact with their hosts which have frustrated efforts to design drugs effective against different *Trypanosoma* spp [27 – 29]. Eflornithine is the only new molecule registered for the treatment of human African trypanosomiasis over the last 50 years [33]. It is the drug used mainly as a back-up for melarsoprol refractory *Trypanosoma brucei gambiense* cases [33]. Although this drug is effective, anemia due to bone marrow suppression is reported as an important adverse effect [33].

D. Anemia and Toxoplasma

Introduction to Toxoplasmosis

Toxoplasmosis is a zoonotic protozoal disease, caused by an obligatory intracellular parasite of the genus Toxoplasma [34]. The disease is widely distributed affecting more than a billion million people, worldwide [34].

The main species, Toxoplasma gondii, is a widespread protozoan parasite that infects all nucleated cell types of warm-blooded vertebrates [35]. Concerning human toxoplasmosis, the disease potentially highly affects two groups of patients: fetus and immunosuppressed patients [36]. Toxoplasmosis is considered to be viscerotropic in adults and children and neurotropic in fetal and newborn children [34]. Toxoplasma exists in three forms: oocysts, tissue cysts and tachyzoites [37]. The definitive hosts of Toxoplasma are members of the cat family: they shed unsporulated oocysts in the feces. After sporulation, oocysts become infectious [37]. Tachyzoites are crescent-shaped forms responsible for manifestations of acute *Toxoplasma* spp infection in the intermediate host [37]. Raising sheep and cattle, handling and eating raw meat, interaction with domestic cats and climate conditions play an important role in the distribution of the disease [36].

Concerning the pathogenesis of toxoplasmosis, parasite motility is regulated by polymerization of new actin filaments that provide a substrate for the small myosin TgMyoA [35]. Interaction between the cytoplasmic tails of parasite adhesins and the actin-binding protein aldolase links these cell surface proteins with the cytoskeleton. Translocation of adhesins coupled to extracellular receptors allows the parasite to glide across the substrate, and this conserved system is important for active penetration into host cells and tissue migration by *T. gondii* [35]. Entry into the host cell is accompanied by dramatic remodeling of the intracellular vacuole that the parasite resides in and this compartment resists fusion with host cell endocytic organelles, yet recruits mitochondria and endoplasmic reticulum in order to gain access to host cell nutrients [35]. *Toxoplasma* spp is therefore considered an important intracellular parasite.

An accurate and fast diagnosis of the toxoplasmosis is highly important, particularly in pregnant women, since the results may affect both the mother and her fetus [34]. The determination of diagnosis and therapy on the basis of a single serum examination is very important; it is possible on the basis of a single serum sample [36, 38]. In most cases, it is possible to differentiate between recent and latent infections using a combination of suitable methods, which permit us to confirm particular antibody classes [36, 38].

The present diagnostic methods consist of a combination of basic and supplemented diagnostic methods [38]. Basic tests which include the detection of total antibodies with CFT or IFT and specific classes of IgM and IgG antibodies by ELISA should be performed [38]. In addition, the potential activity of toxoplasma infection can be determined by supplementary methods such as IgG avidity antibodies, establishment of IgA antibodies, western blotting method and monitoring of antibodies production [38]. Concerning the blood smear interpretation, it is useless in diagnosis due to very low sensitivity.

Anemia in Toxoplasmosis

Anemia is an important manifestation of toxoplasmosis. Generally, postnatally acquired toxoplasmosis is a consequence of infection from cysts (by ingestion of undercooked meat of infected animals), oocysts (by ingestion of soil, fruits, vegetables contaminated by cat feces) and tachyzoites (by blood transfusion) while congenital *Toxoplasma* spp infection causes congenital toxoplasmosis [37]. Concerning congenital toxoplasmosis, Hrnjakovic-Cvjetkovic *et al.* noted that clinical manifestations of this condition include chorioretinitis and other ocular findings, central nervous system abnormalities (such as microcephaly, hydrocephalus, encephalomyelitis, seizures and mental retardation), icterus, hepatosplenomegaly, rash, anemia, erythroblastosis, thrombopenia [37]. Wiwanitkit also proposed that congenital toxoplasmosis is an important differential diagnosis for congenital anemia and jaundice [39]. Concerning the acquired toxoplasmosis, the general manifestation is mild and usually asymptomatic except for the immunocompromised hosts. The hematological manifestations of acquired toxoplasmosis include anemia [40] and disturbance of platelet [41]. Those anemic disorders in acquired toxoplasmosis was demonstrated as hemolytic anemia type and usually co-presented with fever and splenomegaly [42].

However, a severe form known as hemophagocytic syndrome (HPS), a combination between febrile hepatosplenomegaly, pancytopenia, hypofibrinemia, and liver dysfunction is described [43 - 44]. The benign HPS in acquired toxoplasmosis is defined by bone marrow and organ infiltration by activated, nonmalignant macrophages phagocytizing blood cells [43 - 44]. In the toxoplasmosis cases with HPS, severe anemia can be seen. Luckily, the HPS in acquired toxoplasmosis is rare [43 – 44].

Management of Anemia Due to Toxoplasmosis

The management of anemia due to toxoplasmosis must follow the principles of management for anemia and infection. Since most anemic cases in acquired toxoplasmosis are mild and in congenital toxoplasmosis are fatal resulting in abortion, the blood transfusion is rarely indicated. In general acquired toxoplasmosis cases, chemotherapy is indicated. El-On and Peiser mentioned that both *Toxoplasma* spp and *Plasmodium* spp belonged to the Phylum Apicomplexa, and were, therefore, almost similarly sensitive to anti-malarial drugs [34]. Pyrimethamine combined with sulfonamide becomes a widely recommended therapeutic of choice for those acquired toxoplasmosis cases. However, general practitioners should realize that megaloblastic anemia is a secondary complication due to pyrimethamine treatment [45 - 46].

E. Anemia and Theileria

Theileria is an important protozoa for animals, causing a disease called theileriosis. Theileriosis manifests itself in the form of Corridor disease (CD), caused by *Theileria parva lawrencei*, and East Coast fever (ECF), caused by *Theileria parva parva* [47 – 48]. This disease is a tick-borne disease [47 – 48]. Concerning cattle at present, intensive acaricidal tick control can now be supplemented by an attenuated schizont vaccine against T.annulata, while immunization against East Coast fever is carried out on a limited scale using virulent sporozoite infection and treatment [47]. Anemia can be seen in the animal infected with *Theileria* spp. In 2004, Shiono *et al.* reported that the low levels of IgG-bound RBC before the development of anemia were triggered in proportion with the progression of anemia and parasitaemia [49]. They suggested an accelerated destruction of RBC in anaemic cattle by IgG-dependent phagocytosis [49].

At present, this disease is prevalent in the tropics. Recently, Magona *et al.* reported an occurrence of concurrent trypanosomosis, theileriosis, anaplasmosis and helminthosis in the cattle in Uganda [50]. They proposed that theileriosis was an important veterinarian public health problem [50].

Concerning human theileriosis, Euzeby proposed the possibility of the occurrence of this disease, which could be a new important emerging infectious disease [51].

Anemia Due to Intestinal Protozoa

As already mentioned, most intestinal protozoa themselves do not directly lead to anemia. The secondary anemia resulting from the nutritional disorder as the primary result of intestinal protozoa infestation is mentioned. Curtale *et al.* studied the intestinal parasitic infestations among school age students in Egypt and found that among the protozoa, *Giardia intestinalis* was significantly correlated with low haemoglobin levels [52]. Weigel *et al.* studied the outcome of pregnancy corresponding to the intestinal parasitic infestations and found that high *Entamoeba histolytica* load was associated with decreased maternal serum hemoglobin and hematocrit levels, iron deficiency anemia, and indicators of diminished intrauterine growth including a decreased ponderal index, mid-arm circumference, and mid-arm/head circumference ratio [53]. A summation on the anemia in some important intestinal protozoa was described as the following:

Entamoeba

Entamoeba spp infection was reported by Weigel *et al.* relating to iron deficiency anemia [53]. Similarly, they reported that there was an association between anemia and intestinal *E. histolytica* infestation in children, particularly in rural areas. They also noted that correlation between anemia and mixed infestation of *E. histolytica*, *G. intestinalis* and *Ascaris lumbricoides* reached a highly significant level [54]. However, the *Entamoeba* spp has been reported as a direct cause of anemia as well. In 1984, McKinney reported the hemolytic-uremic syndrome accompanied *Entamoeba histolytica* infection. This report implied that the hemolytic anemia can be seen in Entamoeba infection [55].

Extra-intestinal infestation of *E. histolytica* is also reported as the cause of anemia. Amebic liver abscess is an extra-intestinal manifestation of *E. histolytica* and is usually mentioned for its association with anemia [56]. Chaves *et al.* studied 56 cases of amebic liver abscess and found that anemia and an elevated erythrocyte sedimentation rate, frequently without an elevated leucocyte count, were the most frequent hematologic findings [57]. Wiwanitkit also discovered a similar finding in Thai patients as well [58].

Giardia

G. intestinalis is reported for its association to anemia [52]. Sackey *et al.* indicated that *G. intestinalis* infection had an adverse impact on child linear growth and hemoglobin [59]. Akkad *et al.* postulated that *G. lamblia* might be a relevant cause of fever, anemia and weight loss in some elderly cases [60]. Shubair *et al.* performed a study in Gaza and found that *G. lamblia* and *E. histolytica* are associated with anemia and malnutrition [61]. These several reports confirmed that importance of anemia as a secondary complication of *Giardia* spp infestation and the main corresponding pathogenesis is due to the chronic diarrhea.

Trichomonas

The data on the correlation between *Trichomonas* spp infestation and anemia is limited. However, there is a report describing that phagocytosed erythrocytes can also be seen in the cytoplasm of *T. vaginalis*, a non-intestinal protozoa, suggesting the need for the patient to be tested for anemia [62].

Cryptosporidium

The main pathogenesis of anemia in cryptosporidiasis is believed to be due to the chronic diarrhea similar to giardiasis. According to the study of Chen *et al.* in China, routine blood examination and immunoassay performed on blood samples from some of the children with cryptosporiadiasis indicated that more than half of them had anemia and lower cellular immunity [63]. However, *Cryptosporidium* spp as the cause of hemolytic anemia, in hemolytic uremic syndrome has also been described [64 – 65].

References

[1] Rosenmund A. Blood parasitosis--mechanisms and limitations of a species-alien coexistence. *Schweiz Med Wochenschr* 1991;121:1669-74.

[2] Frisancho Velarde O. Intestinal parasitosis: physiopathologic aspects. *Rev Gastroenterol Peru* 1993;13:45-9.

[3] Krause PJ. Babesiosis. *Med Clin North Am* 2002;86:361-73.

[4] Gray J, von Stedingk LV, Granstrom M. Zoonotic babesiosis. *Int J Med Microbiol* 2002;291 Suppl 33:108-11.

[5] Montenegro-James S. Prevalence and control of babesiosis in the Americas. *Mem Inst Oswaldo Cruz* 1992;87 Suppl 3:27-36.

[6] Hunfeld KP, Brade V. Zoonotic Babesia: possibly emerging pathogens to be considered for tick-infested humans in Central Europe. *Int J Med Microbiol.* 2004 Apr;293 Suppl 37:93-103.

[7] Krause PJ. Babesiosis diagnosis and treatment. *Vector Borne Zoonotic Dis* 2003;3:45-51.

[8] Weiss LM. Babesiosis in humans: a treatment review. *Expert Opin Pharmacother* 2002;3:1109 – 15.

[9] Reine NJ. Infection and blood transfusion: a guide to donor screening. *Clin Tech Small Anim Pract 2004*;19:68-74.

[10] Hatcher JC, Greenberg PD, Antique J, Jimenez-Lucho VE. Severe babesiosis in Long Island: review of 34 cases and their complications. *Clin Infect Dis* 2001;32:1117-25.

[11] Rosner F, Zarrabi MH, Benach JL, Habicht GS. Babesiosis in splenectomized adults. Review of 22 reported cases. *Am J Med* 1984;76:696-701.

[12] Clark IA, Jacobson LS. Do babesiosis and malaria share a common disease process? *Ann Trop Med Parasitol* 1998;92:483-8.

[13] Slovut DP, Benedetti E, Matas AJ. Babesiosis and hemophagocytic syndrome in an asplenic renal transplant recipient. *Transplantation.* 1996;62:537-9.

[14] Cahill KM, Benach JL, Reich LM, Bilmes E, Zins JH, Siegel FP, Hochweis S. Red cell exchange: treatment of babesiosis in a splenectomized patient. *Transfusion* 1981;21:193-8.

[15] Jacoby GA, Hunt JV, Kosinski KS, Demirjian ZN, Huggins C, Etkind P, Marcus LC, Spielman A. Treatment of transfusion-transmitted babesiosis by exchange transfusion. *N Engl J Med* 1980;303:1098-100.

[16] Ok UZ, Balcioglu IC, Taylan Ozkan A, Ozensoy S, Ozbel Y. Leishmaniasis in Turkey. *Acta Trop* 2002;84:43-8.

[17] Stefaniak J, Paul M, Kacprzak E, Skoryna-Karcz B. Visceral leishmaniasis. *Przegl Epidemiol* 2003;57:341-8.

[18] Herwaldt BL. Leishmaniasis. *Lancet* 1999;354: 1191-9.

[19] Singh S, Sivakumar R. Recent advances in the diagnosis of leishmaniasis. *J Postgrad Med* 2003;49:55-60.

[20] Elnour IB, Akinbami FO, Shakeel A, Venugopalan P. Visceral leishmaniasis in Omani children: a review. *Ann Trop Paediatr* 2001;21:159-63.

[21] Kafetzis DA. An overview of paediatric leishmaniasis. *J Postgrad Med* 2003;49:31-8.

[22] Collin S, Davidson R, Ritmeijer K, Keus K, Melaku Y, Kipngetich S, Davies C. Conflict and kala-azar: determinants of adverse outcomes of kala-azar among patients in southern Sudan. *Clin Infect Dis* 2004;38:612-9.

[23] Werneck GL, Batista MS, Gomes JR, Costa DL, Costa CH. Prognostic factors for death from visceral leishmaniasis in Teresina, Brazil. *Infection* 2003;31:174-7.

[24] Grech V, Mizzi J, Mangion M, Vella C. Visceral leishmaniasis in Malta--an 18 year paediatric, population based study. *Arch Dis Child* 2000;82:381-5.

[25] Haidar NA, Diab AB, El-Sheik AM. Visceral Leishmaniasis in children in the Yemen. *Saudi Med J* 2001;22:516-9.

[26] Sundar S, Rai M. Advances in the treatment of leishmaniasis. *Curr Opin Infect Dis* 2002;15:593-8.

[27] Barrett MP, Burchmore RJ, Stich A, Lazzari JO, Frasch AC, Cazzulo JJ, Krishna S. The trypanosomiases. *Lancet* 2003;362:1469-80.

[28] Aksoy S, Gibson WC, Lehane MJ. Interactions between tsetse and trypanosomes with implications for the control of trypanosomiasis. *Adv Parasitol* 2003;53:1-83.

[29] Cattand P, de Raadt P. Laboratory diagnosis of trypanosomiasis. *Clin Lab Med* 1991;11:899-908.

[30] Lejon V, Buscher P. Stage determination and follow-up in sleeping sickness. *Med Trop* (Mars) 2001;61:355-60.

[31] Rickman WJ, Cox HW. Association of autoantibodies with anemia, splenomegaly, and glomerulonephritis in experimental African trypanosomiasis. *J Parasitol* 1979;65:65-73.

[32] Rickman WJ, Cox HW. Immunologic reactions associated with anemia, thrombocytopenia, and coagulopathy in experimental African trypanosomiasis. *J Parasitol* 1980;66:28-33.

[33] Burri C, Brun R. Eflornithine for the treatment of human African trypanosomiasis. *Parasitol Res.* 2003 Jun;90 Supp 1:S49-52.

[34] el-On J, Peiser J. Toxoplasma and toxoplasmosis. *Harefuah* 2003;142:48-55.

[35] Sibley LD. Toxoplasma gondii: perfecting an intracellular life style. *Traffic.* 2003;4:581-6.

[36] Ondriska F, Jalili NA, Catar G. Laboratory diagnosis of toxoplasmosis. *Bratisl Lek Listy* 2000;101:294-301.

[37] Hrnjakovic-Cvjetkovic I, Jerant-Patic V, Cvjetkovic D, Mrdja E, Milosevic V. Congenital toxoplasmosis. *Med Pregl* 1998;51:140-5.

[38]   Montoya JG. Laboratory diagnosis of Toxoplasma gondii infection and toxoplasmosis. *J Infect Dis* 2002;185 Suppl 1:S73-82.

[39]   Wiwanitkit V. Laboratory investigation in neonatal jaundice. *Med J Ubon Hosp* 2001; 22: 231 –9.

[40]   Fleming AF. Haematological manifestations of malaria and other parasitic diseases. *Clin Haematol* 1981;10:983-1011.

[41]   Wiwanitkit V, Soogarun S, Suwansaksri J. Platelet parameters in Toxoplasma gondii IgG-seropositive subjects. *Lab Hematol* 2003;9:248-9.

[42]   Michelson AD, Lammi AT. Haemolytic anemia associated with acquired toxoplasmosis.: *Aust Paediatr J* 1984;20:333-5.

[43]   Karras A, Thervet E, Legendre C; Groupe Cooperatif de transplantation d'Ile de France. Hemophagocytic syndrome in renal transplant recipients: report of 17 cases and review of literature. *Transplantation* 2004;77:238-43.

[44]   Rivas de la Lastra E, Sagel E, Acevedo D, Arias J, Sierra I. Benign hemophagocytic syndrome. First confirmed case in Panama. *Rev Med Panama* 1989;14:38-43.

[45]   Avello Sanchez JL, Pila Perez R. Megaloblastic anemia secondary to pyrimethamine treatment. *Rev Clin Esp* 1987;181: 55.

[46]   Deihl K, Berlinger R. Pyrimethamine-induced megaloblatic anemia in florid toxoplasmosis. *Med Welt* 1976;27:315-9.

[47]   Nambota A, Samui K, Sugimoto C, Kakuta T, Onuma M. Theileriosis in Zambia: etiology, epidemiology and control measures. *Jpn J Vet Res* 1994;42:1-18.

[48]   Uilenberg G, Dobbelaere DA, de Gee AL, Koch HT. Progress in research on tick-borne diseases: theileriosis and heartwater. *Vet Q* 1993;15:48-54.

[49]   Shiono H, Yagi Y, Kumar A, Yamanaka M, Chikayama Y. Accelerated binding of autoantibody to red blood cells with increasing anemia in cattle experimentally infected with Theileria sergenti.: *J Vet Med B Infect Dis Vet Public Health* 2004 ;51:39-42.

[50]   Magona JW, Mayende JS. Occurrence of concurrent trypanosomosis, theileriosis, anaplasmosis and helminthosis in Friesian, Zebu and Sahiwal cattle in Uganda. *Onderstepoort J Vet Res* 2002;69:133-40.

[51]   Euzeby J. The fate of parasites of animal origin transmitted to humans. *Med Trop* (Mars) 1997;57(3 Suppl):16-22.

[52]   Curtale F, Nabil M, el Wakeel A, Shamy MY. Anemia and intestinal parasitic infections among school age children in Behera Governorate, Egypt. Behera Survey Team. *J Trop Pediatr* 1998;44:323-8.

[53]   Weigel MM, Calle A, Armijos RX, Vega IP, Bayas BV, Montenegro CE. The effect of chronic intestinal parasitic infection on maternal and perinatal outcome. *Int J Gynaecol Obstet* 1996; 52:9-17.

[54]   al-Agha R, Teodorescu I. Intestinal parasites infestation and anemia in primary school children in Gaza Governorates--Palestine. *Roum Arch Microbiol Immunol* 2000;59:131-43.

[55]   McKinney RE Jr. Hemolytic-uremic syndrome and Entamoeba histolytica infection. *Pediatr Infect Dis* 1984 ;3:371.

[56]   Mayet FG, Powell SJ. Anemia associated with amebic liver abscess. *Am J Trop Med Hyg* 1964;13:790-3.

[57] Chaves FJ, Cruz I, Gomes C, Domingues W, da Silva EM, Veloso FT. Hepatic amebiasis-analysis of 56 cases. II. Laboratory and chest x-ray findings. *Am J Gastroenterol* 1977;68:273-77.

[58] Wiwanitkit V. A note on clinical presentations of amebic liver abscess: an overview from 62 Thai patients. *BMC Fam Pract* 2002;3:13.

[59] Sackey ME, Weigel MM, Armijos RX. Predictors and nutritional consequences of intestinal parasitic infections in rural Ecuadorian children. *J Trop Pediatr* 2003;49:17-23.

[60] Akkad T, Kirchgatterer A, Kranewitter W, Aschl G, Hobling W, Knoflach P. Fever and weight loss as leading symptoms of infection with giardia lamblia. *Z Gastroenterol* 2002;40:73-6.

[61] Shubair ME, Yassin MM, al-Hindi AI, al-Wahaidi AA, Jadallah SY, Abu Shaaban N al-D. Intestinal parasites in relation to haemoglobin level and nutritional status of school children in Gaza. *J Egypt Soc Parasitol* 2000;30:365-75.

[62] Demirezen S, Safi Z, Beksac S. The interaction of trichomonas vaginalis with epithelial cells, polymorphonuclear leucocytes and erythrocytes on vaginal smears: light microscopic observation. *Cytopathology* 2000;11:326-32.

[63] Chen YG, Yao FB, Li HS, Shi WS, Dai MX, Lu M. Cryptosporidium infection and diarrhea in rural and urban areas of Jiangsu, People's Republic of China. *J Clin Microbiol* 1992;30:492-4.

[64] Sehgal R, Mahajan RC, Thapa BR, Ganguly NK. Cryptosporidium causing chronic diarrhea. *Indian J Pediatr* 1989;56:129-31.

[65] Berthier M, Lacroix C, Agius G, Nivet H, Boufassa S, Jacquemin JL, Hoppeler. Haemolytic uraemic syndrome associated with cryptosporidium oocysts. *Eur J Pediatr* 1988;147:213.

Chapter 4

Hookworm Anemia and other Intestinal Helminth-Induced Anemia

Intestinal Helminth Infestation and Anemia

Intestinal helminth infestation is a common public health problem in developing tropical countries. These intestinal parasites cause significant morbidity and mortality. Several studies mention the correlation between intestinal helminth infestation and anemia. In 2001, Gilgen *et al.* conducted a randomized clinical intervention trial over 24 weeks on a tea estate in northeast Bangladesh to investigate the effect of iron supplementation and anthelmintic treatment on the labour productivity of adult female workers [1]. According to this study, there was a negative association for all three worms (*Ascaris lumbricoides*, *Trichuris trichiura* and hookworms) between the intensity of helminth infections (eggs/faeces) and all measures of labor productivity [1]. In addition, lower haemoglobin values and anemia were both associated with lower labor productivity and more days sick and absent [1]. Chakma *et al.* performed another study among school-going children (6-14 years) of Baiga, Abuihmadia and Bharia tribes of Madhya Pradesh to assess the prevalence of anemia and intestinal parasitic infestation among themselves [2]. In this study, a total of 776 school-going children were included in the study of whom blood samples of all and stool samples of 409 were collected and the results revealed that 30.3% of the children had severe anemia and 50% children had intestinal parasites [2]. Chakma *et al.* found that the most common parasites were hookworms (16.3%) and *A. lumbricoides* (18.5%) [2]. Chakma *et al.* concluded that though hookworm ova loads indicated mild to moderate infestation in most of the children, the continued presence of worms in marginally nourished children could contribute significantly to blood loss in the intestine with resultant anemia [2]. According to those studies, the important effects of intestinal helminth infestation on anemia can be confirmed.

In 1998, Triteeraprapab *et al.* studied the prevalence and the relationship between eosinophilia, anemia and parasitism in 169 Thai-Karens from Mae Lamung and Mae Chan subdistricts, Umphang district, Tak Province, Thailand using an automated complete blood counter, and microscopic examination for intestinal parasites and microfilaria [3]. According to this study, in Mae Chan, 5 individuals were microfilaremic, 72% of individuals examined were infected with at least one kind of intestinal parasite, and 50% were anemic, with normal mean red cell volume (MCV) and in Mae Lamung, 46% were parasitized but none was microfilaremic or anemic. In addition, eosinophilia was prevalent in both populations (77%) [3]. Of interest, Triteeraprapab *et al.* noted that hookworm infection was found to be significantly associated with eosinophilia, but not anemia nor microcytosis of red cells [3]. Triteeraprapab *et al.* noted that the parasites' relationship with anemia and eosinophilia had been rarely reported due to limited health care access, especially in rural areas and there is need for further investigations [3]. The correlation between the intestinal helminth infestations and anemia is therefore still an interesting topic in tropical medicine. In this chapter, hookworm anemia and other intestinal helminth-induced anemia are presented.

Hookworm Anemia

1. What Is Hookworm and Hookworm Infestation?

Hookworm is a parasitic roundworm. Hookworm infestation is an infection of one of two different 7 to 13 mm long roundworms, *either Ancylostoma duodenale or Necator americanus*. Generally, harboring hookworm infestation does not present any symptoms. However, the route of hookworm infestation starts from the skin to the blood, to the lungs and then, eventually, to the intestines; thus, there may be symptoms from the infection in any of these places. Concerning the hookworm lifecycle, the transmission of this infestation begins with the infected human passing the parasite eggs into the soil due to poor toilet habits and those eggs, in proper humidity, can hatch into the infective stage larva. Those larva may survive several months in warm, damp soil. Then those larva subsequently penetrate the skin of other humans who do not wear shoes and migrate through the body to the intestines, where the median survival time of the hookworm is one year (figure 4.1).

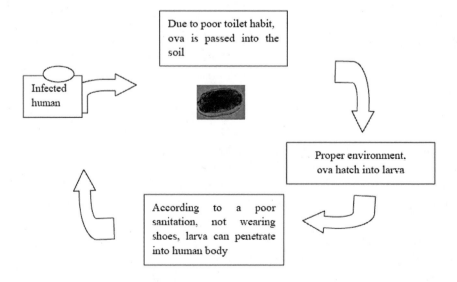

Figure 4.1. Life cycle of hookworm

According to the hookworm lifecycle, the two major contributing factors for the transmission is poor sanitation and proper soil environment. Of interest, these two factors are common in the tropics, therefore, there is no doubt that the hookworm infestation is a common public health problem for tropical countries. Concerning poor sanitation, Moraes *et al.* performed a study in Brazil and suggested that sewerage and drainage could have a significant effect on intestinal nematode infections, by reducing transmission occurring in the public domain [4]. In addition, according to the study of Olsen *et al.* in Kenya, the multiple logistic regression analysis revealed that the absence of latrines was a significant predictor for hookworm infection with an odds ratio (OR) of 1.9 [5]. Considering the soil environment factor, hookworm is a good example of soil transmitted helminthiasis. Bakta *et al.*, who studied the hookworm infestation in Bali, Indonesia and found that the condition and humidity of soil was an important determinant for the prevalence of hookworm infection [6].

Recently Hosain *et al.* found that the dog hookworm larva responded to environmental and host stimuli with four behavioral phases of host-finding: (1) Snake-like movement was stimulated by warmth and by defined vibrations of the substratum, (2) Waving behavior was a prerequisite for the passive change-over to hairs and was stimulated by heat radiation and by the CO2 content, warmth, and humidity of an air stream, (3) Creeping direction: the larvae were attracted by heat in temperature gradients as weak as 0.04 degrees C mm-1 and by hydrophilic skin surface extracts, but not by skin lipids or serum and (4) Penetration into agar was stimulated by heat and serum [7]. These results are believed to be the model for other hookworm species.

2. Hookworm and Anemia

Molecular and Genetic Basis of Hookworm Anemia

Hookworms are a leading cause of iron deficiency anemia in the tropics [8]. Del Valle noted that these parasites have evolved potent mechanisms of interfering with mammalian hemostasis, presumably for the purpose of facilitating bloodfeeding, the underlying process for chronic blood loss and subsequent anemia [8]. They noted that adult *Ancylostoma caninum* worm extracts contained an activity that inhibits platelet aggregation and adhesion by blocking the function of two cell surface integrin receptors, Glycoprotein IIb/IIIa and GPIa/Iia [8]. According to their study, a cDNA corresponding to the purified hookworm platelet inhibitor (HPI) protein has been cloned from adult A. caninum RNA, and the translated amino acid sequence shows significant homology to Neutrophil Inhibitory Factor and Ancylostoma Secreted Proteins, suggesting that these related hookworm proteins represent a novel class of integrin receptor antagonists [8]. They also noted that HPI was secreted by the adult stage of the parasite at the site of intestinal attachment [8]. A similar study was performed by Harrison *et al.* [9]. In their study, the major anticoagulant inhibitor of coagulation factor Xa had been identified as the hookworm parasite *A. ceylanicum* using reverse transcription PCR and 3'-rapid amplification of cDNA ends [9]. However, these studies are only in vitro experiments. Recently, the in vivo effect of hookworm infestations on human platelet was proposed by Wiwanitkit *et al.* [10]. According to that study, the effects of hookworm infestations on platelet parameters were noted [10].

Population Epidemiology of Hookworm Anemia

Hookworm infestation can be seen worldwide but a high prevalence is reported in tropical countries. In Asia, hookworm anemia is common in South Asia and Southeast Asia. Concerning South Asia, the prevalence of this geohelminthiasis is very high. According to the study of Traub *et al.* in India, the individual prevalence of hookworm was 43% [11]. In this study, the strongest predictors for the intensity of geohelminths using multiple regression were socioeconomic status, age, household crowding, level of education, religion, use of footwear when outdoors, defecation practices, pig ownership and water source [11]. Yadla also reported a similarly high prevalence in their study in India as well [12]. In this study, the overall prevalence rate of hookworm infestation was found to be 34% and men had significantly higher rates of infestation at all ages [12]. In addition, prevalence rates increased with age as well [12]. Although there are a lot of reports confirming the high prevalence of hookworm infestations in South Asia, there are only a few reports on the hookworm anemia. An interesting study was performed by Sampathkumar and Rajaratnam *et al.* [13]. This study investigated the prevalence of both anemia and hookworm infestation among 197 female adolescents in India's Tamil Nadu State [13]. According to this study, the prevalence of anemia was 76.6% and 63% of the 130 girls who provided stool samples had hookworm. When questioned about personal hygiene practices, 48.5% of girls reported they did not wear slippers when they went outside, confirming that the poor sanitation is the main contributing factor to hookworm infestation [13]. Srinivasan *et al.* performed another similar study in South India. In that study, evidence of hookworm infection was present in 92%, 77% having a count of under 100 epg, 11% a count of 1000 to 1999 epg, and 4% having counts between 2000 and 12,000 epg. while hemoglobin was also estimated: 80% of adult males, 87% of adult females and 90% of children were anemic [14]. Srinivasan *et al.* found that there was a significant negative association between ova load and hemoglobin level, and the decrease in hemoglobin for a doubling of the ova load was estimated by regression analysis to be 0.18, 0.29 and 0.16 g/dl in adult males, adult females and children, respectively [14].

Concerning Southeast Asia, Sagin *et al.* performed a study in Malyasia and found that anemia was more common among males > 40 years and among adolescents and young reproductive females, as well as elderly females > 61 years old [15]. In this study, 6.0% and 3.6% of the 83 anemic individuals had *Trichuris trichiura* or hookworm respectively; however there was no clear association with intestinal worm infection [15]. Another cross sectional study was conducted in Bali by Bakta and Budhianto to assess some characteristics of hookworm anemia among the adult population [16]. In this study, 15 cases of hookworm anemia were found among 454 total samples (3.3%), or among 123 cases of iron deficiency anemia (12.2%) [16]. Bakta and Budhianto concluded that hookworm anemia was characterized by iron deficiency anemia with eosinophilia, high serum total IgE level, hypoalbuminemia and moderate to severe hookworm infection [16]. Concerning West Asia, the prevalence of hookworm anemia is very low because of the dry climate. Nazari and Massoud found that the anemia produced by hookworm infection in Khuzestan was not significant [17].

In Africa, the hookworm anemia can be seen as well. Guyatt *et al.* indicated that the prevalence of anemia was high (54%) among schoolchildren in Tanzania, particularly those with high intensities of hookworm [18]. In this study, attributable fraction analysis suggested that hookworm was responsible for 6% of anemia cases [18]. Levi *et al.* retrospectively studied the medical records of all Ethiopians over the age of 18, who immigrated to Israel in the early 90's [19]. They found that 64% had evidence of *A. duodenale* infection [19]. Levi *et al.* found that the patients infected with *A. duodenale* had significantly lower mean corpuscular volume (MCV) and serum iron, and were likely to have eosinophilia and hypoalbuminemia [19].

Pathophysiology and Clinical Presentation of Hookworm Anemia

As already mentioned, hookworm anemia is usually found in the chronic hookworm infestations. This type of anemia is remarkable as a hypochromic microcytic anemia. Pathophysiologically, the adult parasites attached to the villi of the small intestines will suck blood causing abdominal discomfort, diarrhea and cramps, anorexia, weight loss, and in advanced disease, anemia [20]. Georgiev noted that hookworm infections in man, especially in children, are one of the leading causes of iron-deficiency anemia resulting directly from intestinal capillary blood loss following the feeding activities of fourth-stage (L4) larva and adult worms [20]. Crompton and Whitehead said that hookworms contribute significantly to iron-deficiency anemia through the feeding activities of intestinal stages leading to chronic blood loss into the gut. They also presented a mathematical model to explain how human iron metabolism may respond to hookworm infection in a variety of intensity. According to their work, the two considerable contributing factors for development of hookworm anemia are intensity of worm load and period of infestation [21].

Gottstein *et al.* performed an experimental infectious dog model for hookworm infestation. In this study, eosinophilia, erythroblastosis and microcytic, hypochromic anemia developed in all puppies during their first four weeks [22]. The hookworms, *A. duodenale* and *N. americanus*, cause significant gastrointestinal blood loss. In clinical studies, greater blood losses have been reported with *A. duodenale* [22].

Albonico *et al.* studied 492 children with hookworm positive fecal cultures, hemoglobin and ferritin concentrations decreased with increasing proportions of *A. duodenale* [23].

Diagnosis and Management for Hookworm Anemia

The diagnosis of hookworm anemia requires confirmation of co-presentation of anemia by hemoglobinometry and hookworm infestation by stool examination for the presence of the characteristic hookworm ova, thin-walled eggs containing few blastomeres (Figure 4.1). However, it should be noted that not all cases with both anemia and hookworm infestation have hookworm anemia since anemia can be a common co-presentation with intestinal helminth infestation in the tropics. Although the anemia is confirmed to be microcytic it can be the manifestation of another type of tropical anemia, especially for thalassemia [24].

A good method of diagnosis is the therapeutic trial, the antihelminthic drug, albendazole (200 mg/day for 3 consecutive days, repeated 1 month later), prescription as well as iron supplementation (60 mg elemental iron/day) is recommended. This treatment protocol was recently proved effective for the treatment of hookworm anemia by Dossa *et al.* [25]. In this study, no significant difference in changes in anthropometric parameters was observed between study groups (albendazole with iron supplementation, iron supplementation, albendazole and placebo), and also not in a sub-sample of stunted and anemic subjects [25].

However, changes in hemoglobin were highest in the iron-treated subjects at the end of the 3-month intervention period and hookworm infections decreased significantly in albendazole-treated subjects [25]. Concerning treatment for hookworm anemia, Brentlinger *et al.* noted that anemic women should be offered stool testing whether hookworm was present, and should be considered for antihelminthic treatment even if pregnant in any infestment cases [26].

Concerning severe hookworm anemia, a blood transfusion is sometimes indicated [27]. However, the role of a blood transfusion is limited and is not recommended. According to the study of Williams and Naraqi in the severe anemic patients in the area with high prevalence of malarial and hookworm anemia, Papua New Guinea, blood transfusion did not appear to be necessary in this group of patients despite a very low hemoglobin level [28]. On the other hand, Holzes *et al.* performed an interesting study in Tanzania [29]. According to this study, 116 children were randomized to receive either treatment for malaria and hookworm alone or, in addition, a transfusion of whole blood which had tested negative for antibodies against the human immunodeficiency virus (HIV) [29]. In this study, there was a trend towards more hospital admissions and deaths in the no transfusion group [29]. Fleming concluded that because of the risk of transmission of HIV, it was more important than ever to prevent severe anemia, and to give blood transfusion only as a life-saving treatment [30].

Prevention of Hookworm Anemia

Hookworm infestation and associated anemia is an important public health problem in the tropics that needs specific effective disease prevention and control. Albonico and Savioli noted that hookworms infected approximately 1.3 billion people worldwide, and 96 million suffer from associated morbidity, including also insidious effects on nutritional status and on physical and intellectual development [31]. De Silva said that mass chemotherapy appears to give maximal returns in terms of improved health in areas where hookworm is a major problem and albendazole is used regularly, along with iron supplements; in children it improves physical growth and iron stores, and in pregnant women it reduces the prevalence of iron-deficiency anemia [32]. In addition, Albonico and Savioli mentioned that periodic chemotherapy should be implemented in the context of ongoing improvement of sanitation and promotion of health education for the control of transmission of hookworm infection [31]. They concluded that chemotherapy with new, single dose broad spectrum, safe anthelminthic drugs as the mainstay of control strategy to reduce intensity of infection, iron-deficiency anaemia and other morbidity indicators associated with hookworm infections should be recommended [31]. They also mentioned that these elements should be integrated into the prevailing system of primary health care and must be based on multisectoral collaboration to ensure sustainability of control programs [31]. Similarly, Gilles noted that to control measures for hookworm, anemia should include chemotherapy to reduce the intensity of infection and the transmission potential and sanitation [33].

Other Intestinal Helminth-Induced Anemia

1. Diphyllobotrium Latum and Megaloblastic Anemia

Diphyllobotrium latum, known as fish tapeworm, is a well-known tapeworm that can induce anemia. The fish tapeworm infestation is mentioned as a possible cause of megaloblastic anemia, known as tapeworm pernicious anemia. The main pathogenesis of the fish tapeworm induced megaloblastic anemia is due to the pernicious anemia and vitamin B12 metabolism disturbance [34 - 35]. Von Bonsdorff B and Gordin said that the *D. latum*, attached to the proximal portion, jejunum, of the intestine, absorbed the vitamin B12 contained in the food, thus preventing vitamins from binding to the intrinsic factor of the gastric juice from reaching the receptors in the distal portions of the small intestine of the host [36]. If the infestation is chronic, the megaloblastic anemia can occur. The cobalamin malabsorption due to fish-tapeworm infestation is also mentioned for the *Giardia lamblia* infestation [37]. However, since the fish-tapeworm is endemic in Scandinavia, not in the tropics, therefore, the detail of diagnosis and management for fish-tapeworm anemia is hereby not mentioned.

2. Anemia in Strongyloidiasis

Strongyloidiasis is an intestinal parasitic disease caused by a parasitic roundworm namely *Strongyloides stercoralis* [38]. Basically, detecting larva of *S. stercoralis* in feces makes a definitive diagnosis [38]. In the AIDS era, the severe infestation of *S. stercoralis*, hyperinfection or disseminated strongyloidiasis, becomes an important superimposed infection [38]. In those cases with disseminated strongyloidiasis, weight loss, gastrointestinal symptoms, hypoproteinemia, and anemia are the main clinical presentations [39]. According to the recent study of Abedayo *et al.*, the anemia is common in patients with hyperinfective strongyloidiasis [39]. Concerning another study of Lemos *et al.*, anemia resulted from the immune process that can be seen in the patient with hyperinfective strongyloidiasis [40].

3. Anemia in Schistosomiasis

Molecular and Genetic Basis of Schistosomiasis – Related Anemia

Chronic infestation with *Schistosoma mansoni* commonly manifests with the relatively asymptomatic intestinal form of the disease, whereas a small minority develops hepatosplenism characterized by severe hepatic disease with portal hypertension [41]. In 1993, Henderson *et al.* performed an animal model, inbred male CBA/J mice, to predict a spectrum of disease [41]. Pathologically and immunologically, moderate splenomegaly syndrome (MSS) and hypersplenomegaly syndrome (HSS) remarkably parallel the intestinal and hepatosplenic clinical forms, respectively, in humans [41]. Henderson *et al.* found that HSS affected approximately 20% of these mice and consists of massive splenomegaly, ascites, thymic atrophy, severe anemia, and cachexia and the remaining majority of mice with

MSS develop moderate splenomegaly only [41]. In this study, histopathological features of HSS include 1) relatively extensive hepatic fibrosis and granulomatous inflammation, 2) splenic congestion, 3) lymph node plasmacytosis, and 4) worms and eggs in the pulmonary vasculature [41]. Henderson *et al.* said that the idiotypes present on antisoluble egg antigen antibodies from HSS mice were distinct from those from mice with acute infections or the chronic MSS infection and these idiotypic differences are similar to those observed in patients with intestinal and hepatosplenic forms of the disease and might have regulatory importance [41].

Population Epidemiology of Schistosomiasis – Related Anemia

In addition to hookworm anemia, anemia in schistosomiasis is another important public health problem, especially for those tropical countries in Africa. Leenstra *et al.* said that malaria and schistosomiasis were the main risk factors for anemia in younger girls (12-13 yr), while menstruation was the principal risk factor in older girls (14-18 yr) in Western Kenya [42]. Urbani *et al.* reported the first epidemiological survey on intestinal parasitic infections in Mauritania and the first study on *S. mansoni* on the Mauritanian side of the Senegal River [43]. According to this study, overall prevalence was 38.1% for intestinal parasitic infection, 7.1% for intestinal schistosomiasis [43]. Measurement of hemoglobin levels showed that 50.4% of children were anemic and that there was a correlation between anemia and infection by *S. haematobium* [43].

Pathophysiology and Clinical Presentation of Schistosomiasis – Related Anemia

Schistosomiasis or bilharziasis is a group of helminthic infestations caused by blood flukes of the Schistosoma genus. The pathology of schistosomosis is mostly brought about by ova trapped in the tissues. Three important forms of schistosomiasis; intestinal, urinary and hepatic are described [44]. The intestinal and urinary forms of schistosomiasis are the two common forms relating to anemia. Stephenson noted that there are several negative effects of urinary and intestinal schistosomiasis on the following nutritional parameters in humans: urinary and fecal blood and iron loss, anaemia and haemoglobin levels, proteinuria, child growth and adult protein-energy status, physical fitness and physical activity [45]. Fleming said that S. mansoni caused blood loss in 7 Egyptian patients of 7.5- 25.9 ml/day [46]. At present, it is accepted that a late stage of intestinal schistosomiasis can be a cause a severe anemia due to iron deficiency [47]. In 1989, Abou-Taleb et al. carried a study on 60 male patients, 20 have simple intestinal mansoniasis, 20 have simple urinary bilharziasis and 20 have hepatosplenic mansoniasis [48]. According to this study, latent iron deficiency anaemia, defined as those having normal Hb content (greater than 13 g/dl) and low serum ferritin (less than 15 ng/mL) was found in 35% of cases with simple mansoniasis, 20% of cases with simple urinary bilharziasis but not in any case with hepatosplenic mansoniasis [48]. This study can confirm the importance of anemia as a complication of intestinal and urinary schistosomiasis [48].

Pathophysiologically, the underlying mechanism for anemia in schistosomiasis is chronic blood loss via stool or urine. Concerning S. mansoni infestation, the main corresponding agent for intestinal and hepatic schistosomiasis, the blood loss is usually via stool. In 1991,

Ndamba et al. studied a total of 315 workers with S. mansoni infection and lack of anti-schistosomal chemotherapy during the previous three years [49]. According to this study, stool overt and occult blood in stool was detected in a significantly high number of infected people compared to the control subjects, however, the blood loss was found to have no anemia-producing effect as determined by hemoglobin and red blood cell counts [49]. Concerning S. haematobium, the main corresponding agent for urinary schistosomiasis, the blood loss is usually via urine. In 1992, Praul et al. studied the relationship between iron status and degree of infection by S. haematobium in 174 schoolchildren from Niger in an area endemic for urinary schistosomiasis [50]. In this study, hematuria and proteinuria were found in 76.4% and 79.9% of the children, respectively, while 95.4% excreted eggs [50]. In addition, anemia was observed in 59.7% of the subjects, iron deficiency equaled 47.1%, and anemia was associated with iron deficiency in 57.7% of the cases [50]. Praul et al. found that the hemoglobin level and transferrin saturation decreased significantly when the degree of hematuria increased, while prevalence of anemia and prevalence of iron deficiency increased significantly [50]. In addition, the hemoglobin level and the hematocrit were negatively correlated with egg count, while prevalence of anemia increased with increasing egg count [50]. Praul et al. concluded that this inverse relationship between degree of infection by S. haematobium and iron status showed a deleterious consequence of urinary schistosomiasis on nutrition and hematopoietic status, which should be considered in the design of nutrition intervention programs [50].

Diagnosis and Management for Schistosomiasis – Related Anemia

The diagnosis of anemia in schistosomiasis requires confirmation of co-presentation of anemia by hemoglobinometry and blood fluke infestation by stool or urinary examination for the presence of the blood fluke ova. However, it should be noted that not all cases with both anemia and blood fluke infestation have anemia as a result of blood fluke infestation since anemia can be a common co-presentation with helminth infestation in the tropics. The other causes of iron deficiency anemia, especially for hookworm infestation should be evaluated. Indeed, the co-infestation between hookworm and blood fluke are reported in many African countries [51].

Similar to hookworm anemia, management of anemia in schistosomiasis is usually started with an antihelminthic drug. Beasley *et al.* suggested that single-dose anthelminthic treatment distributed in schools in the endemic area achieved haematological benefits in nearly half of children infected with S. *haematobium* [52].

The recommended drug for treatment of schistosomiasis infestation is praziquantel (40 mg/kg), similar to other fluke infestations. In addition, the nutritional supplementation therapy should be similar to hookworm anemia. However, since praziquantel does not reduce the hookworm intensity of infection, another major cause of anemia in the endemic area, changes in the prevalence of anemia in the population should be due only to the elimination of *Schistosoma* spp infestation. Therefore, in the area with high prevalence of co-infestation of hookworm and blood fluke, combined antihelminthic drugs for the two infestations is recommended [53]. Recently, Friis *et al.* found that multi-micronutrient supplementation and anthelminthic treatment increased Hb independently and the effects were also independent of baseline Hb and general nutritional status. The treatment effect was due to reductions in S.

mansoni and hookworm intensities of infection [53]. Taylor *et al.* noted that in areas with schistosomiasis and hookworm infection, combination treatment with praziquantel, triple-dose albendazole, plus iron supplementation, is likely to improve the population's health and hemoglobin levels [54].

Prevention on Schistosomiasis – Related Anemia

Stephenson noted that community-level treatment and control of schistosomiasis in areas where the infection, protein-energy malnutrition, and anemia are common are to be encouraged and are likely to improve child growth, appetite, physical fitness and activity levels and to decrease anemia and symptoms of the infestation [45]. Hence, the screening test and early management of detected cases are proper strategies in preventive medicine for schistosomiasis – related anemia.

4. Anemia in Trichuriasis

Trichuriasis is caused by a parasitic roundworm namely *Trichuris trichiura*. The main mode of transmission for trichuriasis is oro-fecal. Human can get the helminthic egg from the soil and then ingest it due to poor sanitation, no hand washing before a meal [55]. The endemicity of this helminth is similar to those of other intestinal helminthes in tropical countries. This helminth infestation is frequently reported in the same setting to the hookworm infestation and anemia [55 - 56]. However, the direct effect of this helminthic infestation as the cause of anemia, such as induction of hemolytic anemia, is rarely reported [57].

References

[1]   Gilgen DD, Mascie-Taylor CG, Rosetta LL. Intestinal helminth infections, anaemia and labour productivity of female tea pluckers in Bangladesh. *Trop Med Int Health* 2001;6:449-57.

[2]   Chakma T, Rao PV, Tiwary RS. Prevalence of anaemia and worm infestation in tribal areas of Madhya Pradesh. *J Indian Med Assoc.* 2000;98:567, 570-1.

[3]   Triteeraprapab S, Nuchprayoon I. Eosinophilia, anemia and parasitism in a rural region of northwest Thailand. *Southeast Asian J Trop Med Public Health* 1998;29:584-90.

[4]   Moraes LR, Cancio JA, Cairncross S. Impact of drainage and sewerage on intestinal nematode infections in poor urban areas in Salvador, Brazil. *Trans R Soc Trop Med Hyg* 2004;98:197-204.

[5]   Olsen A, Samuelsen H, Onyango-Ouma W. A study of risk factors for intestinal helminth infections using epidemiological and anthropological approaches. *J Biosoc Sci* 2001;33:569-84.

[6]   Bakta IM, Widjana ID, Sutisna P. Some epidemiological aspects of hookworm infection among the rural population of Bali, Indonesia. *Southeast Asian J Trop Med Public Health* 1993;24:87-93.

[7]   Hosain GM, Saha S, Begum A. Impact of sanitation and health education on intestinal parasite infection among primary school-aged children of Sherpur, Bangladesh. *Trop Doct* 2003;33:139-43.

[8]   Del Valle A, Jones BF, Harrison LM, Chadderdon RC, Cappello M. Isolation and molecular cloning of a secreted hookworm platelet inhibitor from adult Ancylostoma caninum. *Mol Biochem Parasitol* 2003;129:167-77.

[9]   Harrison LM, Nerlinger A, Bungiro RD, Cordova JL, Kuzmic P, Cappello M. Molecular characterization of Ancylostoma inhibitors of coagulation factor Xa. Hookworm anticoagulant activity in vitro predicts parasite bloodfeeding in vivo. *J Biol Chem* 2002;277:6223-9.

[10] Wiwanitkit V, Soogarun S, Saksirisampant V, Suwansaksri J. Platelet parameters in subjects infected with hookworm. *Platelets* 2003;14:391-3.

[11] Traub RJ, Robertson ID, Irwin P, Mencke N, Andrew Thompson RC. The prevalence, intensities and risk factors associated with geohelminth infection in tea-growing communities of Assam, India. *Trop Med Int Health* 2004;9:688-701.

[12] Yadla S, Sen HG, Hotez PG. An epidemiological study of ancylostomiasis in a rural area of Kanpur district Uttar Pradesh, India. *Indian J Public Health.* 2003 ;47:53-60.

[13] Sampathkumar V, Rajaratnam A. Prevalence of anaemia and hookworm infestation among adolescent girls in one rural block of TamilNadu. *Indian J Matern Child Health* 1997;8:73-5.

[14] Srinivasan V, Radhakrishna S, Ramanathan AM, Jabbar S. Hookworm infection in a rural community in south India and its association with haemoglobin levels. *Trans R Soc Trop Med Hyg* 1987;81:973-7.

[15] Sagin DD, Ismail G, Mohamad M, Pang EK, Sya OT. Anemia in remote interior communities in Sarawak, Malaysia. *Southeast Asian J Trop Med Public Health* 2002;33:373-7.

[16] Bakta IM, Budhianto FX. Hookworm anemia in the adult population of Jagapati village, Bali, Indonesia. *Southeast Asian J Trop Med Public Health* 1994;25:459-63.

[17] Nazari MR, Massoud J. Hookworm infection and blood changes in the rural population of Dezful area in Khuzestan, South-West of Iran. *Bull Soc Pathol Exot Filiales* 1980;73:108-11.

[18] Guyatt HL, Brooker S, Kihamia CM, Hall A, Bundy DA. Evaluation of efficacy of school-based anthelmintic treatments against anaemia in children in the United Republic of Tanzania. *Bull World Health Organ* 2001;79:695-703.

[19] Levi I, Gaspar N, Riesenberg K, Porath A, Yerushalmi R, Gilad J, Schlaeffer F. Iron-deficiency anemia related to ancylostoma duodenale infection among Ethiopian immigrants to Israel. *Harefuah* 2003;142:606-8.

[20] Georgiev VS. Parasitic infections. Treatment and developmental therapeutics. 1. *Necatoriasis. Curr Pharm Des* 1999;5:545-54.

[21] Crompton DW, Whitehead RR. Hookworm infections and human iron metabolism.: *Parasitology* 1993;107 Suppl:S137-45.

[22] Gottstein B, Ising S, Stoye M. Parasitologic, clinical, hematologic and serologic findings in puppies after lactogenic infection with Ancylostoma caninum ERCOLANI 1859 (Ancylostomidae). *Zentralbl Veterinarmed B* 1991;38:111-22.

[23] Albonico M, Stoltzfus RJ, Savioli L, Tielsch JM, Chwaya HM, Ercole E, Cancrini G. Epidemiological evidence for a differential effect of hookworm species, Ancylostoma duodenale or Necator americanus, on iron status of children. *Int J Epidemiol* 1998;27:530-7.

[24] Differentiation of thalassaemia minor from iron deficiency. *Lancet* 1973; 2:155-6.

[25] Dossa RA, Ategbo EA, de Koning FL, van Raaij JM, Hautvast JG. Impact of iron supplementation and deworming on growth performance in preschool Beninese children. *Eur J Clin Nutr* 2001;55:223-8.

[26] Brentlinger PE, Capps L, Denson M. Hookworm infection and anemia in adult women in rural Chiapas, Mexico. *Salud Publica Mex* 2003;45:117-9.

[27] Knight R. The management of hookworm anaemia. *East Afr Med J* 1968;45:746-9.

[28] Williams G, Naraqi S. Severe anaemia in Port Moresby. A review of 101 adult Melanesian patients with haemoglobin level of 4G/100 ml or less. *P N G Med J* 1979;22:29-36.

[29] Holzer BR, Egger M, Teuscher T, Koch S, Mboya DM, Smith GD. Childhood anemia in Africa: to transfuse or not transfuse? *Acta Trop* 1993;55:47-51.

[30] Fleming AF. The aetiology of severe anaemia in pregnancy in Ndola, Zambia. *Ann Trop Med Parasitol* 1989;83:37-49.

[31] Albonico M, Savioli L. Hookworm infection and disease: advances for control. *Ann Ist Super Sanita* 1997;33:567-79.

[32] de Silva NR. Impact of mass chemotherapy on the morbidity due to soil-transmitted nematodes. *Acta Trop* 2003;86:197-214.

[33] Gilles HM. Selective primary health care: strategies for control of disease in the developing world. XVII. Hookworm infection and anemia. *Rev Infect Dis* 1985;7:111-8.

[34] Curtis MA, Bylund G. Diphyllobothriasis: fish tapeworm disease in the circumpolar north.*Arctic Med Res* 1991;50:18-24.

[35] Donoso-Scroppo M, Raposo L, Reyes H, Godorecci S, Castillo G. Megaloblastic anemia secondary to infection by Diphyllobothrium latum. *Rev Med Chil* 1986;114:1171-4.

[36] Von Bonsdorff B, Gordin R. Castle's test (with vitamin B12 and normal gastric juice) in the ileum in patients with genuine and patients with tapeworm pernicious anaemia. *Acta Med Scand.* 1980;208:193-7.

[37] Festen HP. Intrinsic factor secretion and cobalamin absorption. Physiology and pathophysiology in the gastrointestinal tract. *Scand J Gastroenterol Suppl* 1991;188:1-7.

[38] Zaha O, Hirata T, Kinjo F, Saito A. Strongyloidiasis--progress in diagnosis and treatment. *Intern Med* 2000;39:695-700.

[39] Adedayo O, Grell G, Bellot P. Hyperinfective strongyloidiasis in the medical ward: review of 27 cases in 5 years. *South Med J* 2002;95:711-6.

[40] Lemos LB, Qu Z, *Laucirica R, Fred HL. Hyperinfection syndrome in strongyloidiasis: report of two cases. Ann* Diagn Pathol 2003;7:87-94.

[41]   Henderson GS, Nix NA, Montesano MA, Gold D, Freeman GL Jr, McCurley TL, Colley DG. Two distinct pathological syndromes in male CBA/J inbred mice with chronic Schistosoma mansoni infections. *Am J Pathol* 1993;142:703-14.

[42]   Leenstra T, Kariuki SK, Kurtis JD, Oloo AJ, Kager PA, ter Kuile FO. Prevalence and severity of anemia and iron deficiency: cross-sectional studies in adolescent schoolgirls in western Kenya. *Eur J Clin Nutr* 2004;58:681-91.

[43]   Urbani C, Toure A, Hamed AO, Albonico M, Kane I, Cheikna D, Hamed NO, Montresor A, Savioli L. Intestinal parasitic infections and schistosomiasis in the valley of the Senegal river in the Islamic Republic of Mauritania. *Med Trop* (Mars) 1997;57:157-60.

[44]   Onishi K. Schistosomiasis (intestinal, hepatic, urinary tract). *Ryoikibetsu Shokogun Shirizu*. 1999;(24 Pt 2):481-4.

[45]   Stephenson L. The impact of schistosomiasis on human nutrition. *Parasitology* 1993;107 Suppl:S107-23.

[46]   Fleming AF. Iron deficiency in the tropics. *Clin Haematol* 1982;11:365-88.

[47]   Laudage G, Schirp J. Schistosomiasis--a rare cause of iron deficiency anemia. *Leber Magen Darm* 1996;26:216-8.

[48]   Abou-Taleb S, Abbas A, el-Rakayby AA, Teleb S. Latent iron deficiency anaemia in schistosomiasis. *J Egypt Soc Parasitol* 1989;19:211-7.

[49]   Ndamba J, Makaza N, Kaondera KC, Munjoma M. Morbidity due to Schistosoma mansoni among sugar-cane cutters in Zimbabwe. *Int J Epidemiol* 1991;20:787-95.

[50]   Prual A, Daouda H, Develoux M, Sellin B, Galan P, Hercberg S. Consequences of Schistosoma haematobium infection on the iron status of schoolchildren in Niger. *Am J Trop Med Hyg* 1992;47:291-7.

[51]   Olsen A, Magnussen P, Ouma JH, Andreassen J, Friis H. The contribution of hookworm and other parasitic infections to haemoglobin and iron status among children and adults in western Kenya. *Trans R Soc Trop Med Hyg* 1998;92:643-9.

[52]   Beasley NM, Tomkins AM, Hall A, Kihamia CM, Lorri W, Nduma B, Issae W, Nokes C, Bundy DA. The impact of population level deworming on the haemoglobin levels of schoolchildren in Tanga, Tanzania. *Trop Med Int Health* 1999;4:744-50.

[53]   Friis H, Mwaniki D, Omondi B, Muniu E, Thiong'o F, Ouma J, Magnussen P, Geissler PW, Fleischer Michaelsen K. Effects on haemoglobin of multi-micronutrient supplementation and multi-helminth chemotherapy: a randomized, controlled trial in Kenyan school children. *Eur J Clin Nutr* 2003;57:573-9.

[54]   Taylor M, Jinabhai CC, Couper I, Kleinschmidt I, Jogessar VB. The effect of different anthelmintic treatment regimens combined with iron supplementation on the nutritional status of schoolchildren in KwaZulu-Natal, South Africa: a randomized controlled trial. *Trans R Soc Trop Med Hyg* 2001;95:211-6.

[55]   Wiwanitkit V, Waenlor W, Suyaphan A. Contamination of soil with parasites in a tropical hilltribe village in Northern Thailand. *Trop Doct* 2003;33:180-2.

[56]   Ulukanligil M, Seyrek A. Anthropometric status, anaemia and intestinal helminthic infections in shantytown and apartment schoolchildren in the Sanliurfa province of Turkey. *Eur J Clin Nutr* 2004;58:1056-61.

[57] Huicho L. Trichuriasis associated to severe transient Coomb's-negative hemolytic anemia and macroscopic hematuria. *Wilderness Environ Med* 1995;6:247.

Chapter 5

Anemia in Bacterial Infections

Bacterial Infections and Anemia

Bacterial infections can produce several hematological alterations. The hematological changes include white blood cell, red blood cell and platelet abnormality. The bacterial infections may increase or decrease numbers of circulating erythrocytes, leukocytes, and platelets or may induce qualitative changes in these elements, some of which affect their function [1]. In addition, bacterial infections may also produce thrombosis or hemorrhage [1]. Strausbaugh said that the bacterial infections exerted these effects through mechanisms that involved specific microbial virulence factors or host defenses mobilized against the infectious agents [1]. Concerning the microbial virulence, the alterations to hematopoietic cells are usually mediated via the influence of microbial toxins and cytokines on cellular proliferation, differentiation, and activation [2]. Anemia can be the result of the described mechanism. Concerning the host defenses, anemia can sometimes be a result of improper host response such as autoimmunity.

Concerning the type of anemia in bacterial infections, normocytic, microcytic and macrocytic can be found. The hemolytic anemia from many bacterial toxins can be a good example of normocytic anemia in bacterial infections. The iron deficiency anemia from chronic *Helicobacter pyroli* infection can be a good example of microcytic anemia [3]. The vitamin B12 deficiency from chronic *H. pyroli* infection can be a good example of macrocytic anemia [3]. Since the bacterial infection is still an important health problem for the tropics, the anemia in bacterial infections is also a tropical hematological problem. Some important common bacterial infections and their relation to anemia will be presented in this chapter.

Normocytic Anemia in Bacterial Infection

1. Leptospirosis and Anemia

Leptospirosis is an important tropical disease with high prevalence in developing countries [4 – 6]. The main pathogen of leptospirosis is *Leptospira* spp, a bacteria in the spirochete group. Bharti *et al.* said that mortality of leptospirosis remains significant, related both to delays in diagnosis due to lack of infrastructure and adequate clinical suspicion, and to other poorly understood reasons that may include inherent pathogenicity of some leptospiral strains or genetically determined host immunopathological responses [6]. In addition, Wiwanitkit also reported that the people in the rural endemic area of leptospirosis still have some false knowledge on the disease and the participation of people in health volunteer meetings had a significant correlation to the learning of how to prevent diseases among the villagers [7].

Clinically, presenting symptoms for leptospirosis varied with age in children showing primarily fever, vomiting, headache, abdominal and generalized muscle pain and diarrhea whereas adults had fever, headache, anorexia, muscle pain and constipation [8]. Anemia is also an important manifestation of leptospirosis.

Concerning the pathogenesis of anemia in leptospirosis, some believe that erythropoiesis suppression is an important mechanism [9]. However, Avdeeva *et al.* recently performed sternal biopsy for study of the dynamics of medullary hemopoiesis in 20 patients with leptospirosis caused by *L. icterohaemorragiae, L. canicola* and *L. gebdomadis* [10]. They found a moderate activation of erythropoiesis, irritation of the lymphomonocytic sprout as well as oppression of the basophil and neutrophil series were the characteristic features of myelograms at the acute illness stage [10]. They concluded that leptospirosis did not affect the functional ability of the bone marrow, and anemia in the patients with leptospirosis was predominantly the hyperregenerative nature with the normoblastic hemopoiesis type [10]. Avdeeva *et al.* reported another interesting finding: low glucose-6-phosphate dehydrogenase (G-6-PD) activity of erythrocytes on the second week of the illness preceded anemia in 83.3% cases, which could be a prognostic criterion for developing anemic syndrome [11]. Avdeeva *et al.* concluded that anemia was a typical manifestation of leptospirosis during the second week of disease [12]. The type of anemia is normocytic normochromic hyperregeneratory [12]. Avdeeva *et al.* said that the leading pathogenetic mechanism of anemia associated with leptospirosis was erythrocyte hemolysis, whose intensity during the acute period depended on the severity of intoxication and extracorporeal methods of detoxication and persistence of anemia during convalescent period was due to involvement of the kidneys, nephrotic nephritis [12]. The hemolysis in leptospirosis can not only lead to anemia but also jaundice and hemoglobinuria, which can be an indicator for severity of the disease [13].

Concerning management for anemia in leptospirosis, penicillin treatment should be given for getting rid of the pathogen and intravenous fluid supplements should be considered [8]. Close monitoring for the renal complication should be performed. Concerning the severe case, which usually presented with icterohemorrhagic symptoms, the exchange transfusion is recommended [14]. In 2002, Tse *et al.* reported their experience with a patient who developed severe Weil's syndrome, severe leptospirosis with marked conjugated hyperbilirubinemia and oliguric acute renal failure, and these complications persisted despite treatment with penicillin and hemodiafiltration [15]. In this case, plasma exchange was instituted and a favorable result could be derived [15]. Tse *et al.* concluded that plasma exchange should be considered as an adjunctive therapy for patients with severe icterohemorrhagic leptospirosis complicated by acute renal failure who had not shown rapid clinical response to conventional treatment [15].

2. Tuberculosis and Anemia

Tuberculosis is a group of infectious diseases caused by well-known bacteria, Mycobacterium tuberculosis. At present, this infection can be seen all over the world, not limited to the tropics. In addition, other Mycobacterium spp infections become emerging health problems. The possible explanation for these findings is the wide distribution of human immunodeficiency virus (HIV) infection [16]. Singh et al. normocytic normochromic anaemia was the most common hematological abnormality observed in the patients with tuberculosis (disseminated/miliary tuberculosis 84%, pulmonary TB 86%) [17]. Singh et al. also said that the patients of disseminated/miliary tuberculosis with granulomas in the bone marrow had certain significant differences as compared to patients without granulomas [17]. They mentioned that these patients showed severe anaemia, peripheral monocytopenia and bone marrow histiomonocytosis and the hemogram reverted to normal with antituberculosis therapy in these patients [17]. It is believed that a mechanism, underlying anemia in tuberculosis, is due to decrease of red blood cell production. The red blood cell aplasia (normocytic normochromic anemia, reticulocytopenia and marked paucity of erythroid precursors on bone marrow aspiration and biopsy studies) is indicated in tuberculosis [18]. In addition, Wessels et al. noted that a lower mean hemoglobin was the only significantly different hematological parameter in children with tuberculosis compared with the comparison group [19]. Concerning the prevalence of anemia in tuberculosis, the high prevalence is reported in the cases with advanced diseases. According to the study of Mert et al. in the patients with miliary tuberculosis, 76% of the overall patients had anemia [20]

It is indicated that anemia, low body weight, and extensive infiltrates are clinical predictors of early mortality from tuberculosis [21]. Since anemia in the patients with tuberculosis can lead to poor prognosis, therefore, the proper management for these patients is recommended. The treatment of tuberculosis by antituberculosis drug is recommended for all cases with or without anemia. Since some previous reports indicated for the iron deficiency anemia as a possible result from inflammation or as a co-presentation due to the common endemic, iron supplementation has been practiced irrespective of the etiology [22]. Recently, Das et al. suggested that iron supplementation in mild to moderate anemia associated with pulmonary tuberculosis accelerated the normal resumption of hematopoiesis in the initial phases by increasing iron saturation of transferrin [22]. However, they noted that consistent improvement of hematological status was dependent only on the improvement of the disease process [22]. Another important item that should be noted is the hemolytic anemia as the complication of treatment of tuberculosis by antituberculosis drug, especially for rifampicin [23]. These phenomena are sporadically reported. Ahrens et al. reported that rifampicin might stimulate the production of autoantibodies (aab) and/or drug-dependent antibodies (ddab), and that the resulting haemolytic syndrome bears similarities with autoimmune hemolytic anemia (AIHA) [23]. Yeo et al. reported a similar case, mild hemolytic anemia with flu-syndrome in a patient after getting rifampicin for treatment of pulmonary tuberculosis [24].

3. Anemia and *Escherichia Coli* Infection

Shiga toxin (Stx) producing *Escherichia coli* (STEC) is a newly emerged pathogen that has been the focus of immense international research effort driven by its recognition as a major cause of large scale epidemics and thousands of sporadic cases of gastrointestinal illness [25]. Khan *et al.* said that produced a severe bloody diarrhea that is clinically distinct from other types of diarrhoeal diseases caused by other enteric pathogens [25]. Thorpe noted that approximately 5%-10% of people with STEC infection would develop hemolytic-uremic syndrome (HUS), approximately 10% of those who develop HUS would die or have permanent renal failure, and up to 50% of those who developed HUS would develop some degree of renal impairment [26].

Similar to other diarrheal disease, the STEC is common in the tropics. A variety of foods have been identified as vehicles of STEC-associated illness and this makes the organism one of the most serious threats to the food industry in recent years [25].

Khan *et al.* said that the pathogenesis of STEC is multifactorial and involves several levels of interaction between the bacterium and the host [25]. They noted that STEC strains carry a set of virulence genes that encode the factors for attachment to host cells, elaboration of effective molecules and production of two different types of Shiga toxins [25]. These genes are found in the locus of enterocyte effacement (LEE), lamboid phages, and a large virulence associated plasmid [25]. Concerning the mechanism, underlying anemia in STEC infection, the hemolysis is mentioned as the main corresponding cause. E. coli O157:H7 is the main pathogen in STEC group. Stx associated HUS, is now known to be caused by Escherichia coli O157:7, which produces Stxl or the more potent, Stx2 [27]. The renal tubule is the major tissue affected in the course of HUS, and Stx2 is known to be toxic to the renal tubular cells (RTC) [27]. Recently, Lee *et al.* purified Stx2 from the *E. coli* O157:7, which was isolated from a typical diarrhea-associated HUS patient and then tried to compare the cytokine gene expression between the stimulated RTC and un-stimulated RTC using cDNA-array [27]. According to this study, one third of the examined cytokine genes were up regulated at least twice by the addition of Vtx2 and these up-regulated genes represented the chemokines (macrophage related cytokines), fibrosis-related cytokine (TNF, PDGF) and leukemia inhibitory factors [27]. Lee *et al.* suggested that VT2 up-regulated the pro-inflammatory cytokines and fibrosis prone growth factors in RTC and that the inhibition of the activation of these cytokines might ameliorate the renal tubular injury in the HUS caused by E. coli O157:7 [27].

Concerning the hemolysis, Proulx *et al.* said that several factors such as Stx, lipopolysaccharide, the adhesins intimin and *E. coli*-secreted proteins A, B, and D, the 60-

MD plasmid, and enterohemolysin likely contributed to the pathogenesis [28]. In addition, Karpman *et al.* found that Stx1, Stx1B, and a factor or factors in the plasma of patients with HUS activated platelets [29]. The presence of Stx1 at the binding site of platelets to human umbilical vein endothelial cells in this study suggested that Stx may be directly involved in the prothrombotic state seen in HUS [29]

Clinically, STEC associated HUS is characterized by the signs of microangiopathic hemolytic anemia, thrombocytopenia with renal lesions and possible manifestations of transient disturbances in the functions of the central nervous system. Misselwitz *et al.* found that the clinical course ranged from mild uncomplicated HUS to severe HUS complicated by multiorgan involvement [30]. Rivas *et al.* performed a study in Buenos Aires and found that cumulative evidence of STEC infection was found in 19 (86.4%) of 22 HUS patients. In this report, the acute stage of the disease occurred with presentation of pallor, edema, anuria, oliguria, hemolytic anemia, thrombocytopenia and neurological involvement [31]. Rivas *et al.* noted that *E. coli* O157:H7, biotype C, Stx2 producer was the most frequently detected pathogen in their HUS cases [31]. Friedrich *et al.* said that Stx1c-producing *E. coli* strains represented a significant subset of eae-negative human STEC isolates, which belonged to various serotypes and frequently possessed LPA and saa as their putative virulence factors [32]. Presently, this infection is not limited to the tropics. There are reports of outbreaks from other non-tropical countries as well [33 – 34]. As already mentioned, food is the main source of the pathogen. In 2001, Sanath Kumar *et al.* reported that seafoods in India is a main source of STEC, and non-O157 serotype is more common [35].

Optimal management of STEC infection includes intravenous hydration, avoidance of antimotility agents and antimicrobials, and monitoring for sequelae [25 – 26]. It is noted that antimicrobials might have a potentially harmful role, possibly by inducing intestinal production of Shiga toxin during the diarrheal phase of illness and recent clinical trials evaluating an intraluminal Shiga toxin-binding agent to ameliorate HUS had showed no improvement in outcome [25 – 26]. Concerning the severe cases, successful management by peritoneal dialysis and packed red cell transfusion was reported [29]. Rivas *et al.* said that up to 90 % of the patients who received these combined treatments recovered renal function [29]. Since this infection is food and water-borne, food and water sanitation is recommended in control and prevention.

4. Anemia and Syphilis

Syphilis is an old well-known disease caused by bacteria namely *Treponema pallidum*. This bacterial infection is considered a common sexually transmitted disease (STD). The high prevalence of this infection can be seen in the underprivileged populations in developing countries [36 - 37]. However, this infection is not limited to the tropics but widespread all over the world. Anemia is mentioned as an important complication in the patients with syphilis, especially the pediatric and obstetric patients.

Mavrov and Goubenko studied 155 pregnant women infected with syphilis and found that pregnancy pathology was observed in 75 cases (48.8%) and more often appeared as anemia in 49 (31.5%) [38]. They noted that the pregnancy pathology in women with syphilis was considered not pathognomonic [38]. While Hollier *et al.* studied the laboratory manifestation in the fetal syphilis and found that abnormal liver transaminases were found in 88%, anemia in 26%, and thrombocytopenia in 35% [39]. Indeed, syphilis needs to be excluded in infants suspected of haemophagocytic lymphohistiocytosis [40]. Pohl *et al.* reported a previously healthy male infant developed hepatosplenomegaly, severe anemia and thrombocytopenia 5 weeks after birth with marked hemophagocytosis in the bone marrow [40]. In this case, a typical maculopapular rash suggested early congenital syphilis and the diagnosis was confirmed by serology and by the presence of untreated syphilis in both parents [40].

The paroxysmal cold hemoglobinuria (PCH), a rare, acquired hemolytic syndrome caused by cold-active antibodies to antigens of the P blood group system, is another finding that is mentioned in the patients with syphilis [41]. However, syphilis is now an uncommon cause of PCH [41 - 42].

The treatment for anemia in congenital syphilis is indicated. Since it is classified as a symptomatic congenital syphilis of which parenteral antibiotic treatment with 100,000 IU penicillin/kg.day for 15 days is recommended [43]. Hoarau *et al.* noted that a single injection of benzathine-penicillin was a good compromise between simple surveillance and admission to hospital for 10 days of intravenous treatment, and serological surveillance was required to check that IgM disappears from the blood or that the titer of IgG decreases [43]. Concerning the prevention of disease, it is noted that STD screening could prevent needless suffering in many women since 5-15% of pregnant women in some developing countries had syphilis [44].

5. Anemia and Shigellosis

Shigellosis is another common diarrheal disease in the tropics. *Shigella flexneri* is a gram-negative bacterium which causes the most communicable of bacterial dysenteries, shigellosis, resulting in 1.1 million deaths and over 164 million cases each year, with the majority of cases occurring in children in developing nations [45]. *S. sonnei* is another, less frequent, pathogen that leads to shigellosis. The pathogenesis of *S. flexneri* is based on the bacteria's ability to invade and replicate within the colonic epithelium, which results in severe inflammation and epithelial destruction [45]. Complications that can lead to death during shigellosis include intestinal as well as systemic manifestations [46]. The former include intestinal perforation, toxic megacolon, and dehydration, and the latter include sepsis, hyponatremia, hypoglycemia, seizures and encephalopathy, hemolyticuremic syndrome, pneumonia, and malnutrition [46].

Considering hematological alterations in shigellosis, peak granulocytosis can occur during the second week of illness, when the patients are commonly afebrile and diarrhea has ceased or is subsiding [47]. It is noted that more than half of the patients with leukemoid reactions subsequently developed a fall in hematocrit associated with striking erythrocyte fragmentation on blood smears [47]. Koster *et al.* mentioned that severe colitis in shigellosis is associated with circulating endotoxin from the colon producing coagulopathy, renal microangiopathy and hemolytic anemia [48]. Similar to anemia due to STEC, the HUS is a severe anemic complication of shigellosis. In 1989, Kato *et al.* performed a molecular biological study and found that the *S. sonnei* strains carrying both of the ipa locus and the invA locus were active in contact hemolysis and cell invasion assays [49]. Luckily, the prevalence of this complication is low. Kavaliotis *et al.* studied 422 cases of shigellosis and found that 94 patients (22%) had extra-intestinal manifestations, with a case of haemolytic-uraemic syndrome [50]. Kovitangoon *et al.* reported 8 cases of HUS in shigellosis. In this study, all patients had prodromal symptoms of mucous bloody diarrhea and the stool culture was positive for Shigella dysentery type I in one case [51]. At present, this infection is not limited to the tropics. Several non-tropical countries have encountered with this infection [52 – 53].

The treatments of HUS in shigellosis include blood transfusion, peritoneal dialysis, exchange transfusion and supportive treatment [51]. Antibiotic in not effective. In addition, antibiotic treatment for shigellosis can sometimes bring HUS [54 – 55]. Similar to STEC infection, this infection is food and water-borne. Food and water sanitation is recommended in control and prevention.

6. Anemia and Salmonellosis

Salmonellosis, caused by *Salmonella* spp, is a common bacterial infection in the tropics. Salmonellosis has a wide range of clinical manifestation, asymptomatic carrier, intestinal syndromes and extra-intestinal syndromes. The most common form of salmonellosis, typhoid fever is diagnosed on the basis of isolation of *Salmonella typhi* from blood, bone marrow, or bile while *S. typhi* found in stool or urine may reflect chronic asymptomatic carriage [56]. Anemia can be seen in the patients with typhoid fever. Butles *et al.* noted that children from birth through 10 years of age were more anemic [57]. HUS is also reported as a rare complication of typhoid fever [58].

It should be noted that salmonellosis itself can lead to anemia and it also can be the complication of many anemic diseases that have a poor immune nature such as sickle cell anemia and thalassemia [59 - 60]. Concerning the treatment for typhoid fever, although antimicrobial therapy may not eliminate carriage, it is effective for the treatment of clinically evident acute disease [56]. Among the drugs currently available, chloramphenicol is the most widely used. Although chloramphenicol is effective and inexpensive, it is associated with a 3% rate of chronic carriage, a high relapse rate, and, in rare cases, aplastic anemia [56]. Concerning the control of the disease, food and water sanitation is recommended similar to other enteric bacterial induced diseases.

7. Brucellosis and Anemia

Brucellosis is a zoonotic disease of worldwide distribution that mainly affects persons working with domestic animals and animal products [61]. Despite being controlled in many developed countries, the disease remains endemic in many parts of the tropical world, including Latin America, the Middle East, Spain, parts of Africa, and western Asia [61]. The disease is mainly transmitted to humans through the ingestion of raw milk or non-pasteurized cheese contaminated with one of the four *Brucella* spp pathogenic to humans [61]. Memish and Balkhy said that the clinical presentation can vary from asymptomatic infection with seroconversion to a full-blown clinical picture of fever, night sweats and joint manifestations; rarely, there is hepatic, cardiac, ocular or central nervous system involvement [61].

Anemia in brucellosis is a hematological finding in the patients with brucellosis. Namidura *et al.* studied 120 Turkish patients with brucellosis and found that the commonest hematological abnormalities were relative lymphomonocytosis (71.6%) and anemia (36.6%) [62]. According to another study of Martin *et al.* in the patients with brucellosis, the hemogram revealed anemia in 30.3% of all cases [63]. Tsolia *et al.* found that anemia (39%) and monocytosis (31%) were the most common hematological manifestations, followed by lymphopenia (18%) [64]. Concerning the pathogenesis of anemia in brucellosis, the suppression of bone marrow is mentioned. Pancytopenia associated with brucellosis is attributed to hypersplenism, hemophagocytosis, and granulomatous lesions of the bone marrow, which is usually hypercellular [65]. Yildirmak *et al.* mentioned that bone marrow hypoplasia was rarely reported and should be kept in mind in the etiology of aplastic anemia in a country where brucellosis is frequently encountered [65]. However, hemolytic anemia is also mentioned in the patients with brucellosis. Yaramis *et al.* reported a case of severe microangiopathic hemolytic anemia (MAHA) and thrombocytopenia with epistaxis, gross hematuria, hemoglobinuria, and skin purpura in a child with Brucella septicemia proven by culture [66]. Concerning the treatment of brucellosis, the most commonly used therapy consisted of the association tetracycline plus streptomycin [62]. In the cases with relapse, rifampicin is indicated [67].

8. Anemia and Anthrax

Anthrax is a bacterial infection caused by a spore-forming Gram-positive bacilli called *Bacillus anthracis*. Anthrax, a disease of mammals including humans. Anthrax is one of the oldest threats to humanity, and remains endemic in animals in many parts of the world [68]. Although human anthrax has become rare, endemic outbreaks still occur in tropical countries, parts of South America and Asia. The incidence of anthrax has decreased in developed countries, but it remains a considerable health problem in developing countries [68]. The disease is transmitted to humans by contact with sick animals or their products, such as wool, skin and meat [68]. Human anthrax has three major clinical forms: cutaneous, inhalational, and gastrointestinal. The diagnosis is easily established in cutaneous cases, characterized by black eschar [68]. Severe intoxication and collapse during the course of bronchopneumonia or hemorrhagic enteritis should prompt suspicion of anthrax [68].

Although anemia is not common in anthrax, there are some case reports.

Recently, Freedman *et al.* reported a case with cutaneous anthrax developed severe systemic illness despite early treatment with antibiotics [69]. This case displayed severe MAHA with renal involvement, coagulopathy, and hyponatremia [69].

They reported another case of anthrax with laboratory findings as hemoconcentration, anemia and leukocytosis [70].

Microcytic Anemia in Bacterial Infection

1. Anemia and Leprosy

Leprosy is another disease resulting from acid-fast bacilli infection, similar to tuberculosis. This disease can still be found in some developing tropical countries such as India. Sen *et al.* studied a total of 128 Indian leprosy patients for the morphological type of anemia, the underlying disturbances in iron metabolism and patterns of erythropoiesis and other cytomorphological changes in the bone marrow [71]. They found that anemia was a mild to moderate degree in paucibacillary (PB) leprosy, while in multibacillary (MB) leprosy, it was of a severe degree [71]. Impaired iron utilization as observed in an anemia of a chronic disorder was a common finding in MB leprosy (41.7%) and more so in new cases (50%), however, iron deficiency was observed in only a few patients [72]. According to this study, irrespective of the type of disease and duration of treatment, increasing frequency of acid-fast bacilli positivity and granulomas was observed in the bone marrow with an increasing severity of anemia [72].

Similar to tuberculosis, the antileprosy drug, dapsone, is the recommended treatment. Sen *et al.* noted that disturbances in iron metabolism and erythropoiesis were also observed but to a lesser degree in the patients receiving specific antileprosy treatment [71]. However, it should be noted for the effect of antileprosy drug on red blood cells. Dapsone commonly results in not only hemolysis but a significant decrease in hemoglobin concentration and this may have serious clinical implications, especially in endemic areas, where, owing to nutrition, malaria, and intestinal parasitism, the hemoglobin concentration is already compromised [72].

2. Anemia and *H. Pylori* Infection

H. pylori infection is now accepted as an important infection complicating the dyspepsia. The persistent inflammation of the stomach induced by H. pylori infection can have consequences on the rest of the body. H. pylori is also mentioned for the pathogenesis of extra-gastric diseases including vascular diseases, autoimmune diseases, skin diseases, sideropenic anemia, diabetes, Parkinson disease, and bronchiectasis [73].

H. pylori gastric infection has emerged as a new cause of refractory iron deficiency anemia, unresponsive to iron therapy, and not attributable to usual causes such as intestinal losses or poor intake, malabsorption or diversion of iron in the reticulo-endothelial system [74]. Barabino noted that microbiological and ferrokinetic studies seemed to suggest that Helicobacter pylori infected antrum could act as a sequestering focus for serum iron by means of outer membrane receptors of the bacterium, that in vitro are able to capture and utilize for growth iron from human lactoferrin [74]. Concerning the transmission of disease, the principal reservoir is the human stomach, and transmission probably occurs by person-to-person passage [75]. Prevalence rates are generally much higher in developing tropical countries compared to developed countries [75]. Go noted that decreasing prevalence in developed countries or in those with rapidly improving socioeconomic conditions [75].

Hacihanefioglu *et al.* proposed that *H. pylori* infection may be involved in cases of iron deficiency anemia of unknown origin, and the eradication of the infection may improve blood parameters other than serum ferritin levels [76]. Recently, Nahon *et al.* performed a study on 105 patients with unexplained iron deficiency anemia after upper endoscopy, colonoscopy, small bowel radiographic examination and duodenal biopsies. They found that A H. pylori-associated chronic gastritis was identified in 63 cases, higher than in the control group (45 cases) [77]. Nahon *et al.* concluded that *H. pylori* infection and chronic gastritis, especially atrophic gastritis, are significantly associated with unexplained iron deficiency anemia [77].

Concerning the treatment, combination therapy consisting of lansoprosol or omeprazole, clarithromycin and amoxicillin is found to be effective for eradication of *H. pylori* gastric infection and can correct the red blood cell parameter alterations in the patients [76] According to the trial of Hacihanefioglu *et al.*, serum hemoglobin, iron and transferrin saturations of the patients were found to be increased at 20-24 weeks of follow-up after the eradication therapy while serum ferritin levels were not found to be increased [76]. Recently, Russo-Mancuso *et al.* described 9 pediatric patients with a history of long-standing iron deficiency anemia and *H. pylori* infection [78]. In these cases, Anti-*H.pylori* therapy for 2 weeks were prescribed and it found that the eradication of HP was associated with stable normalization of iron stores [78]. Russo-Mancuso *et al.* concluded that *H. pylori* infection may be involved in cases of IDA of unknown origin, and the eradication of *H. pylori* was associated with the resolution of anemia [78].

Macrocytic Anemia in Bacterial Infection

Macrocytic anemia in bacterial infection is not common. However, there are some reports on the macrocytic anemia due to the *H. pylori* infection. Indeed, the gastric infection by *H. pylori* is mentioned as a cause of iron deficiency anemia [78].

However, *H. pylori* infection has also been mentioned for its association with vitamin B12 deficiency. Presotto *et al.* noted that the frequent detection of *H. pylori* infection in subjects with early gastric autoimmunity, indicated by the presence of parietal cell antibodies, suggests that *H. pylori* could have a crucial role in the induction and/or the maintenance of autoimmunity at the gastric level [79].

Shuval-Sudai and Granot mentioned that the higher prevalence of *H. pylori* infection among subjects with serum vitamin B12 levels that were within the lower end of the normal range suggested a causal relationship between *H pylori* infection and vitamin B12 levels in healthy adults [80]. Finally, Marignani *et al.* proposed that *H pylori* infection should be investigated in any unexplained microcytic and macrocytic anemia [81].

Another interesting, non-tropical prevalent condition that should be mentioned is small bowel bacterial overgrowth (SBBO) syndrome, which is associated with excessive numbers of bacteria in the proximal small intestine [82]. Singh and Toskes said that the pathology of this condition involved competition between the bacteria and the human host for ingested nutrients, leading to intraluminal bacterial catabolism of nutrients, often with production of toxic metabolites and injury to the enterocyte [82]. A complex array of clinical symptoms ensues, resulting in chronic diarrhea, steatorrhea, macrocytic anemia, weight loss, and less commonly, protein-losing enteropathy [82]. Therapy is targeted at correction of underlying small bowel abnormalities that predispose to SBBO and appropriate antibiotic therapy. Complete reversion can be expected after treatment [82].

Although the bacterial-induced macrocytic anemia is not common in humans, it is common in animals. Several bacterial infections in animals are reported as a cause of macrocytic anemia such as *Haemobartonella felis* in domestic cats [83] and *Eperythrozoon suis* in piglets [84].

References

[1] Strausbaugh LJ. Hematologic manifestations of bacterial and fungal infections. *Hematol Oncol Clin North Am* 1987;1:185-206.

[2] McKenzie SB, Laudicina RJ. Hematologic changes associated with infection. *Clin Lab Sci* 1998;11:239-51.

[3] Annibale B, Capurso G, Delle Fave G. Consequences of Helicobacter pylori infection on the absorption of micronutrients. *Dig Liver Dis* 2002;34 Suppl 2:S72-7.

[4] Sundharagiati B, Harinasuta C, Photha U. Human leptospirosis in Thailand. *Trans R Soc Trop Med Hyg* 1966;60:361-5.

[5] Tangkanakul W, Tharmaphornpil P, Plikaytis BD, Bragg S, Poonsuksombat D, Choomkasien P, Kingnate D, Ashford DA. Risk factors associated with leptospirosis in northeastern Thailand, 1998. *Am J Trop Med Hyg* 2000 ;63:204-8.

[6] Bharti AR, Nally JE, Ricaldi JN, Matthias MA, Diaz MM, Lovett MA, Levett PN, Gilman RH, Willig MR, Gotuzzo E, Vinetz JM; Peru-United States Leptospirosis Consortium. Leptospirosis: a zoonotic disease of global importance. *Lancet Infect Dis* 2003;3:757-71.

[7] Wiwanitkit V. Knowledge of the villagers towards leptospirosis, a survey in the area with high prevalence, Prakonchai District, Buriram Province. *Presented at the Joint International Tropical Medicine Meeting* 2001, Bangkok Thailand.

[8] Heisey GB, Nimmanitya S, Karnchanachetanee C, Tingpalapong M, Samransamruajkit S, Hansukjariya P, Elwell MR, Ward GS. Epidemiology and characterization of leptospirosis at an urban and provincial site in Thailand. *Southeast Asian J Trop Med Public Health* 1988;19:317-22.

[9] Somers CJ, Al-Kindi S, Montague S, O'Connor R, Murphy PG, Jeffers M, Enright H. Erythroid hypoplasia associated with leptospirosis. *J Infect* 2003;47:85-6.

[10] Avdeeva MG, Moisova DL, Kachanov AV. Bone marrow hematopoiesis in leptospirosis and its role in anemia pathogenesis. *Klin Lab Diagn* 2003;(1):38-40.

[11] Avdeeva MG, Moisova DL, Gorodin VN, Kostomarov AM, Zotov SV, Cherniavskaia OV. The role glucose-6-phosphate dehydrogenase in pathogenesis of anemia in leptospirosis. *Klin Med* (Mosk) 2002;80:42-4.

[12] Avdeeva MG, Moisova DL, Zentsova OA, Kostomarov AM. Hematological parameters in characterization of anemia in leptospirosis. *Klin Lab Diagn* 2001;(5):8-12.

[13] Delacollette C, Taelman H, Wery M. An etiologic study of hemoglobinuria and blackwater fever in the Kivu Mountains, Zaire. *Ann Soc Belg Med Trop* 1995;75:51-63.

[14] Landini S, Coli U, Lucatello S, Bazzato G. Plasma exchange in severe leptospirosis. *Lancet* 1981;2:1119-20.

[15] Tse KC, Yip PS, Hui KM, Li FK, Yuen KY, Lai KN, Chan TM. Potential benefit of plasma exchange in treatment of severe icteric leptospirosis complicated by acute renal failure. *Clin Diagn Lab Immunol* 2002;9:482-4.

[16] Aaron L, Saadoun D, Calatroni I, Launay O, Memain N, Vincent V, Marchal G, Dupont B, Bouchaud O, Valeyre D, Lortholary O. Tuberculosis in HIV-infected patients: a comprehensive review. *Clin Microbiol Infect* 2004;10:388-98.

[17] Singh KJ, Ahluwalia G, Sharma SK, Saxena R, Chaudhary VP, Anant M. Significance of haematological manifestations in patients with tuberculosis. *Assoc Physicians India* 2001;49:788, 790-4.

[18] Sinha AK, Agarwal A, Lakhey M, Ansari J, Rani S. Pure red cell aplasia--report of 11 cases from eastern Nepal. *Indian J Pathol Microbiol* 2003;46:405-8.

[19] Wessels G, Schaaf HS, Beyers N, Gie RP, Nel E, Donald PR. Haematological abnormalities in children with tuberculosis. *J Trop Pediatr* 1999;45:307-10.

[20] Mert A, Bilir M, Tabak F, Ozaras R, Ozturk R, Senturk H, Aki H, Seyhan N, Karayel T, Aktuglu Y. Miliary tuberculosis: clinical manifestations, diagnosis and outcome in 38 adults. *Respirology*. 2001;6:217-24.

[21] Sacks LV, Pendle S. Factors related to in-hospital deaths in patients with tuberculosis. *Arch Intern Med* 1998;158:1916-22.

[22] Das BS, Devi U, Mohan Rao C, Srivastava VK, Rath PK, Das BS. Effect of iron supplementation on mild to moderate anaemia in pulmonary tuberculosis. *Br J Nutr* 2003;90:541-50.

[23] Ahrens N, Genth R, Salama A. Belated diagnosis in three patients with rifampicin-induced immune haemolytic anaemia. *Br J Haematol* 2002;117:441-3.

[24] Yeo CT, Wang YT, Poh SC. Mild haemolysis associated with flu-syndrome during daily rifampicin treatment--a case report. *Singapore Med J* 1989;30:215-6.

[25] Khan A, Datta S, Das SC, Ramamurthy T, Khanam J, Takeda Y, Bhattacharya SK, Nair GB. Shiga toxin producing Escherichia coli infection: current progress and future challenges. *Indian J Med Res* 2003;118:1-24.

[26] Thorpe CM. Shiga toxin-producing Escherichia coli infection. *Clin Infect Dis* 2004;38:1298-303.

[27] Lee JE, Kim JS, Choi IH, Tagawa M, Kohsaka T, Jin DK. Cytokine expression in the renal tubular epithelial cells stimulated by Shiga toxin 2 of Escherichia coli O157:H7. *Ren Fail* 2002;24:567-75.

[28] Proulx F, Seidman EG, Karpman D. Pathogenesis of Shiga toxin-associated hemolytic uremic syndrome. *Pediatr Res* 2001;50:163-71.

[29] Karpman D, Papadopoulou D, Nilsson K, Sjogren AC, Mikaelsson C, Lethagen S. Platelet activation by Shiga toxin and circulatory factors as a pathogenetic mechanism in the hemolytic uremic syndrome. *Blood* 2001;97:3100-8.

[30] Misselwitz J, Karch H, Bielazewska M, John U, Ringelmann F, Ronnefarth G, Patzer L. Cluster of hemolytic-uremic syndrome caused by Shiga toxin-producing Escherichia coli O26:H11. *Pediatr Infect Dis J* 2003;22:349-54.

[31] Rivas M, Balbi L, Miliwebsky ES, Garcia B, Tous MI, Leardini NA, Prieto MA, Chillemi GM, de Principi ME. Hemolytic uremic syndrome in children of Mendoza, Argentina: association with Shiga toxin-producing Escherichia coli infection. *Medicina* (B Aires) 1998;58:1-7.

[32] Friedrich AW, Borell J, Bielaszewska M, Fruth A, Tschape H, Karch H. Shiga toxin 1c-producing Escherichia coli strains: phenotypic and genetic characterization and association with human disease. *J Clin Microbiol* 2003;41:2448-53.

[33] Yamamota T, Wakisaka N. Status of emerging drug resistance in Shiga toxin-producing Escherichia coli in Japan during 1996: a minireview. *Nippon Rinsho* 1998;56:2718-29.

[34] Brooks JT, Bergmire-Sweat D, Kennedy M, Hendricks K, Garcia M, Marengo L, Wells J, Ying M, Bibb W, Griffin PM, Hoekstra RM, Friedman CR. Outbreak of Shiga toxin-producing Escherichia coli O111:H8 infections among attendees of a high school cheerleading camp. *Clin Infect Dis* 2004;38:190-8.

[35] Sanath Kumar H, Otta SK, Karunasagar I, Karunasagar I. Detection of Shiga-toxigenic Escherichia coli (STEC) in fresh seafood and meat marketed in Mangalore, India by PCR. *Lett Appl Microbiol* 2001;33:334-8.

[36] Wiwanitkit V. Prevalence of VDRL seroreactive in Myanmar migrators in a rural area of Thailand. *Sex Disab* 2003; 21: 85-88.

[37] Wiwanitkit V. An Overview of VDRL Serology Screening Checkup Program in Thailand: Part II *Sex Disab* 2003; 21: 151-153.

[38] Mavrov GI, Goubenko TV. Clinical and epidemiological features of syphilis in pregnant women: the course and outcome of pregnancy. *Gynecol Obstet Invest* 2001;52:114-8.

[39] Hollier LM, Harstad TW, Sanchez PJ, Twickler DM, Wendel GD Jr. Fetal syphilis: clinical and laboratory characteristics. *Obstet Gynecol* 2001;97:947-53.

[40] Pohl M, Niemeyer CM, Hentschel R, Duffner U, Bergstrasser E, Brandis M. Haemophagocytosis in early congenital syphilis. *Eur J Pediatr* 1999;158:553-5.

[41] Kumar ND, Sethi S, Pandhi RK. Paroxysmal cold haemoglobinuria in syphilis patients. *Genitourin Med* 1993;69:76.

[42] Patel M, Durao H, Govender Y. Paroxysmal cold haemoglobinuria coexisting with cold agglutinins in a patient with syphilis resulting in peripheral gangrene: a case report. *East Afr Med J* 1993;70:526-7.

[43] Hoarau C, Ranivoharimina V, Chavet-Queru MS, Rason I, Rasatemalala H, Rakotonirina G, Guyon P. Congenital syphilis: update and perspectives. *Sante* 1999;9:38-45.

[44] How prenatal care can improve maternal health. *Safe Mother* 1993;(11):4-5.

[45] Jennison AV, Verma NK. Shigella flexneri infection: pathogenesis and vaccine development. *FEMS Microbiol Rev* 2004;28:43-58.

[46] Bennish ML. Potentially lethal complications of shigellosis. *Rev Infect Dis* 1991;13 Suppl 4:S319-24.

[47] Rahaman MM, JamiulAlam AK, Islam MR, Greenough WB 3rd. Shiga bacillus dysentery associated with marked leukocytosis and erythrocyte fragmentation. *Johns Hopkins Med J* 1975;136:65-70.

[48] Koster F, Levin J, Walker L, Tung KS, Gilman RH, Rahaman MM, Majid MA, Islam S, Williams RC Jr. Hemolytic-uremic syndrome after shigellosis. Relation to endotoxemia and circulating immune complexes. *N Engl J Med* 1978;298:927-33.

[49] Kato J, Ito K, Nakamura A, Watanabe H. Cloning of regions required for contact hemolysis and entry into LLC-MK2 cells from Shigella sonnei form I plasmid: virF is a positive regulator gene for these phenotypes. *Infect Immun* 1989;57:1391-8.

[50] Kavaliotis J, Karyda S, Konstantoula T, Kansouzidou A, Tsagaropoulou H. Shigellosis of childhood in northern Greece: epidemiological, clinical and laboratory data of hospitalized patients during the period 1971-96. *Scand J Infect Dis* 2000;32:207-11.

[51] Kovitangkoon K, Kirdpon S, Pirojkul C, Sripa B. Hemolytic uremic syndrome associated with Shigellosis: a report of 8 cases. *J Med Assoc Thai* 1990;73:401-5.

[52] Kernland KH, Laux-End R, Truttmann AC, Reymond D, Bianchetti MG. How is hemolytic-uremic syndrome in childhood acquired in Switzerland? *Schweiz Med Wochenschr* 1997;127:1229-33.

[53] Houdouin V, Doit C, Mariani P, Brahimi N, Loirat C, Bourrillon A, Bingen E. A pediatric cluster of Shigella dysenteriae serotype 1 diarrhea with hemolytic uremic syndrome in 2 families from France. *Clin Infect Dis* 2004;38:e96-9.

[54] Al-Qarawi S, Fontaine RE, Al-Qahtani MS. An outbreak of hemolytic uremic syndrome associated with antibiotic treatment of hospital inpatients for dysentery. *Emerg Infect Dis* 1995;1:138-40.

[55] Bin Saeed AA, El Bushra HE, Al-Hamdan NA. Does treatment of bloody diarrhea due to Shigella dysenteriae type 1 with ampicillin precipitate hemolytic uremic syndrome? *Emerg Infect Dis* 1995;1:134-7.

[56] Gilman RH. General considerations in the management of typhoid fever and dysentery. *Scand J Gastroenterol Suppl* 1989;169:11-8.

[57] Butler T, Islam A, Kabir I, Jones PK. Patterns of morbidity and mortality in typhoid fever dependent on age and gender: review of 552 hospitalized patients with diarrhea. *Rev Infect Dis* 1991;13:85-90.

[58] Albaqali A, Ghuloom A, Al Arrayed A, Al Ajami A, Shome DK, Jamsheer A, Al Mahroos H, Jelacic S, Tarr PI, Kaplan BS, Dhiman RK. Hemolytic uremic syndrome in association with typhoid fever. *Am J Kidney Dis* 2003;41:709-13.

[59] Wanachiwanawin W. Infections in E-beta thalassemia. *J Pediatr Hematol Oncol.* 2000;22:581-7.

[60] Diebold P, Humbert J, Djientcheu Vde P, Gudinchet F, Rilliet B. Salmonella epidural abscess in sickle cell disease: failure of the nonsurgical treatment. *J Natl Med Assoc* 2003;95:1095-8.

[61] Memish ZA, Balkhy HH. Brucellosis and international travel. *J Travel Med* 2004;11:49-55.

[62] Namiduru M, Gungor K, Dikensoy O, Baydar I, Ekinci E, Karaoglan I, Bekir NA. Epidemiological, clinical and laboratory features of brucellosis: a prospective evaluation of 120 adult patients. *Int J Clin Pract* 2003;57:20-4.

[63] Barroso Garcia P, Rodriguez-Contreras Pelayo R, Gil Extremera B, Maldonado Martin A, Guijarro Huertas G, Martin Salguero A, Parron Carreno T. Study of 1,595

brucellosis cases in the Almeria province (1972-1998) based on epidemiological data from disease reporting. *Rev Clin Esp* 2002;202:577-82.

[64] Tsolia M, Drakonaki S, Messaritaki A, Farmakakis T, Kostaki M, Tsapra H, Karpathios T. Clinical features, complications and treatment outcome of childhood brucellosis in central Greece. *J Infect* 2002;44:257-62.

[65] Yildirmak Y, Palanduz A, Telhan L, Arapoglu M, Kayaalp N. Bone marrow hypoplasia during Brucella infection. *J Pediatr Hematol Oncol* 2003;25:63-4.

[66] Yaramis A, Kervancioglu M, Yildirim I, Soker M, Derman O, Tas MA. Severe microangiopathic hemolytic anemia and thrombocytopenia in a child with Brucella infection. *Ann Hematol* 2001;80:546-8.

[67] Colak H. Brucellosis: clinical and laboratory findings and treatment in 40 patients. *Mikrobiyol Bul* 1987;21:110-6.

[68] Oncu S, Oncu S, Sakarya S. Anthrax--an overview. *Med Sci Monit* 2003;9:RA276-83.

[69] Freedman A, Afonja O, Chang MW, Mostashari F, Blaser M, Perez-Perez G, Lazarus H, Schacht R, Guttenberg J, Traister M, Borkowsky W. Cutaneous anthrax associated with microangiopathic hemolytic anemia and coagulopathy in a 7-month-old infant. *JAMA* 2002;287:869-74.

[70] Winter H, Pfisterer RM. Inhalation anthrax in a textile worker: non-fatal course. *Schweiz Med Wochenschr* 1991;121:832-5.

[71] Sen R, Yadav SS, Singh U, Sehgal P, Dixit VB. Patterns of erythropoiesis and anaemia in leprosy. *Lepr Rev* 1991;62:158-70.

[72] Byrd SR, Gelber RH. Effect of dapsone on haemoglobin concentration in patients with leprosy. *Lepr Rev* 1991;62:171-8.

[73] Richy F, Megraud F. Helicobacter pylori infection as a cause of extra-digestive diseases: myth or reality? *Gastroenterol Clin Biol* 2003;27(3 Pt 2):459-66.

[74] Barabino A. Helicobacter pylori-related iron deficiency anemia: a review. *Helicobacter* 2002;7:71-5.

[75] Go MF. Review article: natural history and epidemiology of Helicobacter pylori infection. *Aliment Pharmacol Ther* 2002;16 Suppl 1:3-15.

[76] Hacihanefioglu A, Edebali F, Celebi A, Karakaya T, Senturk O, Hulagu S. Improvement of complete blood count in patients with iron deficiency anemia and Helicobacter pylori infection after the eradication of Helicobacter pylori. *Hepatogastroenterology* 2004;51:313-5.

[77] Nahon S, Lahmek P, Massard J, Lesgourgues B, Mariaud de Serre N, Traissac L, Bodiguel V, Adotti F, Delas N. Helicobacter pylori-associated chronic gastritis and unexplained iron deficiency anemia: a reliable association? *Helicobacter* 2003;8:573-7.

[78] Russo-Mancuso G, Branciforte F, Licciardello M, La Spina M. Iron deficiency anemia as the only sign of infection with Helicobacter pylori: a report of 9 pediatric cases. *Int J Hematol* 2003;78:429-31.

[79] Presotto F, Sabini B, Cecchetto A, Plebani M, De Lazzari F, Pedini B, Betterle C. Helicobacter pylori infection and gastric autoimmune diseases: is there a link? *Helicobacter* 2003;8:578-84.

[80] Shuval-Sudai O, Granot E. An association between Helicobacter pylori infection and serum vitamin B12 levels in healthy adults. *J Clin Gastroenterol* 2003;36:130-3.

[81] Marignani M, Delle Fave G, Mecarocci S, Bordi C, Angeletti S, D'Ambra G, Aprile MR, Corleto VD, Monarca B, Annibale B. High prevalence of atrophic body gastritis in patients with unexplained microcytic and macrocytic anemia: a prospective screening study. *Am J Gastroenterol* 1999;94:766-72.

[82] Singh VV, Toskes PP. Small bowel bacterial overgrowth: presentation, diagnosis, and treatment. *Curr Gastroenterol Rep* 2003;5:365-72.

[83] Foley JE, Harrus S, Poland A, Chomel B, Pedersen NC. Molecular, clinical, and pathologic comparison of two distinct strains of Haemobartonella felis in domestic cats. *Am J Vet Res* 1998;59:1581-8.

[84] Henderson JP, O'Hagan J, Hawe SM, Pratt MC. Anaemia and low viability in piglets infected with Eperythrozoon suis. *Vet Rec* 1997;140:144-6.

Chapter 6

Anemia in Fungal Infections

Fungal Infections and Anemia

Fungal infections can produce several hematological alterations. The hematological changes include white blood cell, red blood cell and platelet abnormality. Similar to bacterial infections, the fungal infections may increase or decrease numbers of circulating erythrocytes, leukocytes, and platelets or may induce qualitative changes in these elements, some of which affect their function [1]. In addition, fungal infections may also produce thrombosis or hemorrhage [1].

Strausbaugh said that the fungal infections exerted these effects through mechanisms that involved specific fungal virulence factors or host defenses mobilized against the infectious agents [1]. Similar to bacterial infection, anemia can be the result of the described mechanisms due to fungal infection. In addition, due to the fact that fungal infections are more common in the immunocompromised host, the manifestation of anemia in the fungal disease is usually associated with the presentation of immunodeficiency. However, the nature of fungal disease is a chronic disease, therefore, the acute anemic manifestation as seen in anemia due to bacterial infections is rare. Classified by site of infection, anemia is more common in deep than in superficial fungal infections. Many deep fungal infections such as histoplasmosis, cryptococcosis and penicillosis are responsible for anemia.

Concerning the type of anemia in fungal infections, normocytic, microcytic and macrocytic can be found. The hemolytic anemia from many fungal toxins or aplastic anemia due to marrow infiltration by fungus can be good examples of normocytic anemia in fungal infections. The iron deficiency anemia from chronic candidiasis can be a good example of microcytic anemia. Pernicious anemia due to moniliasis can be a good example of macrocytic anemia. Since the fungal infection is still an important health problem for the tropics, the anemia in fungal infections is also a tropical hematological problem. Some important common fungal infections and their relation to anemia will be presented in this chapter.

Anemia in Some Important Fungal Diseases

1. Anemia and Histoplasmosis

Histoplasmosis is a common infection endemic in many regions of America, Asia, India and Africa, with sporadic cases also occurring throughout the world [2]. This infection became more widely spread in the acquired immonodeficiency syndrome (AIDS) era. Disease manifestations range from asymptomatic infection in the normal host with low-inoculum exposure to a rapidly fatal, disseminated infection in the severely immunocompromised host, emphasizing the importance of cellular immunity in the defense against *Histoplasma capsulatum* [3]. Wheat said that the diagnosis of histoplasmosis depended on a high index of suspicion, knowledge of the clinical and epidemiologic features of the infection, and a thorough understanding of the uses and limitations of fungal cultural and serological laboratory procedures [3]. However, clinicians and laboratory directors in developing countries usually face up with the uses and limitations of serologic and mycological tests to accurately diagnose histoplasmosis [2]. The routine laboratory examination such as a blood smear examination can provide poor diagnostic activity for histoplasmosis [4]. Recently, there are several attempts to develop rapid diagnosis based on detection of a polysaccharide antigen in body fluids of patients with histoplasmosis [2 – 3]. However, a new cost-effective approach to the diagnosis of histoplasmosis is still the area of present research interest.

Hepatosplenomegaly, anemia, leucopenia, thrombocytopenia, increased transaminases, and diffuse interstitial pulmonary infiltration are mentioned in the patients with disseminated histoplasmosis. There are some previous reports concerning the prevalence of anemia in the patients with histoplasmosis: most are from the patient with human immune deficiency virus (HIV) infection. Kurtin *et al.* studied the bone marrow and peripheral blood specimens in 13 patients with AIDS and progressive disseminated histoplasmosis (PDH) [5]. They found anemia, leukopenia, and thrombocytopenia in 12, 10, and 7 patients, respectively [5]. Morphologically, the marrow specimens showed one of four patterns: (1) no morphologic evidence of infection (two patients, one with a positive marrow culture); (2) discrete granulomas (two patients, both with positive marrow cultures); (3) lymphohistiocytic aggregates (six patients, four with positive marrow cultures); and (4) diffuse macrophage infiltrates (three patients, all with positive marrow cultures) [5]. Neubauer *et al.* studied 23 patients hospitalized with the diagnosis of AIDS and disseminated histoplasmosis [6]. Of these 23 cases, clinical signs and symptoms included fever (91%), cough (65%), and weight loss (48%) [6]. Concerning the laboratory investigation, anemia (39%), leukopenia (65%), and thrombocytopenia (52%) were common, and 22% had pancytopenia [6]. Fernandez Andreu *et al.* studied the clinical histories of 12 AIDS pediatric patients whose histoplasmosis diagnosis had been confirmed by histopathological studies and found that it appeared as a febrile and waste disease with an elevated hepatomegaly frequency and generalized adenopathies in every case [7]. Fernandez Andreu *et al.* found that more than 50% of the patients had anemia and an accelerated erythrocyte sedimentation [7].

The pathogenesis of anemia in historplasmosis is believed to be due to bone marrow lesion. In most cases, bone marrow aspiration often reveals a hypercellular marrow with reversed M:E ration, dyserythropoesis, reticulum cell hyperplasia, a plentiful golden yellow pigment, and clumps of *H. capsulatum* [8]. However, the reactive hemophagocytic syndrome (RHPS) secondary to disseminated histoplasmosis was mentioned [9]. Koduri *et al.* noted that the combination of fever, cytopenia, elevated serum LDH level (> 1,000 IU/L), and/or hyperferritinemia (ferritin level of > 10,000 ng/mL) was a clue to the diagnosis of RHPS and disseminated histoplasmosis [9]. They also mentioned that a bone marrow biopsy was valuable in establishing the diagnosis [9]. Immune hemolytic anemia is another type of anemia reported in the patients with histoplasmosis [10 - 11]. In 1983, Weinberg *et al.* reported 9 cases of histoplasmosis with presenting manifestations such as obstructive airway disease; subacute parotitis; unilateral cervical lymphadenopathy; anterior mediastinal mass-simulating neoplasm; immune hemolytic anemia; a cutaneous lesion with regional lymphadenopathy; mediastinal mass and pericardial effusion; pulmonary infarction; and a symptom complex of cervical lymphadenopathy, CSF pleocytosis, arthritis, and interstitial nephritis [10].

Concerning the treatment of histoplasmosis, amphotericin B remains the preferred treatment for more severe forms of histoplasmosis, particularly in the immunocompromised host, but oral treatment with ketoconazole or newer imidozoles appears to be effective in less severe infections in non-immunocompromised individuals [2 – 3]. However, monitoring of anemia as a result of treating the HIV infected patients with histoplasmosis with amphotericin B is recommended. Amphotericin B is reported to induce in the permeability properties of erythrocytes and the subsequent effect of procaine on sickling of erythrocytes, and their potential interaction with specific membrane components [12]. In addition, most AIDS patients have zidovudine as an antiretroviral drug, which can induce anemia as well. Therefore, an anemia can be seen in the AIDS patients with histoplasmosis and on a combination treatment between amphotericin B and zidovudine. In these cases, the use of recombinant erythropoietin is reported to be useful [13].

2. Anemia and Penicillosis

Penicillosis is a fungal infection caused by *Penicillium marneffei*, which is endemic to Southeast Asia, especially in the northern part of Thailand, and the southern part of China where specific rodents harboring the fungi live [14]. Until present, *P. marneffei* is the only *Penicillium* species, which is dimorphic and can cause systemic mycosis in human beings. With the increasing incidence of HIV seropositivity, penicillosis marneffei emerged as one of the major problems [14]. It becomes an important tropical fungal infection that general practitioners should know and manage properly. Imwidthaya said that the common presenting signs of histoplasmosis were fever, anemia, hepatomegaly, lymphadenopathy, productive cough and a common skin manifestation known as molluscum contagiosum-like lesions [14]. Huynh *et al.* reported a series of 12 HIV-infected adults with disseminated *P. marneffei* infection in Vietnam [15]. They noted that the clinical signs of these patients were related to the reticuloendothelial system involvement: common clinical features included fever, cutaneous manifestations, lymphadenopathy, hepatomegaly, splenomegaly, and marked anemia [15]. Ranjana *et al.* studied 36 Indian patients with penicillosis and found that common clinical symptoms included fever (97%), weight loss (100%), weakness (86%), anemia (86%), and characteristic skin lesions (81%) [16]. Kurup *et al.* studied 5 cases of penicillosis in Singapore, imported from Thailand, and found that weight loss, anaemia and papular skin lesions were common clinical manifestations in these patients [17]. Duong studied 155 cases of penicillosis and found that *P. marneffei* could infect various organs, particularly the lung, liver, and skin [18]. They found that the most common clinical features include fever, weight loss, and anemia [18]. Supparatpinyo *et al.* studied 80 patients with histoplasmosis in Chiangmai, the biggest province in the north of Thailand [19]. They found that the most common presented symptoms and signs were fever (92%), anaemia (77%), weight loss (76%), and skin lesions (71%) [19].

To diagnose this infection, Sirisanthana noted that the bone marrow culture was the most sensitive (100%), followed by a culture of specimens obtained from skin biopsy (90%) and blood culture (76%) [20]. Similar to histoplasmosis, the main pathogenesis of anemia in penicillosis is believed to be due to the marrow lesion. The marrow infiltration by the fungus can lead to severe anemia.

Concerning the treatment of penicillosis, antifungal drug remains the preferred treatment. The fungus was sensitive to amphotericin B, itraconazole, and ketoconazole [20]. Sirisanthana recommended giving amphotericin B for 2 weeks, followed by itraconazole 400 mg/day orally for the next 10 weeks [20]. After the initial treatment, the patient is given itraconazole 200 mg/day as secondary prophylaxis for life [20]. Sirisanthana and Sirisanthana reported that the response rate in those penicillosis patients who were treated with appropriate antifungal therapy (amphotericin B, fluconazole or ketoconazole) was 82% [21]. Since the disease is potentially curable, prompt diagnosis and treatment will lead to better prognosis [14].

3. Anemia and Candidiasis

Candidiasis is a group of fungal infections, caused by the Candida spp. It is one of the well-known fungal infections that can be seen all over the world, not specific to the tropics. It can be seen in both immunocompenent and immunocompromised host although it is more common in the latter group. Candidiasis is often observed in patients with leukemia and aplastic anemia, all of whom show immunodeficiency. Candida spp can infect many organs from superficial cutaneous to viscera. With the increasing incidence of HIV seropositivity, candidiasis becomes an important opportunistic infection seen in AIDS patients. Furuta said that the incidence of candidiasis had steadily increased with the number of patients who have opportunistic infection [22]. Furuta also mentioned that the number isolated was greater in the order of C. albicans followed by C. glabrata then C. tropicalis then C. parapsilosis and then C. krusei. and C. albicans, which was detected with the most frequently, isolated from 60-70% of all samples every year [22]. Furuta noted that isolated frequencies of C. albicans were 66-77% from sputum, 43-70% from urine, and 62-72% from vaginal swabs [22].

Furuta mentioned that the cases with deep-seated candidiasis often showed low values or levels of lymphocyte, neutrophil, hemoglobin, hemoglobin total protein and total cholesterol [22]. The pathogenesis of anemia in candidiasis is a complicated one. The anemia can manifest as normochromic, microcytic or macrocytic types. Concerning normocytic anemia, the anemia due to the bone marrow disturbance is not common. The Candida spp itself rarely infiltrates into the marrow. However, the candidiasis is a common complication in patients with bone marrow transplantation. Goodrich et al. proposed that the important factors that increased candidiasis in the patients with bone marrow transplantation included age, acute graft-versus-host disease, and donor mismatch [23]. While the anemia due to hemolysis is sometimes reported in the patients with candidiasis. In 1994, Oyefara et al. presented the first report of the association of AIHA with chronic mucocutaneous candidiasis [24]. They reported three patients with AIHA associated with candidiasis, the first case had positive direct antiglobulin tests, and the first patient had both immunoglobulin G (IgG) and IgM erythrocyte autoantibodies, while the remaining two patients had only IgG autoantibody [24]. Oyefara et al. suggested that all patients with chronic mucocutaneous candidiasis should be screened periodically for erythrocyte autoantibodies [24]. They also proposed that the occurrence of erythrocyte autoantibodies in mucocutaneous candidiasis may be related to immunoregulatory disorders in this disease [24]. However, the non – immune hemolysis is also mentioned. Luo et al. examined some species of Candida for their respective responses to an in vitro hemolytic test [25]. They found that only alpha hemolysis was detectable in four Candida species, viz., C. famata, C. guilliermondii, C. rugosa, and C. utilis, while C. parapsilosis and C. pelliculosa failed to demonstrate any hemolytic activity after incubation for 48 hours or longer [25]. Concerning C. albican, they said that the hyphal cells, not yeast cell of C. albicans used hemoglobin as a source of iron [26]. Calderone et al. said that mannan from C. albicans might provide a host recognition function for C. albicans and recent experiments indicated that mannan binds to band 3protein of human red blood cells and causes hemolysis [27]. They noted that this activity might be associated with the ability of the organism to utilize hemoglobin and iron [27]. These mechanisms are believed to be corresponding for the pathogenesis of hemolytic anemia in candidiasis. Concerning treatment for the AIHA with candidiasis, Oyefara et al. proposed that plasmapheresis, a safe ancillary procedure in the management of AIHA, might be life-saving in some cases [24].

Concerning the microcytic anemia, the iron deficiency anemia is mentioned in the patients with chronic candidiasis. Rennie et al. performed a study in a rat model. According to this study, those rats with iron deficiency anemia, in comparison with normal rats, showed no significant difference in susceptibility to experimental infection with C. albicans although anaemic rats had a significantly greater incidence of persistent infection [28]. Rennie et al. suggested that patients with chronic candidosis should be investigated for iron deficiency [28]. Challacombe reported that the prevalences of sideropenia (14.0%), folate deficiency (4.7%) and vitamin B12 deficiency (3.1%) were increased in the patients with oral candidiasis as compared with controls [29]. Chronic mucocutaneous candidiasis is sometimes reported in association with iron deficiency [30]. The defect in the mucosa and impaired iron absorption is believed to be associated with anemia [30]. Heymann et al. said that the human fungal pathogen C. albicans contained a close homologue of yeast siderophore transporters, designated Sit1p/Arn1p [31]. They suggested that siderophore uptake by Sit1p/Arn1p was required in a specific process of C. albicans infection, namely epithelial invasion and penetration, while in the blood or within organs other sources of iron, including heme, might be used [31]. According to these studies, the general practitioners should not overlook the importance of iron deficiency anemia in the patients with candidiasis [32]. The treatment for candidiasis by an antifungal drug is recommended and iron supplementation is useful as well [32 – 33]. However, Williamson and Gordon noted that correction of iron deficiency anemia did not lead to alleviation of candidiasis [34].

Concerning the macrocytic anemia, the pernicious anemia due to candidiasis is reported. It is postulated that in chronic candidiasis and polyendocrinopathy a defect may exist in immunologic cellular surveillance for recognition and destruction of aberrant cells [35]. Pernicious anemia is a component of polyendocrinopathy associated with chronic candidiasis [35]. A defect in immunohomeostasis is mentioned to bring the combination of thymoma, pure red cell aplasia, pernicious anaemia and candidiasis [36]. Autoimmune polyendocrinopathy-candidiasis-ectodermal dystrophy (APECED) is an autosomal-recessive syndrome defined by two of the following conditions: chronic mucocutaneous candidiasis, hypoparathyroidism, or Addison's disease [37]. In addition, other autoimmune conditions may be associated, such as hypothyroidism, hypogonadism, insulin-dependent diabetes mellitus, chronic active hepatitis, pernicious anemia, vitiligo, alopecia, biliary cirrhosis, and ectodermal dysplasia [37]. Genetically, APECED is caused by mutations in the autoimmune regulator gene, mapping to 21q22.3 [37]. In APECED, the antibody to intrinsic factor leading to pernicious anemia is reported [38].

In addition to the pernicious anemia due to the candidiasis endocrinopathy, Junca et al. also mentioned the possible correlation between esophageal candidiasis and pernicious anemia [39].

4. Anemia and Cryptococcosis

Cryptococcosis can be seen all over the world, not limited to the tropics. At present, it is a common deep fungal infection due to the widespread incidence of AIDS. This fungal infection usually manifests as a central nervous system (CNS) infection. *Cryptococcus neoformans* is the main pathogenic fungal causing cryptococcosis. Birds' dung is mentioned as an important source of these fungi and humans can get infection by contact with birds. The microscopic diagnosis of this fungus is rather unique: identification of the capsulated organism by the simple indian ink preparation. The presence of immunological tests to detect the cryptococcal antigen helps general practitioners confirm the diagnosis. Some researchers tried to study this organism by the automated flow cytometer cell count. According to a recent study of Wiwanitkit and Soogarun, this organism manifests mimicking to the basophil in the hemogram by the automated flow cytometry hematology analyzer, Technicon [40].

The anemia in cryptococcosis is mentioned. Concerning the anemia in cryptococcosis, the most common type is hemolytic anemia. AIHA is mentioned in patients with cryptococcosis, both intra CNS [41] and extra CNS [42] infections. In addition, Pozniak *et al.* reported a case of hemolytic uremic syndrome (HUS) in patients with cryptococcosis as well [42]. The combination between hemolytic and uremic manifestations is seen in this case [42]. Treatment of cryptococcosis with amphotericin B and flucytosine was very effective, there being no more growth of fungi in cultures for most cases [43]. However, adverse reactions to the drugs used occurred frequently and consisted mainly of anemia, hepatosis and fever. Therefore, anemia as a complication of cryptococcosis treatment must not be overlooked by the general practitioners [44], and it might be more common than cryptococcosis – induced anemia.

5. Anemia and Aspergillosis

Invasive aspergillosis is generally a life-threatening invasive opportunistic mycosis affecting principally the upper and lower respiratory tract [45]. High mortality rates of aspergillosis are mentioned in bone marrow transplant, liver transplant and patients with aplastic anemia or AIDS [45]. As invasive Aspergillus infections are usually acquired by inhalation of *Aspergillus conidia*, symptoms of a pulmonary infection such as cough, rales and marked pleuritic chest pain can be noted early in the course, whereas hemoptysis typically comes late after neutrophil recovery [46]. Aspergillus infections of the upper respiratory tract may also involve the nasal cavity or sinuses resulting in nasal obstruction, epistaxis, facial pain, periorbital swelling and even palate destruction [46]. Primary cutaneous infections present as non-purulent ulcerations and may be seen in association with implantable intravenous devices [46].

Anemia is mentioned in patients with aspergillosis. Lahoz *et al.* reported a case of aspergillosis of the maxillary antrum, and systemic affectation including anemia, anorexia and fever [47]. After surgical removal of aspergilloma in this case, those symptoms fully recovered [47]. Niyo *et al.* performed a rabbit model experimental study on the influence of immunosuppression by T-2 mycotoxin on the fungal disease aspergillosis [48]. According to this study, changes caused by T-2 toxin included leukopenia, marginal anemia, and increased number of and morphologic changes in nucleated erythrocytes by day 21, followed by a regenerative hematological response [48]. An important form of anemia in patients with aspergillosis is microangiopathic hemolytic anemia (MAHA) [49]. Nishiura *et al.* reported a case of aspergillus vegetative endocarditis complicated with schizocytic hemolytic anemia in a patient with acute lymphocytic leukemia [50]. In this case, severe hemolytic anemia with red cell fragmentation can be seen [50]. Nishiura *et al.* also noted that every leukemic patient suffering from aspergillosis was susceptible to the valvular complication after, rather than during, the period of severe myelosuppression, because platelets play an important role in the formation of thrombotic lesions [50]. It can be noted that anemia in the patients with aspergillosis is not common. However, aspergillosis is one of the common complications in the patients who have bone marrow transplantation due to aplastic anemia and other hematological disorders. Similar to other fungal infections, antifungal drug is recommended for the treatment of aspergillosis.

6. Anemia and Mucormycosis

Zygomycosis is an opportunistic infection of fungi in the two orders, Mucorales and Entomophthorales, in class Phycomycetes or Zygomycetes [51]. Generally, mucormycosis, caused by Mucorales, can manifest five different forms: rhinocerebral, pulmonary, gastrointestinal, cutaneous and the disseminated forms [52 - 53]. Similar to aspergillosis, mucormysis is an invasive fungal infection. The anemia in mucormycosis is rare but there are some case reports. Caraveo *et al.* described a diabetic patient who presented with profound anemia and thrombocytopenia [54]. In this case, extensive bone marrow necrosis was demonstrated and he also had a large renal cyst that contained hyphae later identified as Mucor species [54]. Caraveo *et al.* postulated that the marrow necrosis was a direct or indirect result of Mucor infection [54]. Kubota *et al.* reported a case of intraventricular thrombosis by disseminated mucormycosis in a patient with myelodysplastic syndrome during deferoxamine therapy. This patient is a possible case of MAHA, with the pathogenesis similar to those seen with aspergillosis [55].

References

[1]   Strausbaugh LJ. Hematologic manifestations of bacterial and fungal infections. *Hematol Oncol Clin North Am* 1987;1:185-206.

[2]   Joseph Wheat L. Current diagnosis of histoplasmosis. *Trends Microbiol* 2003;11:488-94.

[3]   Wheat LJ. Diagnosis and management of histoplasmosis. *Eur J Clin Microbiol Infect Dis* 1989;8:480-90.

[4]   Wiwanitkit V, Chaiwong T. Blood smear examination for disseminated histoplasmosis in 50 HIV seropositive patients in Chulalongkorn Hospital. *Srinagarind Med J* 2003; 18: 27-29.

[5]   Kurtin PJ, McKinsey DS, Gupta MR, Driks M. Histoplasmosis in patients with acquired immunodeficiency syndrome. Hematologic and bone marrow manifestations. *Am J Clin Pathol* 1990;93:367-72.

[6]   Neubauer MA, Bodensteiner DC. Disseminated histoplasmosis in patients with AIDS. *South Med J* 1992;85:1166-70.

[7]   Fernandez Andreu CM, Varona CC, Martinez Machin G, Rodriguez Barreras ME, Ruiz Perez A. Progressive disseminated histoplasmosis in AIDS patients. *Rev Cubana Med Trop* 1996;48:163-6.

[8]   Amayo EO, Riyat MS, Okelo GB, Adam AM, Toroitich K. Disseminated histoplasmosis in a patient with acquired immunodeficiency syndrome (AIDS): a case report. *East Afr Med J* 1993;70:61-2.

[9]   Koduri PR, Chundi V, DeMarais P, Mizock BA, Patel AR, Weinstein RA. Reactive hemophagocytic syndrome: a new presentation of disseminated histoplasmosis in patients with AIDS. *Clin Infect Dis* 1995;21:1463-5.

[10] Weinberg GA, Kleiman MB, Grosfeld JL, Weber TR, Wheat LJ. Unusual manifestations of histoplasmosis in childhood. *Pediatrics* 1983;72:99-105.

[11] Beeman EA, Chang PL. Disseminated histoplasmosis with laryngeal involvement and acquired hemolytic anemia: report of a case. *Med Ann Dist Columbia* 1965;34:275-80.

[12] Abu-Salah KM. Inhibition of erythrocyte membrane ATPases with antisickling and anaesthetic substances and ionophoric antibiotics. *Life Sci* 1996;58:187-93.

[13] Kuehl AK, Noormohamed SE. Recombinant erythropoietin for zidovudine-induced anemia in AIDS. *Ann Pharmacother* 1995;29:778-9.

[14] Imwidthaya P. Update of Penicillosis marneffei in Thailand. Review article. *Mycopathologia* 1994;127:135-7.

[15] Huynh TX, Nguyen HC, Dinh Nguyen HM, Do MT, Odermatt-Biays S, Degremont A, Malvy D. Penicillium marneffei infection and AIDS. A review of 12 cases reported in the Tropical Diseases Centre, Ho Chi Minh City (Vietnam). *Sante* 2003; 13:149-53.

[16] Ranjana KH, Priyokumar K, Singh TJ, Gupta ChC, Sharmila L, Singh PN, Chakrabarti A. Disseminated Penicillium marneffei infection among HIV-infected patients in Manipur state, India. *J Infect* 2002;45:268-71.

[17] Kurup A, Leo YS, Tan AL, Wong SY. Disseminated Penicillium marneffei infection: a report of five cases in Singapore. *Ann Acad Med Singapore* 1999;28:605-9.

[18] Duong TA. Infection due to Penicillium marneffei, an emerging pathogen: review of 155 reported cases. *Clin Infect Dis* 1996;23:125-30.

[19] Supparatpinyo K, Khamwan C, Baosoung V, Nelson KE, Sirisanthana T. Disseminated Penicillium marneffei infection in southeast Asia. *Lancet* 1994;344:110-3.

[20] Sirisanthana T. Infection due to Penicillium marneffei. *Ann Acad Med Singapore* 1997;26:701-4.

[21] Sirisanthana V, Sirisanthana T. Disseminated Penicillium marneffei infection in human immunodeficiency virus-infected children. *Pediatr Infect Dis J* 1995;14:935-40.

[22] Furuta I. Candida. *Rinsho Byori* 2000;48:1044-50.

[23] Goodrich JM, Reed EC, Mori M, Fisher LD, Skerrett S, Dandliker PS, Klis B, Counts GW, Meyers JD. Clinical features and analysis of risk factors for invasive candidal infection after marrow transplantation. *J Infect Dis* 1991;164:731-40.

[24] Oyefara BI, Kim HC, Danziger RN, Carroll M, Greene JM, Douglas SD. Autoimmune hemolytic anemia in chronic mucocutaneous candidiasis. *Clin Diagn Lab Immunol* 1994;1:38-43.

[25] Luo G, Samaranayake LP, Yau JY. Candida species exhibit differential in vitro hemolytic activities. *J Clin Microbiol* 2001;39:2971-4.

[26] Tanaka WT, Nakao N, Mikami T, Matsumoto T. Hemoglobin is utilized by Candida albicans in the hyphal form but not yeast form. *Biochem Biophys Res Commun* 1997;232:350-3.

[27] Calderone R, Suzuki S, Cannon R, Cho T, Boyd D, Calera J, Chibana H, Herman D, Holmes A, Jeng HW, Kaminishi H, Matsumoto T, Mikami T, O'Sullivan JM, Sudoh M, Suzuki M, Nakashima Y, Tanaka T, Tompkins GR, Watanabe T. Candida albicans: adherence, signaling and virulence. *Med Mycol* 2000;38 Suppl 1:125-37.

[28] Rennie JS, Hutcheon AW, MacFarlane TW, MacDonald DG. The role of iron deficiency in experimentally-induced oral candidosis in the rat. *J Med Microbiol*. 1983;16:363-9.

[29] Challacombe SJ. Haematological abnormalities in oral lichen planus, candidiasis, leukoplakia and non-specific stomatitis. *Int J Oral Maxillofac Surg* 1986;15:72-80.

[30] Garcia MP, Puig L, Perez M, de Moragas JM. Chronic mucocutaneous candidiasis. *Med Cutan Ibero Lat Am* 1988;16:445-9.

[31] Heymann P, Gerads M, Schaller M, Dromer F, Winkelmann G, Ernst JF. The siderophore iron transporter of Candida albicans (Sit1p/Arn1p) mediates uptake of

ferrichrome-type siderophores and is required for epithelial invasion. *Infect Immun* 2002;70:5246-55.

[32] Tattersall P. Iron deficiency and candida infection. *Practitioner* 1990;234:326.

[33] Higgs JM. Chronic mucocutaneous candidiasis: iron deficiency and the effects of iron therapy. *Proc R Soc Med* 1973;66:802-4.

[34] Williamson MM, Gordon RD. Severe chronic mucocutaneous candidiasis. Favourable response to oral therapy with ketoconazole. Med J Aust 1983;1:276-8.

[35] Richman RA, Rosenthal IM, Solomon LM, Karachorlu KV. Candidiasis and multiple endocrinopathy. With oral squamous cell carcinoma complications. *Arch Dermatol* 1975;111:625-7.

[36] Robins-Browne RM, Green R, Katz J, Becker D. Thymoma, pure red cell aplasia, pernicious anaemia and candidiasis: a defect in immunohomeostasis. *Br J Haematol* 1977;36:5-13.

[37] Buzi F, Badolato R, Mazza C, Giliani S, Notarangelo LD, Radetti G, Plebani A, Notarangelo LD. Autoimmune polyendocrinopathy-candidiasis-ectodermal dystrophy syndrome: time to review diagnostic criteria? *J Clin Endocrinol Metab* 2003;88:3146-8.

[38] Perniola R, Falorni A, Clemente MG, Forini F, Accogli E, Lobreglio G. Organ-specific and non-organ-specific autoantibodies in children and young adults with autoimmune polyendocrinopathy-candidiasis-ectodermal dystrophy (APECED). *Eur J Endocrinol* 2000;143:497-503.

[39] Junca J, Oriol A, Vela D, Ribera JM. Esophageal candidiasis and possible relationship with pernicious anemia. *Med Clin* (Barc) 1994;103:396-7.

[40] Wiwanitkit V, Soogarun S. Flow cytometry pattern in the diagnosis of cryptococcal meningitis in HIV-infected patients. *Songkhanagarind Med J* 2002; 20: 155 – 8.

[41] Egawa M, Tsushima H, Kataoka K, Yamura T, Imanaka H, Shimamoto H, Oda S. Case of autoimmune hemolytic anemia associated with chromomycosis, cryptococcal meningitis and alternarial subcutaneous abscess. *Nippon Hifuka Gakkai Zasshi* 1982;92:965-70.

[42] Pozniak AL, Lucas SB, Miller RF. Haemolytic uraemic syndrome complicated by disseminated extraneural cryptococcosis. *Genitourin Med* 1997;73:410-4.

[43] Weinke T, Rogler G, Sixt C, de Matos-Marques B, Pohle HD, Staib F, Seibold M. Cryptococcosis in AIDS patients: observations concerning CNS involvement. *J Neurol* 1989;236:38-42.

[44] Stevens DA. Overview of amphotericin B colloidal dispersion (amphocil). *J Infect* 1994;28 Suppl 1:45- 9.

[45] Denning DW. Treatment of invasive aspergillosis. *J Infect* 1994;28 Suppl 1:25-33.

[46] Schwartz S, Thiel E. Clinical presentation of invasive aspergillosis. *Mycoses* 1997;40 Suppl 2:21-4.

[47] Lahoz T, Abenia JM, Valero J, Camara F. Sinus aspergillosis with impact on the general health status. *Acta Otorrinolaringol Esp* 1993;44:130-2.

[48] Niyo KA, Richard JL, Niyo Y, Tiffany LH. Pathologic, hematologic, and serologic changes in rabbits given T-2 mycotoxin orally and exposed to aerosols of Aspergillus fumigatus conidia. *Am J Vet Res* 1988;49:2151-60.

[49] Robboy SJ, Salisbury K, Ragsdale B, Bobroff LM, Jacobson BM, Colman RW. Mechanism of Aspergillus-induced microangiopathic hemolytic anemia. *Arch Intern Med* 1971;128:790-3.

[50] Nishiura T, Miyazaki Y, Oritani K, Tominaga N, Tomiyama Y, Katagiri S, Kanayama Y, Yonezawa T, Tarui S, Yamada T, et al. Aspergillus vegetative endocarditis complicated with schizocytic hemolytic anemia in a patient with acute lymphocytic leukemia. *Acta Haematol* 1986;76:60-2.

[51] Aikvanich T, Niampradit N. Mucormycosis: a report of two cases. *Thai J Dermatol* 1990; 6: 113-7.

[52] Puangpornsri P, Prakitlittanon W, Eauananta Y. Mucormycosis: one case report. Khon Kaen *Med J* 1987; 11: 39-42.

[53] Sitthiwong W, Mahaisavariya P, Chaiprasert A, Manonukul J. Chronic subcutaneous zygomycosis: three cases of entomophthoromycosis basidiobolae. *Thai J Dermatol* 2000; 15: 154-61.

[54] Caraveo J, Trowbridge AA, Amaral BW, Green JB 3rd, Cain PT, Hurley DL. Bone marrow necrosis associated with a Mucor infection. *Am J Med* 1977;62:404-8.

[55] Kubota N, Miyazawa K, Shoji N, Sumi M, Nakajima A, Kimura Y, Oshiro H, Ebihara Y, Ohyashiki K. A massive intraventricular thrombosis by disseminated mucormycosis in a patient with myelodysplastic syndrome during deferoxamine therapy. *Haematologica* 2003;88:EIM13.

Chapter 7

Anemia in Viral Diseases

Viral Diseases and Anemia

Viral infections can produce several hematological alterations. The hematological changes include white blood cell, red blood cell and platelet abnormality. Similar to bacterial and fungal infections, the viral infections may increase or decrease numbers of circulating erythrocytes, leukocytes, and platelets or may induce qualitative changes in these elements, some of which affect their function. Similar to bacterial and fungal infections, anemia can be the result of viral infection. Several viral infections are mentioned as an underlying cause of anemia.

Concerning the type of anemia in viral infections, normocytic, microcytic and macrocytic can be found, however, the first type is more common than the other two. Aplastic and hemolytic anemia due to viral infections can be good examples of normocytic anemia in viral infections. Since the viral infection is still an important health problem for the tropics, anemia in viral infections is also a tropical hematological problem. Some important common viral infections and their relation to anemia will be presented in this chapter.

Anemia in Some Important Viral Diseases

1. Cytomegalovirus Infection

Cytomegalovirus (CMV) infection is a viral infection usually found in patients with a defect of immune status. At present, this viral infection is not limited to the tropics but can be seen all over the world. In the AIDS era, it became an important opportunistic infection in the patient with an advanced stage of human immunodeficiency virus (HIV) infection. Anemia is a manifestation in patients with CMV infection. Recently, He *et al.* investigated the mechanism and suppression effect of human CMV on hematopoietic system [2]. They found that CMV AD169 strains inhibited the differentiation and proliferation of CFU-GM, CFU-E, CFU-Mix and CFU-MK by the infection of the hematopoietic progenitors [2]. They proposed that CMV might cause the suppression of hematopoiesis by direct infection, which is thought to be one of the reasons of CMV infection associated with thrombocytopenia, neutropenia and anemia [2]. According to this study, the main pathogenesis of anemia in the CMV infection is believed to be due to the disturbance of erythropoiesis. Indeed, CMV infection is mentioned as a possible underlying factor contributing to aplastic anemia. On the other hand, CMV infection itself is an important opportunistic infection in patients receiving bone marrow transplantation.

Another mechanism underlying anemia in patients with CMV infection is hemolysis. Both immune and non-immune hemolytic anemia can be seen in CMV infection. Concerning the immune hemolytic anemia, Murray *et al.* said that endogenous anti-CMV IgG antibodies were the pathogenic antibodies leading to hemolysis, implicating a possible causal relationship between AIHA and CMV infection [3]. They suggested that investigation for the presence of CMV in infantile AIHA was warranted and that CMV immune globulin should be considered as a therapeutic option [3]. Pemde *et al.* studied 9 patients with congenital CMV infection and found that significant pallor, thrombocytopenia and evidence of hemolysis were present in 8 (89%), 4 (44%) and 4 (44%) patients, respectively [4]. However, Salloum and Lundberg said that because CMV serology was not routinely obtained as a part of hemolysis work-up, the true incidence of this complication might be underestimated [4]. Salloum and Lundberg noted that CMV infection should be considered in the differential diagnosis of hemolytic anemia in adults [5]. Treatment with ganciclovir (5 mg/kg b.i.d.) for 10 days and prednisolone (2 mg/kg/day) for more than 3 months are suggested for the CMV-infected cases with AIHA [6]. Recently, Riechsteiner *et al.* studied the patients undergoing transplantation therapy and proposed that the hemolytic phenomenon was less often in the patients receiving immunosuppressive therapy with mycophenolate mofetil and prophylaxis for cytomegalovirus disease with intravenous immune globulin [7]. Concerning non-immune hemolysis in the patients with CMV infection, the occurrence is much less common than immune hemolysis but there are some case reports. In 1998, Siddiqui and Khan reported a case with acute hemolytic anemia secondary to acute viral hepatitis A and a coexisting acute cytomegalovirus infection [8].

2. Ebstein-Barr Virus Infection

Similar to CMV infection is the Ebstein-Barr virus (EBV), is another viral infection usually found in patients with defect of immune status. It can be found all over the world at present. EBV infection results in many diseases. Li et al. noted that the most common disease caused by EBV infection was a respiratory tract infection known as acute infections mononucleosis (40.5%), followed by infectious mononucleosis (17.9%), Kawasaki disease (6.3%), idiopathic thrombocytopenic purpura (5.8%), viral myocarditis (2.6%), viral encephalitis (2.6%), hemophagocytic syndrome (1.6%), rheumatoid arthritis (1.0%), acute lymphadenitis (1.0%), facial neuritis (1.0%), Evans syndrome (0.5%), systemic lupus erythematosus (0.5%), subacute necrotizing lymphadenitis (0.5%), non-Hodgkin's lymphoma (0.5%), acute aplastic anemia (0.5%) and infantile hepatitis syndrome (0.5%) [9]. Similar to CMV infection, EBV infection is mentioned as a possible underlying factor contributing to aplastic anemia. The International Association for Studying Agranulocytosis and Aplastic

Anemia reported that in 4% of patients, EBV can cause agranulocytosis even a year after the occurrence of acute disease [10]. In the aplastic anemia due to EBV infection, Lau et al. said that the EBV genome was demonstrated in the bone marrow cells and EBV-specific serology suggested reactivation of EBV infection [11].

Concerning the infectious mononucleosis, it is a benign lymphoproliferative, usually a self-limiting disease [10]. Brkic et al. noted that complications are relatively rare, but they may occur, especially hematological and the most common in those cases are AIHA and thrombocytopenia, and they respond to corticoid therapy [10].

Recently, Hernandez-Jodra et al. studied the in vitro production of red cell autoantibodies (RBC AuAbs) for better understanding of the pathogenesis of AIHA [12]. They found that the quantity of RBC AuAb after a 24-hour culture of EBV-transformed B cells was significantly greater in cultures from four patients who had AIHA than in cultures from normal persons [12]. The combination between AIHA and pure red cell aplasia in the patients with EBV infection was also reported [13]. Katayama et al. reported a case of a 53-year old man with systemic lymphadenopathy and hepatosplenomegaly , diagnosed with diffuse large B cell-lymphoma after an inguinal lymph node biopsy [13]. In this case, anemia was noted, direct and indirect Coombs tests were positive, and the haptoglobin level was low, however, the bone marrow aspirate revealed erythroid aplasia [13]. In this case, co-existing autoimmune hemolytic anemia (AIHA) and pure red cell aplasia (PRCA) were diagnosed [13].

3. Herpes Virus Infection and Chicken Pox

Herpes simplex virus (HSV) and varicella-zoster virus (VZV) are both common human alpha-herpes viruses [14]. They are capable of establishing latent infections in neural tissues and to reactivate from these sites, determining the clinical features of the disease [14]. These herpes virus infections are common. Tropical habitats also have been subject to major ecologic changes in the last few decades, exposing humans to direct contact with these viruses and allowing the correlated viral diseases [15]. Concerning HSV infection, the clinical spectrum is wide, ranging from trivial labial blisters to the most severe fatal sporadic encephalitis and neonatal infection [15]. This infection, in its typical form characterized by grouped vesicles, is frequently inapparent or atypical in both primary and recurrent diseases [15]. Concerning VZV infection, the two main manifestations are chicken pox and herpes zoster.

The anemia in the local HSV infection and herpes zoster is rarely mentioned due to the localization of the disease. However, in chicken pox, the disseminated pathology can sometimes be related with anemia. Hemolytic anemia in the patients with chicken pox is mentioned [16]. It is a very rare complication of chickenpox and usually characterized by anti-Pr cold agglutinin with hemolytic anemia after the onset of chickenpox [16 - 17]. However, the hemolytic anemia associated with an anti-I cold agglutinin during the incubation period of chickenpox was also reported by Terada et al. [16]. In addition, paroxysmal cold hemoglobinuria (PCH), an autoimmune disorder characterized by intravascular haemolysis causing haemoglobinuria is also reported [17]. PCH is believed to be due to a biphasic hemolysin known as the Donath-Landsteiner antibody, which binds specifically to the P antigen of red blood cells at low temperatures, leading to complement activation and red cell lysis at 37 degrees C [17]. Herpes virus infection not only lead to anemia but also can be a complication in anemic diseases. Recently, Bhattarakosol et al. reported a high prevalence of herpes virus – 6 seropositive in the Thai thalssemic patients and proposed for the possible cause of superimposed clinical manifestation in those cases [18].

4. Parvovirus Infection

Parvovirus infection is a viral infection that can lead to anemia. Parvovirus B19, a member of the Erythrovirus genus, is the only member of the Parvoviridae family known to cause pathology in humans. Human parvovirus B19 (B19) infection causes human bone marrow failure, by affecting erythroid-lineage cells which are well-known target cells for B19 [20]. The anemia induced by B19 infection is of minor clinical significance in healthy children and adults, however, it becomes critical in those afflicted with hemolytic diseases [20]. Lee et al. studied Taiwanese patients with parvovirus B19 infection and said that human parvovirus B19 has a strong tissue tropism for erythroid progenitor cells and is a causative agent for anemia [21]. They also indicated that the patients with hematological disease had higher seropositive rates for B19 than occur in normal controls and that study of occult parvovirus B19 infection was recommended in patients with hematological disease [21].

Concerning the anemia with hemolysis in the patients infected withn parvovirys B19, this condition is called transient aplastic crisis, and the pathogenesis is explained by the short life-span of red blood cells [20]. Similarly, fetuses are thought to be severely affected by B19-intrauterine infection in the first and second trimester, as the half-life of red blood cells is apparently shorter than RBC at the bone marrow hematopoietic stage [20]. Al-khan et al. said that the development of an acute parvovirus B-19 infection during pregnancy could cause pregnancy complications ranging from early pregnancy loss to nonimmune hydrops and there was no treatment, but preventive measures could be used to decrease perinatal mortality [22]. They noted that if the fetus exhibited hydrops in the latter part of pregnancy, the main treatment options included either correcting the associated anemia with intrauterine blood transfusion or birth with extrauterine management [22]. According to the recent study of Sant'Anna et al. on the prevalence of anti-human parvovirus B19 IgG antibodies in sera from 165 chronic hemolytic anemia patients in Brazil, Anti-B19 IgG antibodies were detected in 32.1% of the patients [23]. In addition, Badr performed another study in Saudi Arabia and noted that parvovirus B19 could be considered as one of the predisposing factors of hemolytic crisis in patients with chronic hemolytic disease [24].

Concerning the pathogenesis, the deficiencies of appropriate immune responses to B19 impair viral elimination in vivo, which results in enlargement of B19-infected erythroid-lineage cells and the subsequent B19-associated damage of erythroid lineage cells is due to cytotoxicity mediated by viral proteins [20]. Chisaka et al. noted that B19-infected erythroid-lineage cells showed apoptotic features, which are thought to be induced by the non-structural protein, NS1, of B19 [20]. In addition, they also mentioned that B19 infection induced cell cycle arrested at the G(1) and G(2) phases; the G(1) arrest was induced by NS1 expression prior to apoptosis induction in B19-infected cells, while the G(2) arrest was induced not only by infectious B19 but also by UV-inactivated B19, which lacked the ability to express NS1 [20]. Qian et al. studied the presence of human parvovirus B19 DNA in the peripheral blood samples of 60 patients with aplastic anemia and 30 healthy controls by nested polymerase chain reaction (PCR) assay [25]. According to this study, 16 (26.7%) of 60 aplastic anemia cases were human parvovirus B19 DNA positive, while all the samples in the control group were negative for human parvovirus B19 [25]. They proposed that human parvovirus B19 infection was not only correlated with the occurrence of children's acute aplastic anemia and chronic aplastic anemia, but also with adult acute aplastic anemia and chronic aplastic anemia, and might be an important viral cause for aplastic anemia in humans [25].

In addition, human parvovirus B19 infection could cause acute pure red cell aplasia not only in the patients with hemolytic anemia but also in the patients with iron deficiency anemia or after acute bleeding [26]. Tsuda et al. suggested that pancytopenia often observed on HPV infection could be at least partly caused by hemophagocytic syndrome [26]. In conclusion, in individuals with underlying haemolytic disorders, B19 infection causes transient aplastic crisis; in immunocompromised patients, persistent B19 infection may develop that manifests as pure red cell aplasia and chronic anemia; B19 infection in utero may result in fetal death, hydrops fetalis, or congenital anemia [27]. Diagnosis is usually based on examination of bone marrow and B19 virological studies and treatment of persistent infection with immunoglobulin leads to a prompt resolution of anemia [27].

5. Hepatitis Virus Infection

Hepatitis virus infection is a group of viral infection consisting of many types of diseases including hepatitis A, hepatitis B, hepatitis C, hepatitis D, hepatitis E and other minor types. The Hepatitis virus infection is an important public health problem in the developing world. The high prevalence of several types of hepatitis virus infections is mentioned in the underprivileged rural populations in the tropical countries [28 - 29]. Anemia in the hepatitis virus infection is well described in medicine. Here, anemia in the three most common viral hepatitis infections, hepatitis A, hepatitis B and hepatitis C will be summarized.

Concerning hepatitis A, the anemia is a common hematological complication of this viral infection. Acute hemolytic anemia due to the hepatitis A infection is mentioned. Chau et al. noted that hemolytic anemia as a complication of acute hepatitis had been reported in up to 23% of patients [30]. They proposed for a routine hepatitis A immunization in the endemic area [30]. Kusaba et al. recently reported an interesting autopsy case in the patients with hepatitis A infection. In this case, bone marrow revealed severe erythroblastopenia, and a diagnosis of thrombocytopenia due to an autoimmune mechanism was made on the basis of elevated levels of platelet-associated immunoglobulin G (PAIgG) and immune complex [31]. Furthermore, the advanced anemia was complicated by concurrent hemolysis [31]. This case may provide information useful for clarifying the pathogenesis of hematopoietic disorders complicated by hepatitis [31]. According to the report of Ritter et al., IgM antibodies against triosephosphate isomerase IgM (IgM) anti-TPI is assumed to be one of the causative agents of hemolysis in the HAV infection [32]. In addition, the co-manifestation of immune hemolytic anemia and immune hepatitis in hepatitis A infection is also mentioned. Urganci *et al.* reported a case diagnosed as autoimmune hepatitis and AIHA induced by hepatitis A infection and noted that steroid therapy resulted in clinical and laboratory remission [33]. However, not only the immune hemolysis but also non-immune hemolysis can be seen in patients with hepatitis A infection. They noted that mild anemia could occasionally be observed during viral hepatitis, but severe hemolysis had previously only been reported in a few patients with glucose-6-phosphate dehydrogenase (G-6-PD) deficiency [34]

Concerning the hepatitis B infection, anemia is common as well. Hemolytic anemia can be seen in hepatitis B infection, similar to hepatitis A infection. However, Kanematsu *et al.* noted that the prevalence of hemolytic anemia according to hepatitis B infection was lower than hepatitis A infection [35]. Kanematsu *et al.* suggested that there were four mechanisms that cause hemolysis to occur in the patients with viral hepatitis: (1) In the individual who has a predisposition to hemolytic anemia, viral infection accelerated the red cell destruction and hemolysis became obvious. (2) Directly, virus itself injured the red cell membrane. (3) The serious liver failure and hypersplenism induced the hemolysis. (4) AIHA because of immunological abnormality caused by symptomatic viral infection [35]. The AIHA in asymptomatic hepatitis B carrier is also mentioned [36]. In addition, the coexistence of hyperreactive malarious splenomegaly (HMS) syndrome and severe chronic HBV or HCV infection may further aggravate the course of the hemolytic disorder, because of the occurrence of spur cell anemia [37].

Concerning hepatitis C infection, hemolytic anemia is also mentioned.

Recently Ramos-Casals *et al.* studied 35 cases with hepatitis C infection and found the following cytopenias: AIHA (17 cases), severe thrombocytopenia (16 cases), aplastic anemia (2 cases), severe neutropenia (1 case), refractory sideroblastic anemia (1 case), and pure red cell aplasia (1 case) [38]. According to this study, different types of immune-mediated cytopenias might be severe and clinically significant in patients with HCV infection, however, hemolytic anemia and severe thrombocytopenia were the most frequent cytopenias observed [38]. In this study, most patients responded well to corticosteroids, although a higher rate of mortality was observed in those with liver cirrhosis [38]. Not only the hemolytic anemia, but the pure red cell aplasia is also reported in the patients with hepatitis C infection. Al-Awami *et al.* reported a case of pure red cell aplasia associated with hepatitis C infection [39]. This patient also had porphyria cutanea tarda and marked hepatic siderosis but no active hepatitis or cirrhosis [39]. In this case, treatment with cyclophosphamide and prednisone produced complete remission of the pure red cell aplasia [39]. Concerning the laboratory finding, erythroid colony formation was reduced in cultures of bone marrow obtained during relapse but was normal in remission marrow, however, addition of the patient serum, whether collected during relapse or remission, inhibited erythroid colony formation by the patient's bone marrow [39]. Al-Awami *et al.* proposed that these observations, and the known extrahepatic immunologic manifestations of hepatitis C infection, suggested that the pure red cell aplasia occurred because of autoimmune mechanism provoked by the hepatitis C infection [39]. Concerning treatment, the most effective treatment for chronic HCV infection is the combination of either interferon (IFN)-alpha or pegylated IFN-alpha and ribavirin [40]. Dieterich and Spivak noted that treatment adherence and dose maintenance were essential for a sustained virologic response, however, both IFN-alpha and ribavirin induced hematologic toxicity, such as anemia, neutropenia, and thrombocytopenia, which could compromise treatment adherence and dose maintenance and could, therefore, potentially influence outcomes [40]. Dieterich and Spivak also noted that although there were currently no approved treatments for hematologic complications of HCV therapy, studies had shown that hematopoietic growth factors could provide significant benefits [40]. However, it should be noted that the treatment of hepatitis C infection by IFN-alpha sometimes can result as a hematological adverse effect, pernicious anemia [40].

6. Influenza Virus Infection

Influenza virus infection is a common viral disease, leading to the respiratory symptoms. Influenza infections have been observed mainly during the rainy seasons in Asian, African and South American countries [41]. Hemolysis anemia is mentioned in the patients with influenza. Concerning the pathogenesis, it is possible that viral infection altered the immunologic host-parasite equilibrium [42]. The co-hematological manifestation as acute thrombocytopenia and rouleaux formation can also be observed [42]. AIHA can be seen in the patients with influenza virus infection. It is also mentioned as a leading cause of hemolytic uremic syndrome (HUS) [43].

7. Dengue Virus Infection

Dengue infection is a major public health problem, affecting general populations in the Southeast Asia Region [44]. Each year an estimated 50-100 million cases of dengue fever and about 250000-500000 cases of dengue hemorrhagic fever occur worldwide [45]. Similar to malaria, dengue infection is a common mosquito-borne disease. Dengue virus infection produces a broad spectrum of clinical presentations ranging from a nonspecific viral syndrome to severe and fatal hemorrhagic disease [46]. The most common hematologic alteration in the patients with dengue hemorrhagic fever is hemoconcentration [47].

However, anemia in the patients with dengue infection has been reported. Rueda *et al.* reported three cases of hemophagocytic syndrome (HPS) associated with dengue hemorrhagic fever [48]. They recommended that a bone marrow aspiration should be carried out as part of the differential diagnosis study in prolonged fever associated with dengue, as there was a possibility that this complication could be secondary HPS. In addition, the hemolytic anemia in the patient with dengue shock syndrome was also mentioned [49].

8. Rubella

Rubella or German measles is a viral infectious disease, which manifests as a viral exanthem. It has been said that naternal rubella was now rare in many developed countries that had rubella vaccination programmes, however, in many developing countries congenital rubella syndrome (CRS) remained a major cause of developmental anomalies, particularly blindness and deafness [50]. Laboratory differentiation of rubella from other rash-causing infections, such as measles, parvovirus B19, human herpesvirus 6, and enteroviruses in developed countries, and various endemic arboviruses is essential [50].

In medicine, anemia in rubella can be seen. Immune hemolytic anemia in the patients with rubella is mentioned. Konig *et al.* reported a case with a relationship between rubella infection and the cold agglutinin specificity anti-PR, known as cold agglutinin syndrome [51]. A similar case report was published by Brody and Kreysel [52]. In addition to the anemia caused directly by the rubella infection, severe hemolytic anemia, HUS, due to the vaccination by mumps-measles-rubella (MMR) vaccine are mentioned [53 – 54].

9. Mumps

Mumps is another preventable viral infection, which manifests as parotitis. A severe complication as orchi-epididymitis is usually mentioned. Concerning the anemia, it is sometimes reported in the patients with mumps. Similar to many viral infections, hemolytic anemia is mentioned. Ozen *et al.* reported a boy presented with acute hemolytic anemia a few days after mumps infection and the ensuing hemoglobinuria resulted in acute renal failure in this child, which was corrected with fluid and alkali therapy [55]. Ozen *et al.* drew attention to this uncommon complication of mumps and the need for careful evaluation [55]. Similar case was reported by Mulaosmanovic *et al.* In this AIHA case, the patient responded well to the therapy (corticosteroides, immunoglobulines, transfusions of red blood cells without buffy coat) with improvement of general condition and clinical aspect [56]. Finally, as already mentioned, HUS related to the MMR vaccination should be considered [53 - 54].

10. Pilio and Gastroenteritis Viruses Infection

Gastroenteritis viruses infection is an important cause of diarrhea in the tropical countries. Much of the gastroenteritis in children is caused by viruses belonging to four distinct families--rotaviruses, caliciviruses, astroviruses and adenoviruses while other viruses, such as the toroviruses, picobirnaviruses, picornavirus (the Aichi virus), and enterovirus 22, may play a role as well [57]. Of several gastroenteritis virus infections, polio is an infection which can bring severe complications such as paralysis but is preventable by effective oral polio vaccine. Polio, itself, is rarely mentioned as an underlying cause of anemia, however, anemia due to oral polio vaccine is mentioned [58]. In those cases, hemolytic anemia can be detected.

Concerning non-polio enterovirus infection, De Petris *et al.* mentioned that enteroviral infections should not be considered a cause of HUS in Verocytotoxin-producing Escherichia coli (VTEC)-negative children [59].

11. Human Immunodeficiency Virus Infection

Human immunodeficiency virus (HIV) is an important ' became the most important sexually transmitted disease leading the world. HIV infection is not a specific problem for tropic Anemia is a common hematological finding in patients with decreased quality of life and increased morbidity and mor categories of anemia in HIV disease are anemia due to impair anemia due to increased red blood cell destruction, and anemia due to increased red blood cell loss [60]. Here, anemia and HIV infections are briefly summarized.

Buskin and Sullivan studied anemia prevalence in a cohort of HIV-infected persons [61]. Concerning treatment, transfusion was associated with a threefold excess mortality risk, but epoetin alfa prescription was not associated with mortality [61]. According to a recent systematic review by Belperio and Rhew in 2004, the prevalence of anemia in HIV disease varied considerably, ranging from 1.3% to 95%: it depends on several factors, including the stage of HIV disease, sex, age, pregnancy status, and injection-drug use as well as the definition of anemia used [62]. Belperio and Rhew said that as the HIV disease progressed, the prevalence and severity of anemia increased and anemia was also more prevalent in HIV-positive women, children, and injection-drug users than in HIV-negative women, children, and injection-drug users [62]. They also mentioned that anemia had been shown to be a statistically significant predictor of progression to AIDS and is independently associated with an increased risk of death in patients with HIV [62].

The pathogenesis of anemia in the patients with the HIV infection is very complex. HIV, opportunistic infection, host response and treatment can be responsible for anemia in HIV-infected patients. In addition, all types of anemia, normocytic, microcytic and macrocytic anemia can be demonstrated. Davis and Zauli said that the pathogenesis of peripheral blood cytopenias in AIDS patients is clearly multifactorial [63]. Concerning HIV, itself, it has now been convincingly demonstrated that HIV can impair the survival/proliferative capacity of purified haematopoietic progenitor cells [63]. Although a subset of haematopoietic progenitor cells are perhaps susceptible to HIV-1 infection, both in vitro and in vivo, the suppressive effect does not require either active or latent infection and is probably mediated by the interaction of viral or virus-associated proteins with the cell membrane of hematopoietic progenitor cells [63]. Davis and Zauli mentioned that both the viral load and the biological characteristics of the virus play an important role in suppression, since different isolates displayed different inhibitory activity [63]. They said that since the hematopoietic stem cell was the common progenitor to both the myeloid and lymphoid lineages, the capacity of HIV to impair the growth of early hematopoietic progenitor cells could contribute not only to the frequent occurrence of anemia, granulocytopenia and thrombocytopenia in AIDS patients, but also to the inability of the bone marrow to reconstitute a functional pool of mature CD4+ T-cells [63].

Concerning the HIV virus, it leads to an initial activation of the immune system, with a subsequent suppression thereafter due to direct viral infection of cells, inhibitory effects of HIV proteins, an altered microenvironment with cytokine imbalance, and increased apoptosis of both infected and non-infected cells [64]. In the first stages of the disease, increased roduction, consequent to a chronic immune activation, is probably responsible for lodysplastic/hyperplastic alterations observed at the bone marrow level while in more nced stages of the disease, the general decline in immune function, the consequent mbalance in cytokine production, and the increase in viral burden, may contribute to dysregulated hematopoiesis and peripheral blood cytopenias [63]. However, Bain concluded that HIV infection itself caused anemia, probably as a consequence of HIV infection of stromal cells rather than HIV infection of hematopoietic stem cells [64 - 65] Concerning opportunistic infection, several opportunistic infections in HIV-infected patients can lead to anemia. These infections included strongyloidiasis, histoplasmosis, penicillosis, CMV infection and etc. The control of the superimposed infection is believed to be beneficial in management of anemia in HIV-infected patients. Concerning the host-response, abnormal immune response can lead to AIHA in the patients with HIV infection [66]. Concerning treatment, bone marrow suppression by antiretroviral therapy, and hemolytic anemia induced by oxidant drugs are usually mentioned [64 - 65].

Classified by type, normocytic anemia seems the most common anemia in the patients with HIV infection. The common causes of normocytic anemic disorders are due to the marrow suppression and hemolysis. However, anemia due to thrombotic microangiopathy is also reported [66]. This anemia responds well to plasmapheresis [66]. Concerning microcytic anemia, iron deficiency anemia in the patients with HIV infection can be expected. Recently, Eley et al. mentioned that iron depletion and iron deficiency anemia were major problems in HIV-infected children in South Africa [67]. Concerning macrocytic anemia, the antiretroviral drug, especially stavudine [68] , can lead to macrocytic anemia in the patient with HIV infection.

Concerning treatment of anemia in HIV infected patients, resolution of HIV-related anemia has been shown to improve quality of life, physical functioning, energy, and fatigue in individuals with HIV [61]. The principles of management are based on both principles of management for anemia "promotion of red blood cell production in cases that have decrease red blood cell production as basic pathophysiology accompanied with red blood cell replacement and decrease red blood cell destruction in cases that have increase red blood cell destruction as basic pathophysiology" and principles of management for infection "getting rid of source of infection and control of complications from pathogen virulence, host responses and treatment". To promote red blood cell production, treatment of anemia with epoetin-alpha has resulted in significantly fewer patients requiring transfusion as well as decreases in the mean number of units of blood transfused [61]. Concerning red blood cell replacement, it is only occasionally recommended at present since it can lead to high mortality [61]. Concerning decreased red blood cell destruction, the plasmapharesis is indicated in the cases with MAHA [66]. Concerning getting rid of the infection and control of direct complications from HIV, the use of highly active antiretroviral therapy has also been associated with a significant increase in hemoglobin concentrations and a decrease in the prevalence of anemia [61]. Ferri et al. noted that anemia had developed in close to 90% of HIV-infected patients before the introduction of highly active antiretroviral therapy (HAART), and it was still found in up to 46% of patients in the HAART era [69]. In addition, getting rid of the co-infection and opportunistic infection are proved to be useful in management of anemia in HIV-infected cases. Volberding et al. mentioned the good impact of the treatment of hepatitis

C virus coinfection on anemia in HIV-infected patients [70]. Concerning control of complications due to host responses, prednisolone is reported to be effective in the HIV-infected cases with AIHA [71]. Concerning control of complications due to treatment, monitoring for drug-induced anemia in HIV-infected patients who receive HARRT and other drugs is needed. Indeed, there are more details concerning anemia in HIV infection that can be found in many publications.

References

[1] Baranski B, Young N. Hematologic consequences of viral infections. *Hematol Oncol Clin North Am* 1987;1:167-83.

[2] He ZX, Pan SN, Chen JL, Xiong W, Li K, Wang QW, Zou XB, Huang LF, Chen ML, Yang M. Effect of human cytomegalovirus on hematopoietic system. *Zhonghua Er Ke Za Zhi* 2003;41:321-4.

[3] Murray JC, Bernini JC, Bijou HL, Rossmann SN, Mahoney DH Jr, Morad AB. Infantile cytomegalovirus-associated autoimmune hemolytic anemia. *J Pediatr Hematol Oncol* 2001;23:318-20.

[4] Pemde HK, Kabra SK, Agarwal R, Jain Y, Seth V. Hematological manifestations of congenital cytomegalovirus infection. *Indian J Pediatr* 1995;62:473-7.

[5] Salloum E, Lundberg WB. Hemolytic anemia with positive direct antiglobulin test secondary to spontaneous cytomegalovirus infection in healthy adults. *Acta Haematol* 1994;92:39-41.

[6] Gavazzi G, Leclercq P, Bouchard O, Bosseray A, Morand P, Micoud M. Association between primary cytomegalovirus infection and severe hemolytic anemia in an immunocompetent adult. *Eur J Clin Microbiol Infect Dis* 1999;18:299-301.

[7] Riechsteiner G, Speich R, Schanz U, Russi EW, Weder W, Boehler A. Haemolytic anaemia after lung transplantation: an immune-mediated phenomenon? *Swiss Med Wkly* 2003;133:143-7.

[8] Siddiqui T, Khan AH. Hepatitis A and cytomegalovirus infection precipitating acute hemolysis in glucose-6-phosphate dehydrogenase deficiency. *Mil Med.* 1998;163:434-5.

[9] Li ZY, Lou JG, Chen J. Analysis of primary symptoms and disease spectrum in Epstein-Barr virus infected children. *Zhonghua Er Ke Za Zhi* 2004;42:20-2.

[10] Brkic S, Aleksic-Dordevic M, Belic A, Jovanovic J, Bogdanovic M. Agranulocytosis as a complication of acute infectious mononucleosis. *Med Pregl* 1998;51:355-8.

[11] Lau YL, Srivastava G, Lee CW, Kwong KY, Yeung CY. Epstein-Barr virus associated aplastic anaemia and hepatitis. *J Paediatr Child Health* 1994;30:74-6.

[12] Hernandez-Jodra M, Hudnall SD, Petz LD. Studies of in vitro red cell autoantibody production in normal donors and in patients with autoimmune hemolytic anemia. *Transfusion* 1990;30:411-7.

[13] Katayama H, Takeuchi M, Yoshino T, Munemasa M, Tada A, Soda R, Takahashi K. Epstein-Barr virus associated diffuse large B-cell lymphoma complicated by

autoimmune hemolytic anemia and pure red cell aplasia. *Leuk Lymphoma* 2001;42:539-42.

[14] Lautenschlager S. Herpes simplex and varicella zoster virus infections. *Ther Umsch* 2003;60:605-14.

[15] Lupi O, Tyring SK. Tropical dermatology: viral tropical diseases. *J Am Acad Dermatol* 2003;49:979-1000.

[16] Terada K, Tanaka H, Mori R, Kataoka N, Uchikawa M. Hemolytic anemia associated with cold agglutinin during chickenpox and a review of the literature. *J Pediatr Hematol Oncol* 1998;20:149-51.

[17] Herron B, Roelcke D, Orson G, Myint H, Boulton FE. Cold autoagglutinins with anti-Pr specificity associated with fresh varicella infection. *Vox Sang* 1993;65:239-42.

[18] Papalia MA, Schwarer AP. Paroxysmal cold haemoglobinuria in an adult with chicken pox. *Br J Haematol* 2000;109:328-9.

[19] Bhattarakosol P, Wiwanitkit V, Boonchalermvichian C, Nuchprayoon I. Human herpes virus 6 antibodies in beta-thalassemia/hemoglobin E pediatric patients. *Southeast Asian J Trop Med Public Health.* 2002;33 Suppl 3:149-51.

[20] Chisaka H, Morita E, Yaegashi N, Sugamura K. Parvovirus B19 and the pathogenesis of anaemia. *Rev Med Virol* 2003;13:347-59.

[21] Lee YM, Tsai WH, You JY, Ing-Tiau Kuo B, Liao PT, Ho CK, Hsu HC. Parvovirus B19 infection in Taiwanese patients with hematological disorders. *J Med Virol.* 2003;71:605-9.

[22] Al-Khan A, Caligiuri A, Apuzzio J. Parvovirus B-19 infection during pregnancy. *Infect Dis Obstet Gynecol* 2003;11:175-9.

[23] Sant'Anna AL, Garcia Rde C, Marzoche M, da Rocha HH, Paula MT, Lobo CC, Nascimento JP. Study of chronic hemolytic anaemia patients in Rio de Janeiro: prevalence of anti-human parvovirus B19 IgG antibodies and the development aplastic crises. *Rev Inst Med Trop Sao Paulo* 2002;44:187-90.

[24] Badr MA. Human parvovirus B19 infection among patients with chronic blood disorders. *Saudi Med J* 2002;23:295-7.

[25] Qian X, Zheng Y, Zhang G, Jiao X, Li Z. Relationship between human parvovirus B19 infection and aplastic anemia. *Chin Med Sci J* 2001;16:172-4.

[26] Tsuda H, Shirono K, Shimizu K, Shimomura T. Postpartum parvovirus B19-associated acute pure red cell aplasia and hemophagocytic syndrome. *Rinsho Ketsueki* 1995;36:672-6.

[27] Brown KE. Haematological consequences of parvovirus B19 infection. *Baillieres Best Pract Res Clin Haematol.* 2000;13:245-59.

[28] Wiwanitkit V. A note in the high prevalence of anti-HCV seropositivity among hilltribers in Mae Jam District, Northern Thailand. *Viral Immunol* 2002;15:645-6.

[29] Wiwanitkit V, Suyaphan A. High prevalence of HBsAg seropositivity in Hilltribers in the Mae Jam district in northern Thailand. *MedGenMed* 2002 ;4:26.

[30] Chau TN, Lai ST, Lai JY, Yuen H. Haemolysis complicating acute viral hepatitis in patients with normal or deficient glucose-6-phosphate dehydrogenase activity. *Scand J Infect Dis* 1997;29:551-3.

[31] Kusaba N, Yoshida H, Ohkubo F, Shimokawa Y, Sata M. Autoimmune thrombocytopenia and erythroid hypoplasia associated with hepatitis A. *Rinsho Ketsueki* 2000;41:739-44.

[32] Ritter K, Uy A, Ritter S, Thomssen R. Hemolysis and autoantibodies to triosephosphate isomerase in a patient with acute hepatitis A virus infection. *Scand J Infect Dis* 1994;26:379-82.

[33] Urganci N, Akyildiz B, Yildirmak Y, Ozbay G. A case of autoimmune hepatitis and autoimmune hemolytic anemia following hepatitis A infection. *Turk J Gastroenterol* 2003;14:204 – 7.

[34] Ibe M, Rude B, Gerken G, Meyer zum Buschenfelde KH, Lohse AW. Coombs-negative severe hemolysis associated with hepatitis A. *Z Gastroenterol* 1997;35:567-9.

[35] Kanematsu T, Nomura T, Higashi K, Ito M. Hemolytic anemia in association with viral hepatitis. *Nippon Rinsho* 1996;54:2539-44.

[36] Yoshioka K, Miyata H. Autoimmune haemolytic anaemia in an asymptomatic carrier of hepatitis B virus. *Arch Dis Child* 1980;55:233-4.

[37] Torres R JR, Magris M, Villegas L, Torres V MA, Dominguez G. Spur cell anaemia and acute haemolysis in patients with hyperreactive malarious splenomegaly. Experience in an isolated Yanomamo population of Venezuela. *Acta Trop* 2000;77:257-62.

[38] Ramos-Casals M, Garcia-Carrasco M, Lopez-Medrano F, Trejo O, Forns X, Lopez-Guillermo A, Munoz C, Ingelmo M, Font J. Severe autoimmune cytopenias in treatment-naive hepatitis C virus infection: clinical description of 35 cases. *Medicine* (Baltimore) 2003;82:87-96.

[39] al-Awami Y, Sears DA, Carrum G, Udden MM, Alter BP, Conlon CL. Pure red cell aplasia associated with hepatitis C infection. *Am J Med Sci* 1997;314:113-7.

[40] Dieterich DT, Spivak JL. Hematologic disorders associated with hepatitis C virus infection and their management. *Clin Infect Dis* 2003;37:533-41.

[41] Shek LP, Lee BW. Epidemiology and seasonality of respiratory tract virus infections in the tropics. : *Paediatr Respir Rev* 2003;4:105-11.

[42] Graves IL, Adams WH, Pyakural S. Recurring hemolytic anemia, babesiasis, and influenza A viruses in a yak at low altitude in Nepal. *Am J Vet Res* 1975;36:843-5.

[43] Asaka M, Ishikawa I, Nakazawa T, Tomosugi N, Yuri T, Suzuki K. Hemolytic uremic syndrome associated with influenza A virus infection in an adult renal allograft recipient: case report and review of the literature. *Nephron* 2000;84:258-66.

[44] Thisyakorn U, Thisyakorn C. Diseases cuased by arboviruses-dengue hemorrhagic fever and Japanese B encephalitits. *Med J Aus* 1994; 160: 22 – 6.

[45] Guzman MG, Kouri G. Dengue and dengue hemorrhagic fever in the Americas: lessons and challenges. *J Clin Virol* 2003;27:1-13.

[46] Guzman MG, Kouri G. Dengue: an update. *Lancet Infect Dis.* 2002;2:33-42.

[47] Wiwanitkit V, Manusvanich P. Can hematocrit and platelet determination on admission predict shock in hospitalized children with dengue hemorrhagic fever? A clinical observation from a small outbreak. *Clin Appl Thromb Hemost* 2004;10:65-7.

[48] Rueda E, Mendez A, Gonzalez G. Hemophagocytic syndrome associated with dengue hemorrhagic fever. *Biomedica* 2002;22:160-6.

[49] Medagoda K, Gunathilaka SB, De Silva HJ. A case of self-limiting Coomb's negative haemolytic anaemia following dengue shock syndrome. *Ceylon Med J* 2003;48:147-8.

[50] Banatvala JE, Brown DW. Rubella. *Lancet* 2004;363:1127-37.

[51] Konig AL, Schabel A, Sugg U, Brand U, Roelcke D. Autoimmune hemolytic anemia caused by IgG lambda-monotypic cold agglutinins of anti-Pr specificity after rubella infection. *Transfusion* 2001;41:488-92.

[52] Brody M, Kreysel HW. Cold agglutinin syndrome after rubella infection. *Kinderarztl Prax* 1992;60:134-6.

[53] Tsimaratos M, Le Menestrel S, Daniel L, Roquelaure B, Almhana T, de Montleon JV, Paut O, Picon G, Casanova P, Sarles J. Hemolytic and uremic syndrome after measles, mumps and rubella vaccination. Fortuitous association? *Arch Pediatr* 1997;4:1261-2.

[54] Karim Y, Masood A. Haemolytic uraemic syndrome following mumps, measles, and rubella vaccination. *Nephrol Dial Transplant* 2002;17:941-2.

[55] Ozen S, Damarguc I, Besbas N, Saatci U, Kanra T, Gurgey A. A case of mumps associated with acute hemolytic crisis resulting in hemoglobinuria and acute renal failure. *J Med* 1994;25:255-9.

[56] Mulaosmanovic V, Sakic M, Ferhatovic M. Secondary autoimmune hemolytic anemia caused by epidemic parotitis virus. *Med Arh* 2002;56 (3 Suppl 1):46-7.

[57] Glass RI, Bresee J, Jiang B, Gentsch J, Ando T, Fankhauser R, Noel J, Parashar U, Rosen B, Monroe SS. Gastroenteritis viruses: an overview. *Novartis Found Symp* 2001;238:5-19.

[58] Pilotti G. Thrombopenia and acute hemolytic anemia in the course of poliomyelitis vaccination. *Minerva Pediatr* 1975;27:637-9.

[59] De Petris L, Gianviti A, Caione D, Innocenzi D, Edefonti A, Montini G, De Palo T, Tozzi AE, Caprioli A, Rizzoni G. Role of non-polio enterovirus infection in pediatric hemolytic uremic syndrome. *Pediatr Nephrol* 2002;17:852-5.

[60] Phillips KD, Groer M. Differentiation and treatment of anemia in HIV disease. *J Assoc Nurses AIDS Care* 2002;13:47-68.

[61] Buskin SE, Sullivan PS. Anemia and its treatment and outcomes in persons infected with human immunodeficiency virus. *Transfusion* 2004;44:826-32.

[62] Belperio PS, Rhew DC. Prevalence and outcomes of anemia in individuals with human immunodeficiency virus: a systematic review of the literature. *Am J Med* 2004;116 Suppl 7A:27S-43S.

[63] Davis BR, Zauli G. Effect of human immunodeficiency virus infection on haematopoiesis. *Baillieres Clin Haematol* 1995 ;8:113-30.

[64] Panoskaltsis N, Abboud CN. Human immunodeficiency virus and the hematopoietic repertoire: implications for gene therapy. *Front Biosci* 1999;4:D457-67.

[65] Bain BJ. Pathogenesis and pathophysiology of anemia in HIV infection. *Curr Opin Hematol* 1999;6:89-93.

[66] Saif MW. HIV-associated autoimmune hemolytic anemia: an update. *AIDS Patient Care STDS* 2001;15:217-24.

[67] Eley BS, Sive AA, Shuttleworth M, Hussey GD. A prospective, cross-sectional study of anaemia and peripheral iron status in antiretroviral naive, HIV-1 infected children in Cape Town, South Africa. *BMC Infect Dis* 2002;2:3.

[68] Martin GJ, Blazes DL, Mayers DL, Spooner KM. Stavudine-induced macrocytosis during therapy for human immunodeficiency virus infection. *Clin Infect Dis* 1999;29:459-60.

[69] Ferri RS, Adinolfi A, Orsi AJ, Sterken DJ, Keruly JC, Davis S, MacIntyre RC. Treatment of anemia in patients with HIV infection, Part 1: The need for adequate guidelines. *J Assoc Nurses AIDS Care* 2001;12:39-51.

[70] Volberding PA, Levine AM, Dieterich D, Mildvan D, Mitsuyasu R, Saag M; Anemia in HIV Working Group. Anemia in HIV infection: clinical impact and evidence-based management strategies. *Clin Infect Dis* 2004;38:1454-63.

[71] Koduri PR, Singa P, Nikolinakos P. Autoimmune hemolytic anemia in patients infected with human immunodeficiency virus-1. *Am J Hematol* 2002;70:174-6.

Chapter 8

Advances in Thalassemia

Introduction to Thalassemia

In tropical countries, thalassemia is an important microcytic anemic disorder, with the second common prevalence following iron deficiency anemia. Thalassemic syndromes, characterized by anemia secondary to genetic defects of hemoglobin, are one of the most common of the genetic blood disorders in the tropics [1 – 3]. Basically, hemoglobin is composed of the heme and globin chains. The fundamental abnormality in thalassemia is impaired production of either the alpha or beta globin chains. The defects in thalassemia might be on alpha globin chain genes or the beta globin chain gene. Alpha thalassemia occurs when one or more of the four alpha chain genes fails to function; beta thalassemia occurs when one or all of the two beta chain genes fails to function [1 – 5]. Compared to alpha thalassemia, beta thalassemia rarely arises from the complete loss of a beta globin gene [1 – 5]. The beta globin gene usually presents, but produces little beta globin protein, therefore, the degree of suppression varies [1 – 5]. In some cases, the affected beta gene makes essentially no beta globin protein (beta-0-thalassemia) while in other cases, the production of beta chain protein is lower than normal, but not zero (beta-(+)-thalassemia) [1 – 3]. Similar to other inherited disorders, the defect can be detected as hemogenicity or heterogenicity (Table 8.1). In addition, the connection between thalassemia and hemoglobinopathy is common and brings anemia to millions of people in the tropics.

Molecular Basis of Thalassemia

The molecular basis of thalassemia is due to the defect of the gene controlling the production of globin chains, which can be either alpha globin or beta globin genes.

Basically, the two chromosomes 11 have one beta globin gene each, for a total of two genes and the two chromsomes 16 have two alpha globin genes each, for a total of four genes. Hemoglobin protein has two alpha subunits and two beta subunits [1 – 7]. Physiologically, each alpha globin gene produces only about half the quantity of protein of a

Table 8.1. Genotype classification of thalassemia

Classification	Brief details
Alpha thalassemia	*One or more of the four alpha chain genes fails to function*
o One-gene deletion alpha thalassemia or silent carriers	o The loss of one gene slightly affects the production of the alpha protein, therefore, this condition looks grossly normal, and as a result can be detected only by special laboratory techniques making it, until recently, under-detected. The affected person is purely a carrier and brings inheritance to their children.
o Two-gene deletion alpha thalassemia	o This type produces a condition with small red blood cells, and at most a mild anemia, which can be accidentally detected by routine laboratory examination. The affected cases usually look and feel normal. Similar to the first type, the affected person is usually a carrier and affects their children.
o Three-gene deletion alpha thalassemia or hemoglobin H disease	o This type brings disease to the affected person. Patients with this condition develop a severe anemia, and often require blood transfusions to survive. The severe imbalance between the alpha chain production and beta chain production causes an accumulation of beta chains inside the red blood cells leading to a generation of an abnormal hemoglobin called hemoglobin H (Hb H).
o Hemoglobin Barts disease	o This type is very severe. Those affected cannot survive and usually die in utero leading to a well-known condition called hydrop fetalis. Due to the depletion of all four alpha chains, the gamma chains produced during fetal life associate in a group of four- pattern to form well-known abnormal hemoglobin called Hemoglobin Barts (Hb Bart).
Beta thalassemia	*One or all of the two beta chain genes fails to function*
o One-gene beta thalassemia	o The affected case has one beta globin gene that is normal, and a second, affected gene with a variably reduced production of beta globin. The red cells are small and a mild anemia may exist. Those affected generally have no symptoms and the problem can be mostly detected by a routine laboratory blood evaluation. Although the degree of imbalance with the alpha globin depends on the residual production capacity of the defective beta globin gene, even when the affected gene produces no beta chain, the condition is mild since the other beta gene still functions normally and the formation of normal alpha-beta combination can still occur.
o Two-gene beta thalassemia	o This type produces a severe anemia and a potentially life-threatening condition. The severity of the disorder depends in part on the combination of genes that have been inherited (beta 0/ beta 0; beta 0/ beta +; beta +/ beta +), therefore, some of those affected can survive and they become the problematic cases.

single beta globin gene, bringing the equality in the production of protein subunits [1 – 7]. Thalassemia occurs when a globin gene fails, and the production of globin protein subunits is imbalanced [1 – 7]. As already described, the abnormality in alpha globin gene results in the whole gene defect while abnormality in the beta globin chain gene can be either the whole or partial gene defect [1 – 7]. However, the association between phenotype and genotype of the thalassmia is complex. Concerning alpha thalassemia, genetic abnormalities causing alpha thalassemia can be classified as alpha 0 or alpha 1 according to whether they caused a lack of two or one alpha globin gene in one chromosome. Leder et al. performed a rat model experiment and found that its phenotype is strongly influenced by the genetic background in which the alpha-thalassemia mutation resides [129(sv/ev)/129(sv/ev) (severe) or 129(sv/ev)/C57BL/6 (mild)] [8]. Further linkage mapping indicates that the modifying gene was very tightly linked to the beta-globin locus (Lod score = 13.3) [8]. In addition, the severity of the phenotype correlated with the size of beta-chain-containing inclusion bodies that accumulate in red blood cells and likely accelerate their destruction [8]. Leder et al. concluded that the variation in severity of the phenotype would not depend on a change in the ratio between alpha- and beta-chains but on the chemical nature of the normal beta-chain, which was in excess [8].

Recently, Igbokwe said that linked duplicate genes in Chromosome 16 conditioned the production not only of alpha-globin chains in the Hemoglobin A (HbA) molecule, but also of the varied forms of alpha thalassemia in human subjects and null allelism, not gene deletion, existed at these gene loci [9]. Basically, two codominant alleles occured at each locus; these are characterized as Gb and Ob at one locus, and as Gc and Oc at the second locus [9]. Gb and Gc are genetically active alleles, and either conditions the production of alpha-globin chain while Ob and Oc are null or genetically inert alleles, and neither conditions the production of alpha-globin chain [9]. Igbokwe said that Gb and Gc are additive in the expression of disease genotype [9]. Igbokwe noted that the number of alpha-globin chains in the HbA molecule, and the absence as well as the varied forms of alpha thalassemia were inherited quantitatively as follows: four alpha-globin chains and the absence of alpha thalassemia result from GbGbGcGc; either GbGbGcOc or GbObGcGc yields three alpha-globin chains and asymptomatic alpha thalassemia minor; any one of three genotypes, GbGbOcOc, GbObGcOc or ObObGcGc, yields two alpha-globin chains and mild alpha thalassemia minor; either GbObOcOc or ObObGcOc yields one alpha-globin chain and severe alpha thalassemia minor; ObObOcOc produces no alpha-globin chain and the fetal alpha thalassemia major [9]. Igbokwe concluded that the inheritance of any combination of active and null alleles, and of the associated forms of alpha thalassemia, was deducible from the alpha-globin as well as the disease phenotypes and/or genotypes of parental subjects [9].

Concerning beta thalassemia, mutations causing beta thalassemia can be classified as beta 0 or beta + according to whether they abolish or reduce the production of beta globin chains. Although most of the molecular lesions involve the structural beta gene directly, some down regulate the gene through in-cis effects at a distance while trans-acting factors are implicated in a few cases [10]. Ho and Thein said that the vast majority of beta thalassemia was caused by point mutations, mostly single base substitutions, within the gene or its immediate flanking sequences and rarely, beta thalassemia was caused by major deletions of the beta globin cluster [11]. They also noted that all these mutations behaved as alleles of the beta locus but in several families the beta thalassemia phenotype segregates independently of the beta globin complex, and were likely to be caused by mutations in trans-acting regulatory factors [11]. Thein said that the remarkable phenotypic diversity in beta thalassemia could be related ultimately to the degree of alpha-globin-beta-globin chain imbalance and arises from variability of mutations affecting the beta gene itself and from interactions with other genetic loci, such as the alpha- and gamma-globin genes [10]. Thein also noted that the presence of other interacting loci was implicated by their interactions in increasing gamma gene expression or by an increased proteolytic capacity of the erythroid precursors [10].

Population Epidemiology of Thalassemia

The prevalence and severity of the thalassemia syndromes are population dependent, with the type of thalassemia seen dependent on racial background. The high prevalence of thalassemia is mentioned in the Mediteranian and Southeast Asia. The well-known Cooley's anemia, first described in Italy, is a classical thalassemic disorder [4]. However, the problems of thalassemia are more complicated in Southeast Asia, especially in Thailand and Laos, at present. The summary of population epidemiology of thalassemia in different tropical countries are described as the following:

Southeast Asia

In Southeast Asia, the reported prevalence for thalassemic diseases and carriers are about 1 % and up to 40 % of the whole population [5]. The highest prevalence is reported in the northeastern region of Thailand, southern region of Laos and northern region of Cambodia [5]. The most common type of thalassemic disorder in this region is alpha thalassemia [5, 12 – 13]. Concerning Thailand, there are several studies on the epidemiology and pattern of thalassemia. Concerning alpha thalassemia, Fucharoen et al. said that SEA deletion is the most common type of alpha 0 thalassemia gene deletion among the Thais in the northeastern region [14]. In 2004, Wiwanitkit summarized the molecular pattern of alpha 0 thalassemia among the Thais and found similar findings [15]. Wanichagoon et al. said that compound heterozygosity for alpha-thalassemia 1 and alpha-thalassemia 2 results in Hb H disease while homozygosity for alpha-thalassemia 1 leads to Hb Bart's hydrops fetalis, the most severe form of thalassemic disease [16]. They also said that three alpha-thalassemic hemoglobinopathies had been detected in Thailand, two of which produce a remarkable reduction in gene product and upon interacting with alpha-thalassemia 1 gene, they could lead to HemH disease [16]. Wanichagoon et al. mentioned that the most common in this group was Hb Constant Spring, which arose from a mutation of the termination codon in the alpha 2-gene resulting in an elongation of the alpha-globin chain [16]. Concerning beta thalassemia, Laig et al. Studied a total of 123 beta-thalassemia genes from northern and northeastern Thailand using five oligonucleotide probes [17]. According to this study, the mutation in 108 genes (88%) was identified: 50 nonsense 17, 49 frameshift 41-42 (-TCTT), 4-28(A----G), 2 IV1 nt5(G----C), 2IVS2 nt654, and 1 deletion removing the entire beta-globin gene and the nonsense 17 mutation (n = 39) was linked to a single haplotype, whereas the frameshift 41-42 mutation occurred with several haplotypes [17]. Nopparatana *et al.* studied a total of 282 beta-thalassemia alleles from southern Thailand, and it was possible to characterize the mutations in 274 (97.2%) alleles studied [18]. According to this study, twelve different point mutations and two different large deletions of the beta-globin gene were identified and seven common mutations, namely 4 bp deletion at codons 41/42. IVS1 position 5 (G-C), codon 19 (AAC-AGC), codon 17 (AAG-TAG), IVS1 position 1 (G-T), position -28 (A-G) and 3.5 kb deletion, accounted for about 91.5% [18].

Concerning other tropical countries, such as Indochina, Laos, Cambodia and Vietnam, there are fewer reports on the thalassemia epidemiology due to limited laboratory resources. In 1988, Dode *et al.* determined alpha+ deletional thalassemia among 143 Southeast Asia refugees (Cambodians, Laotians, and Vietnameses) and found that the gene frequency of alpha+ deletional thalassemia in Vietnameses (0.035) was lower than in Cambodians and Laotians (0.11) [19]. Hurst *et al.* performed hematological evaluations of 254 Southeast Asian refugee children from 163 families and found that the beta-Thalassemia trait was most prevalent in Vietnamese (8%), and less common in Cambodians and Laotians (3%) while alpha-Thalassemia was prevalent in all three groups [20]. Recently Svasti *et al.* studied the beta thalassemia in South Vietnam and found that the two most common mutations were the frameshift at codons 41 - 42 and the nonsense mutation in codon 17 (A-->T) [21], similar to the results of Laig *et al.* in Thailand [17].

South Asia

The prevalence of thalassemia in South Asia is lower than that of Southeast Asia. Both beta- and alpha- thalassemia can be seen. Concerning beta-thalassemia, Nadkami *et al.* performed a study in India and found 11 different beta-thalassemia mutations encountered among 128 beta-thalassemia chromosomes [22]. They found that the nature of the beta-thalassemia mutations was not very different between the beta-thalassemia major and beta-thalassemia intermedia groups in their patients, but co-inheritance of one or more alpha-globin gene deletions and the presence of the XmnI polymorphism were associated with lesser severity of the disease in Indians [22]. Khan and Riazuddin analyzed a representative sample of 602 alleles from six ethnic groups in Pakistan; 99.2% alleles were characterized, while 0.8% remained unidentified [23]. According to this study, the spectrum of mutations is heterogeneous, and we have found 19 different mutations with the four most common mutations as IVS-I-5 (G-->C) (37.7%), codons 8/9 (+G) (21.1%), the 619 bp deletion (12.4%), and IVS-I-1 (G-->T) (9.5%), account for 80.7% of the alleles [23]. Concerning alpha thalassemia, Choubisa *et al.* performed an investigation on a total of 1,647 cord blood samples of newborns in India [24]. According to this study, the incidence of alpha-thalassaemia genes varied from 3.07% in the scheduled tribes, 1.43% in the scheduled castes to 0.77% in the general castes populations giving an overall incidence of 1.88% [24]. In this study, except for 31 (1.88 %) Hb Bart cases, no other cases with mutant hemoglobins were observed. Of those Hb Bart cases, 24 (1.46%) were of alpha-thalassaemia 1 and 7 (0.42%) of alpha-thalassaemia 2 [24].

West Asia

There are some epidemiologic studies of thalassemia in West Asia, especially Saudi Arabia. Al-Awamy said that thalassemia syndromes could be seen in Saudi Arabia: the Beta-Thalassemia genes occured with variable frequency in different regions of Saudi Arabia and both B+ and Bo thalassemia had been reported [25]. el-Hazmi *et al.* said that most commonly encountered mutations in Saudi beta-thalassaemia patients were IVS-I-110, IVS-II-1, CD 39, IVS-I-5 and IVS-I 3' end (-25), while frameshifts at CD 8/9, Cap+1 (A-->C) and CD 6 mutations were identified at a low frequency [26].

Africa

Thalassemia can be seen in Africa. Zorai *et al.* studied the characterization of the molecular spectrum and frequency data of alpha thalassemia defects in Tunisia [27]. They found that the -alpha3.7 deletion was the most common defect (4.5% allele frequency) followed by a polyadenylation (poly A) signal mutation (1.8%), the five nucleotide (nt) deletion and the -alpha4.2 deletion (both 0.9%) [27]. According to this study, the African polymorphism (G-->TCGGCCC at position 7238 and T-->G at 7174) was found with an allele frequency of 11% in the selected group samples, in cases from northeastern Tunisia [27]., Hussein *et al.* studied beta thalassemia in Egypt and found that causative mutation was found in 69 of 71 (97%) beta-thalassemia genes [28]. In this study, 4 mutations accounted for 78% of beta-thalassemia genes in this population; IVS-I-110 (41%), IVS-1 nt 6 (13%), IVS-I-1 (13%), and IVS-II-848 (11%) [28], similar to those reported from Saudi Arabia [26].

Pathophysiology of Thalassemia

Normally, adult hemoglobin (HbA-alpha 2 beta 2), alpha and beta globin are synthesized by genes on different chromosomes, whereas heme is synthesized primarily on mitochondria [29 – 30]. The synthesis of these chains is very tightly coordinated so that the ratio of alpha globin to beta globin, including the beta-like globins delta and gamma, is normally 1 ± 0.05 and specific erythroid proteases are designed to attack and destroy excess alpha or beta globin chains, demonstrating the deleterious impact of the accumulation of excess unmatched globin chains [29 – 30].

Concerning the pathogenesis of thalassemia, the inherited decrease of globin, an important composition of hemoglobin, causes abnormal, fragile red blood cells. In beta thalassemia, production of beta globin decreases and excess alpha globin accumulates and in alpha thalassemia, on the other hand, this process occurs in reverse [29]. Ones with thalassemia will have chronic anemia and other long - term complications [1 – 3]. Schrier said that the thalassemias were extremely heterogeneous in terms of their clinical severity, and their underlying pathophysiology relates directly to the extent of accumulation of excess unmatched globin chains: alpha in beta thalassemia and beta in the alpha thalassemias [29]. Despite discoveries concerning the molecular abnormalities that led to the thalassemic syndromes, it still is not known how accumulation of excess unmatched alpha-globin in beta thalassemia and beta-globin in alpha thalassemia leads to red blood cell hemolysis in the peripheral blood, and in the beta thalassemias particularly, premature destruction of erythroid precursors in marrow or ineffective erythropoiesis [30].

Concerning the effect of thalassemia on red blood cell, Schrier said that the accumulation of each separate globin chain affected red cell membrane material properties and the state of red cell hydration is very different [30]. Schrier said that oxidant injury might cause hemolysis, but there was no evidence that it caused ineffective erythropoiesis [30]. Chakraborty and Bhattacharyya found low activities of reduced glutathione indicating the cell to be in a pro-oxidant state, and decreased activity of catalase favors hydrogen peroxide-mediated lipid peroxidation in beta-thalassemia [31] confirming those mentioned by Schrier [30]. Indeed, ineffective erythropoiesis is proved for thalassemia and believed to be due to the imbalance of production and destruction of red blood cells rather than oxidative stress. Schrier noted that ineffective erythropoiesis now appears to be caused by accelerated apoptosis, in turn caused primarily by deposition of alpha globin chains in erythroid precursors, however, it is not clear how alpha globin deposition causes apoptosis [30]. Clegg and Weatherall said that the thalassemia was believed to provide protection against malaria, as a natural selection process to sickle cell, and it is thought that, in malarial regions of the world, natural selection had been responsible for elevating and maintaining their gene frequencies, an idea first proposed 50 years ago by J.B.S. Haldane [32]. They mentioned that population and molecular genetic analysis of thalassemia variants, and microepidemiological studies of the relationship between alpha-thalassemia and malaria in the southwest Pacific, had provided unequivocal evidence for protection [32]. In addition, some of this protection appeared to derive from enhanced susceptibility in very young thalassemic children to both *Plasmodium falciparum* and, especially, *P. vivax*, and this early exposure appeared to provide the basis for better protection in later life [32].

Concerning anemia in thalassemia, the microcytic type is mentioned for the non-silent carrier cases. The pathogenesis of anemia in thalassemia is complicated: many underlying causes are mentioned. The defect in red blood cell production due to the ineffective erythropoiesis can be seen and the increase of red blood cell destruction due to the hemolytic anemia and the trapping of the abnormal red blood cell by reticuloendothelial system are seen in a case with thalassemia. Concerning the ineffective erythropoiesis, marrow hyperplasia can be seen and markedly expanded marrow space leads to various skeletal manifestations including spine, skull, facial bones, and ribs [33]. In thalassemia, surplus polypeptide chain synthesized by normal globin gene causes harmful effects to skeleton proteins of the erythrocyte membrane, such as spectrin, ankirin and 4.1 protein, via a few different ways and the normal integrity of the membrane is disturbed [34].

Clinical Manifestation of Thalassemia

Clinical characteristics of the thalassemias are ineffective erythropoiesis and hemolytic anemia with microcytic-hypochromic erythrocytes [34]. However, thalassemia is very heterogeneous in the manifestation (Table 8.2). In all thalassemias, clinical features that result from anemia, transfusional, and absorptive iron overload are similar but vary in severity [33]. Briefly, the manifestation of thalassemia can be a hematological system and a non-hematological system manifestation. As already described, the main manifestation in the hematological system is anemia. The important manifestations in a non-hematological system include bone destruction, resulting in a classical sign known as thalassemic face, splenomegaly and growth retardation. Extramedullary hematopoiesis (ExmH), hemosiderosis, and cholelithiasis are among the non-skeletal manifestations of thalassemia [33]. There are also several manifestations due to the complication of thalassemia itself and treatment. Those manifestations included hemochromatosis syndrome and symptoms of several superimposed infections.

The association between the genotype and clinical manifestation of alpha thalassemia is not as complex as beta thalassemia. In spite of seemingly identical genotypes, severity of beta thalassemic patients can vary greatly [35]. Heterogeneity in the clinical manifestation of beta thalassemic diseases may occur from the nature of beta globin gene mutation, alpha thalassemia gene interaction and difference in the amount of Hb F production, which is partly associated with a specific beta globin haplotype [35]. The other co-inherited hemoglobinopathies also affects the manifestation of thalassemia. The combination between hemoglobin E and beta + thalassemia can lead to more severe manifestation.

Diagnosis of Thalassemia

A. Screening Test

Basically, in endemic areas, all cases with hypochromic microcytic anemia should be suspected for thalassemia disorder. The basic laboratory screenings for thalassemia are blood smear interpretation, red blood cell index determination by automated hematology analyzers, mathematical models, osmotic fragility test (OF). Of these methods, the mathematical models [36] and OF [37] are the reliable and recommended tests. However, in the resource-limited settings, the blood smear interpretation is still useful [38]. In Thailand, an endemic country for thalassemic disorder, the hemoglobin electrophoresis and molecular diagnosis is proved not cost – effective [39]. The author recommends a mass screening by simple screening test, especially the combination between OF and DCIP, and further additional definitive diagnosis by electrophoresis or molecular diagnosis in positive cases from screening.

Blood Smear Interpretation
Blood smear interpretation can detect microcytic anemia in most types of thalassemia, expect for the silent alpha thalassemia carrier. The determination of microcytic anemia from routine blood smear examination can lead to the further diagnosis of thalassemia. However, blood smear interpretation gives poor diagnostic property in screening for thalassemia [39].

Table 8.2. Clinical classification of thalassemia

Manifestations	Brief details
Alpha thalassemia	
o Silent carrier state	o The corresponding genotype classification is one-gene deletion alpha thalassemia (alpha 1/ alpha). The cases with this type manifest no symptom and sign, however, can be detected by special investigation such as polymerase chain reaction (PCR) test.
o Mild alpha-thalassemia	o The corresponding genotype classification is two-gene deletion alpha thalassemia (alpha 1/alpha 1 or trans deletion; alpha 0/ alpha or cis deletion). The cases with this type manifest no symptom but abnormal red blood cells can be seen in routine blood smear examination. The blood films of these cases are similar to those of iron deficiency anemia and frequently misdiagnosed resulting in maltreatment. Therefore, in cases suspected for iron deficiency anemia with poor response to iron supplementation, thalassemia should be investigated.
o Hemoglobin H disease	o The corresponding genotype classification is three-gene deletion alpha thalassemia (alpha 0/alpha 1). The cases with this type usually manifest anemic symptoms. The non-hematologic manifestation including bone deformity, striking cheeks and forehead, and huge spleen, up to ten times normal, are common. The blood films reveal many microcye and red cell fragments. Inclusion bodies, Heinz bodies, can be seen by special stain.
o Hb Bart hydrop fetalis	o The corresponding genotype classification is four-gene deletion alpha thalassemia (alpha 0/alpha 0). The cases with this type usually die in utero.
Beta thalassemia	
o Thalassemia minor, or thalassemia trait	o The cases with this type manifest no symptoms but abnormal red blood cells can be seen in routine blood smear examination. The blood films of these cases are similar to those of iron deficiency anemia and frequently misdiagnosed resulting in maltreatment. The primary caution for those with beta-thalassemia trait involves the possible problems that their children could inherit if their spouses also have beta thalassemia trait.
o Thalassemia intermedia	o The cases with thalassemia intermedia have significant anemia, but are able to survive without blood transfusions. It should be noted that this diagnosis is based mainly on clinical symptoms not genotype.
o Thalassemia major	o The cases with thalassemia major have significant anemia and are transfusion dependent: death will occur without transfusions.

Osmotic Fragility Test

Osmotic fragility test is a simple test to determine the fragility of the red blood cell [40]. Basically, the red blood cell osmotic fragility test is based on the measure of the resistance of red blood cells to lysis as a function of decreasing sodium chloride concentration [40 - 41]. Pribush *et al.* said that the erythrocyte swelling is controlled by the initial cell shape, volume, intracellular hemoglobin concentration, and elastic membrane properties, whereas the kinetics of the pore formation depend solely on the resistivity of the stretched membrane of the swollen red blood cell to the osmotic shock [42]. They performed a study and found that the probability of the pore formation in the stretched membrances varied in the following order: thalassemia < control < spherocytosis [42]. Recently, Fernandez-Alberti *et al.* also proposed the osmotic fragility confidence intervals [41]. According to their study, the absorbance of the hemoglobin measured at 540 nm, released by the red blood cells of 40 healthy adult individuals, was fitted to the equation Absorbance=p3 erfc ([NaCl] - p1/p2); p3 measures one half the absorbance produced by maximum red blood cell hemolysis, p1 is the [NaCl] producing 50% red blood cell hemolysis, and p2 is the dispersion in [NaCl] producing red blood cell hemolysis [41].

There are some previous studies concerning the diagnostic property of OF test for screening thalassemia. Recently Wiwanitkit performed a metanalysis on the diagnostic property of OF test for screening thalassemia in Thai pregnants. According to this study, a total of 595 pregnant subjects were screened by OF test and 258 were found to be thalassaemic, giving a prevalence 43.36% [43]. The overall sensitivity, specificity, false positive rate and false negative rate are 91.47%, 81.60%, 18.40% and 8.53%, respectively [43]. Concerning the overall risk for OF positive cases (236/258) to OF negative cases (62/337) to have thalassaemia, the rate 4.97 can be derived [43].

Red Blood Cell Index

Due to the advance in automated hematology analyzer technology, the red blood cell index determination becomes more available. However, similar to blood smear interpretation, only the detection of microcytic and hypochromic usually gives poor diagnostic property in screening for thalassemia. Therefore, the more complicated screening method, mathematical model, is developed.

Mathematical Model

Based on the modern electronic cell counter, quick differential screening of iron deficiency anemia from beta-thalassemia by blood count parameters has been purposed [44 - 46]. Generally, DFs are obtained from a mathematic formula of the parameters, which was first described by Fisher in 1936 [47]. A number of DFs have been proposed since the publication of the first report such as $0.01 \times MCH \times (MCV)^2$ [48], RDW X MCH x $(MCV)^2$/ Hb x 100 [49], MCV/RBC [50] and MCH/RBC [51]. However, these DFs were mostly applied to the differentiation of iron deficiency anemia from beta thalassemia. The screening of the general population by some DFs have been tested and found acceptable results [44, 52]. According to a study of Wiwanitkit *et al.* in using England and Frazer's calculation method in screening for hemoglobin disorder in Thai pregnant subjects, good diagnostic property was received [53]. The mathematical model is mentioned as a cost-effective method in screening for thalassemia [54].

B. Definitive Test

Hemoglobin Electrophoresis

Hemoglobin electrophoresis is a widely used medical electrophoresis. This test can determine the different types of hemoglobin in the blood by an electrical separating process that causes movement of particles in an electric field, resulting in formation of hemoglobin bands that separate toward one end or the other in the field. Quantitative determination of each hemoglobin band by densitometry is then performed (Figure 8.1).

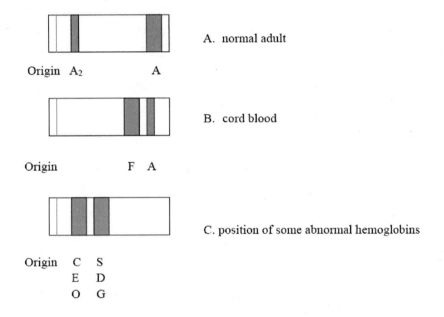

Figure 8.1. Diagram showing the hemoglobin electrophoresis pattern (by alkaline cellulose acetate)

In adults, these hemoglobin molecules make up the total hemoglobin, as follows Hb A_1: 95% to 98%, Hb A_2: 2% to 3% and Hb F: 0.8% to 2% while in children under 6 months, there are more Hb F, in newborn up to 80 %. Abnormal values can vary by lead to diagnosis of thalassemia such as Hgb A_2 up to 4-5.8% in thalassemia minor and under 2% in Hb H disease or Hb F up to 2-5% in thalassemia minor and up to 10-90% in thalassemia major. The hemoglobin electrophoresis is still used as a reference for diagnosis of thalassemia in developing tropical countries. Hemoglobin electrophoresis can not only detect thalassemia but also other hemoglobinopathies such as hemoglobin C, hemoglobin S and hemoglobin J. However, the hemoglobin electrophoresis is still limited for diagnosis of the alpha thalassemia trait.

Hemoglobin Chromatography

Alkaline cellulose acetate and acidic citrate agar electrophoreses are the most widely utilized methods for hemoglobin analysis. However, due to their limited resolution, incorrect or unresolved diagnosis of common hemoglobinopathies are sometimes encountered [55]. Since in hemoglobin electrophoresis, Hb A_2 does not separate as well with densitometric quantitation as it does with the chromatographic method since hemoglobin A_2 is difficult to distinguish from hemoglobin C, as they migrate together. Testing by high performance liquid chromatography (HPLC) allows the actual quantification of A_2 in the presence of Hb C or Hb E. Ou and Rognerud said that the method is capable of separating more than 45 commonly encountered hemoglobin variants including Barts, H, A1C, Raleigh, Hope, I, F, Camden, N-Baltimore, I-High Wycombe, I-Paris, J-Baltimore, N-Seattle, Grade, Fannin-Lubbock, Malmo, South Florida, A, Chicago, G-Georgia, Lepore-Baltimore, P-Galveston, G-Coushatta, Lepore-Boston, E, Zurich, Osu Christiansborg, A2, G-Philadelphia, Korle Bu, Russ, E-Saskatoon, Richmond, D-Punjab, Deer Lodge, Koln, Montgomery, S, Q-Thailand, G-San Jose, A2', Hasharon, Q-India, Tampa, Constant Spring, SG-hybrid, C-Harlem, O-Arab, British Columbia, and C within 12 minutes. They said that this method provides not only the identification of the aforementioned hemoglobin and variants but also an accurate quantitation of their concentrations, particularly Hb F and A2, which are useful for the diagnosis of beta thalassemia [55].

Molecular diagnosis

Molecular diagnosis is the gold standard in diagnosis of thalassemia. The molecular diagnosis can not only determine the type of thalassemia but also the mutations [56]. The recent epidemiologic studies on thalassemia focus on the genetic epidemiology performed by the molecular diagnosis. Tan *et al.* said that non-molecular techniques allow samples to be screened rapidly but these techniques are unable to detect mutations at the gene level while molecular analysis of alpha- and beta-globin genes either by Southern Blotting and radionuclides or DNA amplification using the PCR allows detection of specific mutations and have enabled prenatal diagnosis of the thalassaemias [57].

Management for Anemia in Thalassemia

Anemia is an important manifestation in thalassemia, especially in cases with hemoglobin H disease and thalassemia major. Similar to other anemic diseases, the main principle in management for anemia in thalassemia included an increase in red blood cell production, decrease in red blood cell destruction and red blood cell supplementation. Concerning the increase in red blood cell production, the erythropoietin has been used in a trial on the thalassemic patients. Most trials are focused on the transfusion dependant beta thalassemia. Recently, Chaidos et al. said that recombinant human erythropoietin (rHuEPO or epoetin-alpha) treatment had a beneficial effect in transfusion-dependent beta-thalassemia patients [58]. Makis et al. also reported a similar finding and mentioned that rHuEpo was well tolerated without complications and this treatment could improve the quality of life in beta-thalassemia major [59]. Concerning the thalassemia intermedia, the previous studies mentioned for the benefit of erythropoietin treatment in the patients as well [60 – 61]. Recently, Voulgari et al. reported for the presence of EPO antibodies in the thalassemic patients, which can make the PO treatment in the thalassemic patients more complicated [62].

Concerning the decrease in red blood cell destruction, the main management in the patients with severe anemia due to thalassemia, Cooley's anemia, is splenectomy. Splenectomy is performed in order to decrease the red blood cell trapping, leading to hemolysis, by the reticuloendothelial cells in the spleen [63]. In 2002, Al-Salem and Nasserulla studied the splenectomy in the thalassemic patients and concluded that total splenectomy was beneficial for children with thalassemia and hypersplenism because it reduced their transfusion requirements while partial splenectomy may be beneficial for those with Hb H disease [64]. They noted, however, for those with beta-thalassemia, partial splenectomy was beneficial in reducing their transfusion requirements only as a temporary measure, and it is recommended for children who were less than 5 years of age [64]. The post – splenectomy care is an important management in the splenectomized thalassemic patients. Several superimposed infections in these patients are expected due to the deficit of immune status [65]. Williams and Kaur recommended three types of preventive measures: immunoprophylaxis (vaccines); chemoprophylaxis (antibiotics); and education, ranging from providing a medical alert bracelet to teaching about symptoms of febrile illness to advising immediate treatment [65].

Concerning the red blood cell supplementation, blood transfusion is a classical management for thalassemia with long history. Repeated polytransfusion requirement is the hallmark of the thalassemia major. Prati said that early and regular blood transfusion therapy in patients with homozygous beta-thalassaemia decreases the complications of severe anaemia and prolongs survival [66]. Prati noted that transfusion regimens for beta-thalassaemia have changed substantially during the past four decades, however, Prati recommended that pre-transfusion haemoglobin concentration should not exceed 95 g/l to allow adequate control of anemia, with a relatively low rate of iron accumulation [66]. Due to the huge amount of transfusion, several transfusion complications can be expected. First, the blood – borne infections among the transfusion-dependant thalassemic patients are high, especially in the setting where screening in the blood bank process is poor. In previous days, human immunodeficiency virus (HIV), hepatitis B and hepatitis C infection are common in the thalassemic patients with a history of prolonged blood transfusion therapy. However, in the present day, HIV and hepatitis B screenings are included in the general blood bank process, therefore, hepatitis C becomes the most common transfusion – related infectious problem. For example, according to a recent study of Al-Sheyyab et al. in Jordan in 2001, hepatitis C is the most common post transfusion infectious problem [67].

Second, the non-infectious complication especially the iron overload is mentioned and can be the cause of death in those transfusion thalassemic patients. Prati said that the beneficial effects of transfusions were limited by the organ damage resulting from iron overload, a consequence of the body's limited capacity to excrete iron, and by the complications of infection with blood-borne agents [66]. In order to control and prevent the hemachormatosis due to iron overload, the iron chelation therapy in the thassemic patients as well as the monitoring for the erythropoietic in the transfusion-dependant thalassemic patients are needed. Concerning iron chelation therapy, in 1963, the introduction of desferrioxamine (DFO), a hexadentate chelator, marked a breakthrough in the treatment of beta-thalassemia. DFO significantly reduces body iron burden and iron-related morbidity and mortality [68 – 69]. For a long time, deferoxamine has been the only effective iron-chelating agent and should be given in a daily dose of 40 mg/kg at initiation of the transfusion programa, and administration has been recommended by subcutaneous infusions from 8 to 10 hours per day [68]. The goal of iron-chelating treatment is to maintain serum ferritin levels between 500 and 1,000 ng/ml [68]. However, this long-term treatment is a significant burden for patients, therefore, consideration should be given to alternative treatments such as as oral non-toxic iron-chelating agents as they become available [68, 70]. The tridentate triazoles have been investigated for clinical potential; they are readily absorbed from the gastrointestinal tract and promote iron excretion with high efficacy [70]. In similar fashion, several bidentate hydroxypyridinones have been demonstrated to possess potential as oral chelating agents [70]. Concerning monitoring of erythropoiesis in transfusion treatment, many laboratory investigations are available. Those laboratory investigations include reticulocyte count, erythropoietin, ferritin and transferrin receptor. Among these parameters, reticulocyte is the most simple test and seems cost-effective in the setting with limited resources.

The new advance in management of thalassemia is stem cell transplantion. In 2003, Lawson et al. suggested that allogeneic bone marrow transplantation (BMT) became an important treatment option for children with beta thalassaemia major, particularly when compliance with iron chelation was poor [71]. They studied 57 thalassemic patients who had undergone BMT and found that despite the majority of patients being in class 2 or 3 due to Pesaro risk classification, transplant-related mortality was low (5.4%) [71]. According to their study, the principal complication was graft rejection accompanied by autologous reconstitution that occurred in 13.2% of transplants [71]. Issaragrisil said that bone marrow transplantation offered a high probability of cure when performed in young children but there was a higher risk as the patient becomes older, especially the high incidence of graft rejection [72]. Issaragrisil said that the alternative use of stem cells from cord blood made possible earlier transplants with a better chance of cure, although the engraftment was slower compared to bone marrow transplantation [72]. Until present, BMT is the only method that can cure the thalassemia [72]. However, this method is very expensive and intensive post-tranplantation care is needed.

References

[1]   Lo L, Singer ST. Thalassemia: current approach to an old disease. *Pediatr Clin North Am* 2002;49:1165-91.
[2]   Old JM. Screening and genetic diagnosis of haemoglobin disorders. *Blood Rev* 2003;17:43-53.
[3]   Fucharoen S, Wanichagoon G. Thalassemia and abnormal hemoglobin. *Int J Hematol* 2002;76 Suppl 2:83-9.
[4]   Gabutti V. Current therapy for thalassemia in Italy. *Ann N Y Acad Sci* 1990; 612:268-74.

[5]   Glader BE, Look KA. Hematologic disorders in children from southeast Asia. *Pediatr Clin North Am* 1996;43:665-81.

[6]   Giardina P, Hilgartner M. Update on thalassemia. *Pediatr Rev* 1992;13:55-62.

[7]   Rund D, Rachmilewitz E. Thalassemia major 1995: older patients, new therapies. *Blood Rev* 1995; 9:25-32.

[8]   Leder A, Wiener E, Lee MJ, Wickramasinghe SN, Leder P. A normal beta-globin allele as a modifier gene ameliorating the severity of alpha-thalassemia in mice. *Proc Natl Acad Sci U S A* 1999;96:6291-5.

[9]   Igbokwe EC. Molecular genetics of alpha thalassemia. *Med Hypotheses* 1989;30:75-9.

[10] Thein SL. Beta-thalassaemia. *Baillieres Clin Haematol* 1998;11:91-126.

[11] Ho PJ, Thein SL. Gene regulation and deregulation: a beta globin perspective. *Blood Rev* 2000;14:78-93.

[12] Suwankiri P, Saengkijjaporn S, Samaharn S, Rattanawilaisakul P. Detection for thalassemia and hemoglobinopathy carriers. *Chula Med Tech Bull* 1992; 5: 981-91.

[13] Paritpokee N, Suwansaksri J, Wiwanitkit V, Siritantikorn A. Screening tests forinherited hemoglobin disorders in pregnancies. *Chula Med J* 1999;43: 645-653.

[14] Fucharoen G, Fucharoen S, Wanhakit C, Srithong W. Molecular basis of alpha (0)-thalassemia in northeast of Thailand. *Southeast Asian J Trop Med Public Health* 1995;26 Suppl 1:249-51.

[15] Wiwanitkit V. Overview of molecular deletion patterns of alpha0-thalassemia in Thailand. *Lab Hematol* 2004;10:122-3.

[16] Winichagoon P, Fucharoen S, Wasi P. The molecular basis of alpha-thalassemia in Thailand. *Southeast Asian J Trop Med Public Health*. 1992;23 Suppl 2:7-13.

[17] Laig M, Sanguansermsri T, Wiangnon S, Hundrieser J, Pape M, Flatz G. The spectrum of beta-thalassemia mutations in northern and northeastern Thailand. *Hum Genet* 1989;84:47-50.

[18] Nopparatana C, Panich V, Saechan V, Sriroongrueng V, Nopparatana C, Rungjeadpha J, Pornpatkul M, Laosombat V, Fukumaki Y. The spectrum of beta-thalassemia mutations in southern Thailand. *Southeast Asian J Trop Med Public Health* 1995;26 Suppl 1:229-34.

[19] Dode C, Labie D, Rochette J. Types of alpha+ thalassemia in Southeast Asia refugees. *Ann Genet* 1988;31:201-4.

[20] Hurst D, Tittle B, Kleman KM, Embury SH, Lubin BH. Anemia and hemoglobinopathies in Southeast Asian refugee children. *J Pediatr* 1983;102:692-7.

[21] Svasti ML, Hieu TM, Munkongdee T, Winichagoon P, Van Be T, Van Binh T, Fucharoen S. Molecular analysis of beta-thalassemia in South Vietnam. *Am J Hematol* 2002;71:85-8.

[22] Nadkarni A, Gorakshakar AC, Lu CY, Krishnamoorthy R, Ghosh K, Colah R, Mohanty D. Molecular pathogenesis and clinical variability of beta-thalassemia syndromes among Indians. *Am J Hematol* 2001;68:75-80.

[23] Choubisa SL, Choubisa DK, Khare S. Alpha-thalassaemia (Hb-Bart's) in Rajasthan (India). *Haematologia* (Budap) 2000;30:209-13.

[24] Khan SN, Riazuddin S. Molecular characterization of beta-thalassemia in Pakistan. *Hemoglobin* 1998;22:333-45.

[25] Al-Awamy BH. Thalassemia syndromes in Saudi Arabia. Meta-analysis of local studies. *Saudi Med J* 2000;21:8-17.

[26] el-Hazmi MA, al-Swailem AR, Warsy AS. Molecular defects in beta-thalassaemias in the population of Saudi Arabia. *Hum Hered* 1995;45:278-85.

[27] Zorai A, Harteveld CL, Bakir A, Van Delft P, Falfoul A, Dellagi K, Abbes S, Giordano PC. Molecular spectrum of alpha-thalassemia in Tunisia: epidemiology and detection at birth. *Hemoglobin* 2002;26:353-62.

[28] Hussein IR, Temtamy SA, el-Beshlawy A, Fearon C, Shalaby Z, Vassilopoulos G, Kazazian HH Jr. Molecular characterization of beta-thalassemia in Egyptians. *Hum Mutat* 1993;2:48-52.

[29] Schrier SL. Thalassemia: pathophysiology of red cell changes. Annu Rev Med 1994;45:211-8

[30] Schrier SL. Pathophysiology of thalassemia. *Curr Opin Hematol* 2002;9:123-6.

[31] Chakraborty D, Bhattacharyya M. Antioxidant defense status of red blood cells of patients with beta-thalassemia and Ebeta-thalassemia. *Clin Chim Acta* 2001;305:123-9.

[32] Clegg JB, Weatherall DJ. Thalassemia and malaria: new insights into an old problem. *Proc Assoc Am Physicians* 1999;111:278-82.

[33] Tunaci M, Tunaci A, Engin G, Ozkorkmaz B, Dincol G, Acunas G, Acunas B. Imaging features of thalassemia. *Eur Radiol* 1999;9:1804-9.

[34] Fujita S. Congenital hemolytic anemia--hemoglobin abnormality—thalassemia. *Nippon Rinsho* 1996;54:2454-9.

[35] Fucharoen S, Winichagoon P. Thalassemia and abnormal hemoglobin. *Int J Hematol* 2002;76 Suppl 2:83-9.

[36] Suwansaksri J, Wiwanitkit V, Paritpokee N. Screening for hemoglobin disorders in Thai pregnant women by England and Frazer's calculation method. *Arch Gynecol Obstet 2003 Sep 9* [Epub ahead of print].

[37] Wiwanitkit V, Suwansaksri J, Paritpokee N. Combined one-tube osmotic fragility (OF) test and dichlorophenol-indolphenol (DCIP) test screening for hemoglobin disorders, an experience in 213 Thai pregnant women. *Clin Lab* 2002; 48: 525-528.

[38] Wiwanitkit V. Blood smear interpretation for screening of hemoglobin disorder in Thai pregnant women, is it effective? *Reg 4 Med J* 2000; 19: 91 – 4.

[39] Paritpokee N, SuwansaksriJ, SiritantikornA, Wiwanitkit V. Cost –effective analysis of screening tests for inherited hemoglobin disorders in pregnancies. *Chula Med* J 1999; 43: 883-891.

[40] Fujii H. Osmotic fragility test. *Nippon Rinsho* 1997;55 Suppl 1:153-5.

[41] Fernandez-Alberti A, Fink NE. Red blood cell osmotic fragility confidence intervals: a definition by application of a mathematical model. *Clin Chem Lab Med* 2000;38:433-6.

[42] Pribush A, Hatskelzon L, Kapelushnik J, Meyerstein N. Osmotic swelling and hole formation in membranes of thalassemic and spherocytic erythrocytes. *Blood Cells Mol Dis* 2003;31:43-7.

[43] Wiwanitkit V. Osmotic fragility test for screening for thalassaemia in Thai pregnant subjects: a re-evaluation. *Haema* 2004; 7:205-207.

[44] Ittarat W, Ongcharoenjai S, Rayatong O, Pirat N. Correlation between some discrimination functions and hemoglobin E. *J Med Assoc Thai* 2000 83:259-265.

[45] Cohnson CS, Tegos C, Beutler E. Thalassemia minor: routine erythrocyte measurements and differentiation from iron deficiency. *Am J Clin Pathol* 1983; 80:31-6.

[46] Jimenez CV. Iron-deficiency anemia and thalassemia trait differentiated by simple hematological tests and serum iron concentrations. *Clin Chem* 1993; 39:2271- 2275.

[47] Fisher H, Bowman J. Hemoglobin E, an oxidatively unstable mutation. *J Lab Clin Med* 1975; 85: 531 – 539.

[48] Shine I, Lai S. A strategy to detect α-thalassemia minor. *Lancet* 1977; 1: 692 – 694.

[49] Green R, King R. A new red cell discriminant incorporating volume dispersion for differentiating iron deficiency anemia from thalassemia minor. *Blood Cells* 1989; 15:481-491.

[50] Mentzer W. Differentiation of iron deficiency from thalassemia. *Lancet* 1973; 1: 449 – 452.

[51] Srivastava PC. Differentiation of thalassemia minor from iron deficiency. *Lancet* 1973; 2: 154 – 155.

[52] Kaewborworn U, Bunyaratvej A, Ravivongse R, Thuvasethakul P, Hathirat P.Application of a discriminant function distinguishing iron deficiency anemia and heterozygous beta-thalassemia from other genetic abnormalities. *Birth Defects Orig Artic Ser* 1987 23:177-180.

[53] Wiwanitkit V, Paritpokee N, Suwansaksri J. Screening for hemoglobin disorder in pregnant subjects by England and Frazer calculation method. Presented at the National Meeting on *Biomedical Engineer* 2001. Bangkok: Thailand 2001.

[54] Suwansaksri J, Wiwanitkit V, Paritpokee N. Screening for hemoglobin disorders in Thai pregnant women by England and Frazer's calculation method. *Arch Gynecol Obstet* 2003 Sep 9.

[55] Ou CN, Rognerud CL. Diagnosis of hemoglobinopathies: electrophoresis vs. HPLC. 1: *Clin Chim Acta* 2001;313:187-94.

[56] Gu X, Zeng Y. A review of the molecular diagnosis of thalassemia. *Hematology* 2002;7:203-9.

[57] Tan J, Tay JS, Wong HB. Detection and molecular analysis of alpha and beta thalassaemia genes--recent developments in screening protocols. *J Singapore Paediatr Soc* 1992;34:53-6.

[58] Chaidos A, Makis A, Hatzimichael E, Tsiara S, Gouva M, Tzouvara E, Bourantas KL. Treatment of beta-thalassemia patients with recombinant human erythropoietin: effect on transfusion requirements and soluble adhesion molecules. *Acta Haematol* 2004;111:189-95.

[59] Makis AC, Chaliasos N, Hatzimichael EC, Bourantas KL. Recombinant human erythropoietin therapy in a transfusion-dependent beta-thalassemia major patient. *Ann Hematol* 2001;80:492-5.

[60] Bourantas K, Economou G, Georgiou J. Administration of high doses of recombinant human erythropoietin to patients with beta-thalassemia intermedia: a preliminary trial. *Eur J Haematol* 1997 ;58:22-5.

[61] Nisli G, Kavakli K, Vergin C, Oztop S, Cetingul N. Recombinant human erythropoietin trial in thalassemia intermedia. *J Trop Pediatr* 1996;42:330-4.

[62]   Voulgari PV, Chaidos A, Tzouvara E, Alymara V, Alamanos Y, Drosos AA, Bourantas KL. Antierythropoietin antibodies in thalassemia patients. *Ann Hematol* 2004;83:22-7.

[63]   Piomelli S. The management of patients with Cooley's anemia: transfusions and splenectomy. *Semin Hematol* 1995;32:262-8.

[64]   Al-Salem AH, Nasserulla Z. Splenectomy for children with thalassemia. *Int Surg* 2002;87:269-73.

[65]   Williams DN, Kaur B. Postsplenectomy care. Strategies to decrease the risk of infection. *Postgrad Med* 1996;100:195-8.

[66]   Prati D. Benefits and complications of regular blood transfusion in patients with beta-thalassaemia major. *Vox Sang* 2000;79:129-37.

[67]   Al-Sheyyab M, Batieha A, El-Khateeb M. The prevalence of hepatitis B, hepatitis C and human immune deficiency virus markers in multi-transfused patients. *J Trop Pediatr* 2001;47:239-42.

[68]   de Montalembert M, Guillemot F, Clairicia M, Girot R. Iron chelation in children. *Ann Pediatr* (Paris) 1989;36:533-8.

[69]   Nick H, Acklin P, Lattmann R, Buehlmayer P, Hauffe S, Schupp J, Alberti D. Development of tridentate iron chelators: from desferrithiocin to ICL670. *Curr Med Chem* 2003;10:1065-76.

[70]   Liu DY, Liu ZD, Hider RC. Oral iron chelators--development and application. *Best Pract Res Clin Haematol* 2002;15:369-84.

[71]   Lawson SE, Roberts IA, Amrolia P, Dokal I, Szydlo R, Darbyshire PJ. Bone marrow transplantation for beta-thalassaemia major: the UK experience in two paediatric centres. *Br J Haematol* 2003;120:289-95.

[72]   Issaragrisil S. Stem cell transplantation for thalassemia. *Int J Hematol* 2002;76 Suppl 1:307-9.

Chapter 9

Tropical Hemoglobinopathy

Introduction to Hemoglobinopathy

Apart from thalassemia, the other inherited hemoglobin disorder is hemoglobinopathy. Hemoglobinopathy is a group of inherited hemoglobin disorders where the structure of hemoglobin is abnormal, or where hemoglobin was improperly formed but not due to the depletion of the globin gene. Similar to thalassemia, hemoglobinopathy can lead to anemia and becomes an important anemic health problem in the tropics [1 – 2]. Up to now, there have been more than one hundred hemoglobinopathies documented in the literature. One hemoglobinopathy has its own underlying genetic defect, therefore, has its specific property and manifestation. Here, the details of some hemoglobinopathies relating to anemia in some endemic tropical areas are described.

Table 9.1. Some hemoglobinopathies detected by hemoglobin electrophoresis

Position in electrophoresis (from – to +)	Examples of hemoglobinopathies
Before Hb C	o Hb Constant spring, Hb F Kuala Lumper, Hb F Texas I
Overlap with Hb C	o Hb E Saskatoon, Hb E, Hb C Harten, Hb C Ziquinchor
Between Hb C and Hb S	o Hb O Indonesia, Hb Agenogi, Hb Sabine, Hb Istanbul, Hb Koln, Hb Notthingham, Hb Kenya, Hb Gun Hill, Hb A_2 Babinga, Hb Setif
Overlap with Hb S	o Hb Memphis, Hb Arya, Hb G Norfolk, Hb D Iran, Hb Willamette, Hb Lepore- Baltimore, Hb Carribien
Between Hb S and Hb F	o Hb Sawara, Hb G Szuhu, Hb Kemsey, Hb Tak, Hb Mahidol
Overlap with Hb F	o Hb Tarrant, Hb Deer Lodge, Hb Newcastle
Between Hb F and Hb A	o Hb M Iwate, Hb Waco, Hb Richmond, Hb Rush
Overlap with Hb A	o Hb M Saslatoon, Hb York, Hb Bethesda, Hb Rainier, Hb Creteil
Between Hb A and Hb J	o Hb Jackson, Hb Moscva, Hb Lufkin, Hb Austin, Hb J Bangkok, Hb Pyrgos
Overlap with Hb J	o Hb Hofu, Hb J Toronto, Hb J Cairo
Between HB J and Hb I	o Hb Hikari, Hb N Baltimore, Hb Hajiyama, Hb Anatharaj

Important Hemoglobinopathies in Southeast Asia

Hemoglobinopathies are prevalent in Southeast Asia. A well-known hemoglobinopathy, hemoglobin E is a peak endemic in this area, in northeastern Thailand and Laos [2 - 3]. Due to the recent study of Dode et al., high prevalence of Hb E and alpha-thalassaemia were found among Southeast Asian refugees [4]. However, there are some other hemoglobinopathies, such as Hb Tak, Hb Suandok, Hb Mahidol, in Southeast Asia as well. These hemoglobinopathies become important public health problems for the populations in Southeast Asia.

Hemoglobin E

Heterozygotes and homozygotes for HbE (beta 26, GAG-AAG, Glu-Lys) are microcytic, minimally anemic, and asymptomatic [5]. Hemoglobin E has the same electrophoretic mobility on alkaline cellulose acetate as hemoglobin A2 and hemoglobin C, however, the mobility of these hemoglobins differs on agar gel electrophoresis (pH 6.2) and they can be distinguished by this method. The synthesis of hemoglobin E in reticulocytes of A/E heterozygotes and E/E homozygotes appears to be significantly impaired, seems to be in the production of beta E chains, therefore, the Hb E structural gene may be viewed as a beta-thalassemia-like gene. Rees et al. said that the microcytosis is attributed to the beta thalassemic nature of the beta E gene, whereas the in vitro instability of HbE does not contribute to the phenotype, however, the compound heterozygote state HbE/beta thalassemia results in a variable, and often severe anemia, with the phenotype ranging from transfusion dependence to a complete lack of symptoms [6]. In addition, Schrier said that anemia severity may be related to the extent of oxidant attack on the unstable hemoglobin E [7]. Chotivanich et al. said that HbAE erythrocytes have an unidentified membrane abnormality that renders the majority of the RBC population relatively resistant to invasion by Plasmodium falciparum [8]. Chotivanich et al. said that this would not protect from uncomplicated malaria infections but would prevent the development of heavy parasite burdens and was consistent with the "Haldane" hypothesis of heterozygote protection against severe malaria for hemoglobin E [8].

Similar to thalassemia carrier, heterozygous Hb E without concomitant thalassemia usually presents no or only a few symptoms. These cases are usually mild and can be detected by blood smear on routine laboratory examination. An individual with hemoglobin E as the principal hemoglobin but no hemoglobin A, homozygous Hb E E (E/E) is also non-fatal. They may have a mild to moderate degree of anemia with a slight reduction of red cell survival and a significant reduction in mean corpuscular volume (MCV). However, an individual with concomitant thalassemia (E/beta-thal) is more severe and manifests anemic symptoms. Concerning the combination, if the beta thalassemia is beta 0, the condition becomes fatal and can be classified as thalassemia major. These cases can present marked skeletal abnormalities and retardation of growth and development and there is an increased incidence of infection and this is the most common cause of death from this disease. These patients are transfusion dependent and can be the problematic case. The interaction of HbE/beta + -thalassemia, some hemoglobin A present, results in a milder condition.

Similar to thalassemia, for those patients dependent on blood transfusion, iron-chelating agents are required. Unfortunately, the combination between Hb E and beta thalassemia is the most common form of hemoglobin E in the Southeast Asia.

Concerning the epidemiology of hemoglobin E disorders in Southeast Asia, there are several prevalence studies. Recently, Tanphaichitr *et al.* studied prevalence of hemoglobin E in 1,000 cord bloods in Bangkok [9]. According to this study, among 985 cases studied for Hb typing, 61.92% revealed normal Hb type AF while Hb E was present in 18.68% and Hb Bart's designated alpha-thalassemias were present in 25.18% respectively [9]. Wiwanitkit *et al.* reported the prevalence of hemoglobin E disorder among 213 Thai pregnant equaled to 30 % [11]. Soogarun *et al.* studied Thai medical technologist students and found that about 24 % had Hb E disorders [11]. According to these recent studies, the importance of Hb E disorders among the Thais can be confirmed.

Concerning the laboratory diagnosis of hemoglobin E disorders, there are both screening and definitive tests. Concerning the screening tests, blood smear interpretation and red blood cell index determination are two common tests similar to thalassemia. Concerning blood smear interpretation, the hypochromic microcytic anemia is characterized. Similar to thalassemia, the hallmark abnormal red cell, target cell, can be seen. Brown said that when the underlying cause of hypochromic microcytic anemia was obscure, the serum ferritin concentration should be measured first [12]. If serum ferritin is normal or increased, serum iron and free erythrocyte protoporphyrin levels can be determined [12]. The serum iron level is low in anemias caused by iron deficiency and chronic disease but normal or elevated in those resulting from the thalassemias, hemoglobin E disorders, and lead toxicity and the free erythrocyte protoporphyrin level is elevated with iron deficiency, the anemia of chronic disease, and lead toxicity but normal with thalassemias and hemoglobin E disorders [12]. Marsh *et al.* studied the peripheral smear and automated red blood cell parameters in Southeast Asian immigrants with hemoglobin E and found that homozygosity for Hb E results in an asymptomatic condition similar to thalassemia minor with microcytic RBC, large numbers of target cells, normal or slightly reduced hematocrit and greater than 90 percent Hb E [13]. In addition, people heterozygous for HbE were asymptomatic and have hematologic findings similar to thalassemia minor with slightly reduced or low normal MCV and 25 to 35 percent HbE [13].

The other screening method for hemoglobin E disorders are the mathematical model and dichlorophenol-indolphenol (DCIP) test. Concerning the mathematical model, Ittarat *et al.*performed a study and concluded that identification of Hb E especially the heterozygous form by using parameters from an electronic cell counter was not easy [14]. They said that discriminant functions and red cell indicies might be used as an initial diagnosis but confirmation was needed in all cases [14]. In addition, they mentioned that applying the MCV of 80 fl would miss 5 percent of hemoglobin E carriers but would not miss the homozygous form [14]. Concerning DCIP, this test can be good for hemoglobin E disorders. DCIP based on the principle of dye precipitation of Hb E and other unstable hemoglobin was first proposed by Frischer *et al.* [15]. Basically, the blue dye, 2, 6 dichlorophenolindophenol (DCIP) can be reduced by nonprotein-bound SH groups (of cysteine or GSSG) and by the

protein-bound SH groups at position 112 which have become available in Hb beta4 or Hb H
[15]. It was also noticed that DCIP accelerates the precipitation of Hb E in the hemolysate
and recent evidence indicated that the accelerated precipitability of Hb E by DCIP was most
likely due to weakened alpha1 beta1 contact and the increased dissociation of dimers into
monomers liberates reactive SH groups and these, if oxidized resulted in precipitation of the
protein at physiologic pH [15]. This test became a focused screening test for Hb E in the
present day and recommended in combination with one-tube osmotic fragility test for
screening for hemoglobin disorders in the pregnant [10, 16]. There are several reports on
using DCIP for screening hemoglobin E in general populations. For example, the metanalysis
of those reports in Thailand are presented in Table 9.2. According to Table 9.2, the sensitivity
and specificity of DCIP are 94.4 % and 99.7 %, respectively. Although very good diagnostic
property can be derived, it might be due to the high prevalence in Thailand. Application to
use this test in other tropical countries, where the prevalence of Hb E disorders is lower,
requires caution. The other definitive test is hemoglobin electrophoresis: it will show Hb E
(40%), Hb A (1 - 30%), and a significant increase in Hb F (30 - 50%). However, the
molecular diagnosis is the most reliable diagnostic test, which can not only document the
hemoglobin E disorders but also abnormal hemoglobin disorders.

**Table 9.2. Previous reports on the diagnostic property of DCIP in screening
for Hb E disorders in general Thai population**

Authors	Number	Prevalence (%)	Sensitivity	Specificity
Phawaphutanon Na Mahasarakam et al., 1993 [17]	240	25.8	100	100
Soogarun et al., 2004 [11]	46	23.9	100	100
Tunsaringkarn et al., 2002 [18]	145	23.4	82.6	99.0
Summary	431	24.8	94.4	99.7

Concerning the management of hemoglobin E disorders, anemia is the main problem for
the case with hemoglobin E/ beta thalassemia. These cases are as severe as thalassemia
major. Severe anemia, similar to Cooley's anemia, traps these patients into the repeated
polytransfusion. However, until present, there is no specific protocol for the transfusion
regimen for the patients with hemoglobin E/ beta thalassemia. In Thailand, the transfusion
regimen for thalassemia major is adapted. Briefly, the patients are prescribed for transfusion
every 2 - 4 weeks and receive 12 ml/kg of red blood cells at a rate up to 5 ml/kg/hr. However,
some of the patients receiving this regimen still have hyperstimulation [19]. Similar to the
thalassemia, the complications from repeated polytransfusion, blood borne transmitted
diseases and hemochromatosis, are of medical importance. To prevent hemochromatosis, the
iron chelation and monitoring of the erythropoiesis [20] is needed.

Hemoglobin Suan-Dok

In Thailand, the most common form of hemoglobinopathy is hemoglobin E disorder. This disorder presented its highest prevalence in the Northeastern Region of Thailand. However, there are several other forms of hemoglobinopathy in Thailand. Hemoglobin Suan-Dok is an example of hemoglobinopathy first described in Thailand. In this article, the author presented a summary about this Thai originated hemoglobinopathy. Hb Suan-Dok is an unstable hemoglobin variant associated with alpha-thalassemia. It is first described in Thailand by Sanguansermsri et al. in 1979 [21]. The main abnormality is the replacement of alpha 2 109 (G16) Leu by Arg beta 2 [21]. It is first described in a Thai female patient [21]. Clinically, the quantity in the heterozygote is 8.8% and if found in combination with alpha-thal-1, it can give Hb H disease [21 - 22]. It usually presents as a mild alpha-thalassemia with microcytosis and hypochromia, in the heterozygote form [21]. This hemoglobin moves slower than, slightly behind, Hb F at alkaline pH and amounted to approximately 9% by hemoglobin electrophoresis [21 – 23]. By chromatography, it can be isolated on a DEAE-Sephadex column [21 - 23]. This variant haemoglobin was somewhat unstable under heat denaturation and in the isopropanol test [21].

Suan-Dok is the name of a famous area in a Northern Province of Thailand, Chiangmai. There is a large tertiary hospital, the largest hospital in Northern Thailand, at Suan-Dok. The area of Suan-Dok can be described as a hilly town with a lot of native hilltribers. Of interest, there are still a lot of public health problems for the hilltribers in Thailand in the present day. The high prevalence of malaria and other infectious diseases can be seen in the hilltribe communities of Northern Thailand [24 – 25]. In 1979, Sanguansermsri et al. described an abnormal hemoglobin variant detected in a seven-year old Thai girl [21]. In this girl, the clinical and hematological pictures were indistinguishable from Hb H disease [21]. Upon cellulose acetate electrophoresis at pH 8.5, an abnormal hemoglobin variant was found together with Hb A and H [21]. Globin chain synthesis studies of peripheral blood reticulocytes incubated with tritiated leucine revealed that the total radioactivity ratio alpha-chain + variant alpha-chain/beta-chain was 0.59, while the ratio variant alpha-chain/beta-chain was 0.12 [21]. Structural studies by component isolation, globin chain separation, peptide mapping and amino acid analysis of abnormal peptides showed a new hemoglobin mutant and it was later named Hb Suan-Dok [21].

Concerning the pathogenesis of Hb Suan-Dok, a CTG->CGG mutation at codon 109 of the alpha2 gene is the basic pathology of Hb Suan-Dok [21 – 23]. The nature of the thalassemic defect associated with the alpha SD mutation has been investigated by structural and functional studies [21]. Sequence analysis of the cloned Suan-Dok allele showed a missense mutation (T----G) at codon 109 in an otherwise normal alpha 2-globin gene [21]. When the alpha 2SD-globin gene was introduced into mouse erythroleukemia cells, the steady state alpha-globin messenger RNA (mRNA) level was equivalent to the alpha A-globin gene control. Although in vitro translation of a synthetic alpha 2SD-globin mRNA generated levels of alpha globin equivalent to alpha 2A-globin mRNA at early time points, the ratio of alpha SD to alpha A globin decreased markedly at later time points [21]. In 1990, Hundrieser et al. noted that Hb Suan-Dok mutation can also create a new Sma I restriction site, which is possible to diagnose the mutation by restriction analysis [26]. These data suggest that the thalassemic defect associated with the Suan-Dok mutation results from a significant instability of the alpha SD globin [23]. Conclusively, Hb Suan-Dok has an alpha-thalassemia-like effect due to low production and instability of the altered alpha-globin chain.

After the first presentation of Hb Suan-Dok in 1979, there are only a few sporadic case reports of this hemoglobin disorder in Thailand [26 – 28]. Most cases are from the northern region of Thailand. Conclusively, most cases of Hb Suan-Dok presented to the physician with the picture of Hb H but was accidentally detected by further investigation. The predilection occurrence of this hemoglobinopathy in the northern region of Thailand might reflect on the natural selection process in response to the local biological hazard especially malaria, as described in the general Hb H disease [28]. Conclusively, Hb Suan-Dok (alpha 109Arg) is a rare alpha globin structural mutation that is linked to an alpha-thalassemia (alpha-thal) determinant [23]. When inherited in trans to an alpha-thal-1 mutation (-), it results in Hb H disease associated with low levels (9%) of the Suan-Dok Hb [23]. The endemic area of this hemoglobinopathy is in the northern region of Thailand.

Hemoglobin Constant Spring

Hemoglobin Constant Spring (Hb CS) is a chain variant with an elongated alpha globin chain of 28 to 31 amino acids. This is caused by a mutation that alters the mRNA termination codon. Hb CS is common in Southeast Asia. Laig *et al.* found that The Hb CS gene frequency was 0.033 in northern Thailand and near 0.01 in central Thailand and Cambodia [29]. The gene frequency for alpha cs alpha is about 0.05 for Laotians [30]. In addition, high frequencies, between 0.05 and 0.06, were observed in northeastern Thailand [29]. Similar to other hemoglobinopathies, the hemoglobin electrophoreis is the definitive diagnosis for Hb CS. Concerning the hemoglobin electrophoreis, the mobility is between carbonic anhydrase and Hb A, on cellulose acetate. The percentage is usually about 1% in heterozygote carriers, 5 to 7% in homozygotes, and 3 to 5% in hemoglobin H disease caused by Hb CS with trans two gene deletion alpha thalassemia.

Clinically, heterozygotes with Hb CS and two normal trans at genes are hematologically normal while homozygotes for Hb CS have a mild hemolytic anemia and may have splenomegaly. Similar to the connection between Hb E and beta thalassemia, a case with Hb H disease from Hb CSpr and two-gene deletion alpha thalassemia manifests a more severe disease with more Hb H and Bart's than three- gene deletion alpha thalassemia [31 - 32]. Concerning the diagnosis of Hb CS, the hemoglobin electrophoresis is an important tool, however, Constant Spring protein can sometimes not detect by electrophoresis. Molecular diagnosis is therefore an important tool at present. Recently, Hsia *et al.* reported a new technique for allele specific polymerase chain amplification of the 3'-end of the alpha 2 globin gene improved detection of the alpha cs alpha haemoglobin variant in DNA samples by slot-blot hybridisation [30]. Hb CS is also an important public health problem in Southeast Asia because of the high incidence of cis alpha thalassemia 1 or alpha thalassemia 0 which puts couples at risk for having infants with Hb H disease [31].

Important Hemoglobinopathies in West Asia

Hemoglobin O-Arab

In West Asia, Hb O-Arab is the most well known hemoglobinopathy, relating to anemia. This hemoglobinopathy can be seen in North Africa, Bulgaria, and the eastern Mediterranean area as well. Molecularly, The animo acid substitution is lysine for glutamic acid in the beta 121 position [beta 121(GH4)Glu-->Lys]. Heterozygote carriers have no clinical manifestations. However, Hb O-Arab has significance in sickle syndromes because it interacts with Hb S to produce clinical manifestations approaching the severity of Hb SS disease [32]. Compound heterozygotes for Hb S and HbO-Arab have hemoglobins in the 7 - 8 gm/dl range with reticulocytosis, jaundice, splenomegaly, episodes of pain, and many other complications seen in Hb SS disease [32]. Compound heterozygotes for Hb O-Arab and Beta thalassemia have manifestations similar to thalassemia intermedia [32].

Similar to other hemoglobinopathies, the hemoglobin electrophoreis is the definitive diagnosis for Hb O-Arab. Concerning the hemoglobin electrophoreis, the mobility is in the Hb A, / C position on cellulose acetate and between Hb S and Hb A on citrate agar, pH 6,2. Migration on isoelectric focusing is with Hb E and Hb C Harlem. Joutovsky and Nardi also mentioned that the HPLC method can be the tool for both confirmatory and diagnostic of Hb O-Arab at the same time [33]. However, the molecular diagnosis is the most accurate tool at present. Conclusively, Hb O-Arab is also an important health problem leading to tropical anemia in West Asia because of the potential for interaction with Hb S and beta thalassemia producing significant disease [32].

Important Hemoglobinopathies in Africa

Hemoglobin S

Hemoglobin S (Hb S) is the most well known hemoglobinopathy in medicine.

Hemoglobin S (Hb S) has a substitution of valine for glutamic acid in the sixth position of the Beta globin chain [32]. Hb S occurs in high frequency in Africa in areas previously exposed to falciparum malaria [34]. Heterozygosity for the mutant sickle hemoglobin confers protection from severe *Plasmodium falciparum* infection [35]. Hebbel said that this protection derived from the instability of sickle hemoglobin, which clustered red cell membrane protein band 3 and triggerred accelerated removal by phagocytic cells [35]. The other endemic areas of Hb S are India, the Mediterranean area, and Saudi Arabia [32]. Recently, Adewuyi and Gwanzura studied the frequency of the sickle haemoglobin gene in Zimbabwe [36]. According to this study, 868 samples were analysed and the sickle haemoglobin (Bs) gene frequency at birth was found to be 0.012 [36]. Similar to other hemoglobinopathies, heterozygous Hb S has mild clinical manifestation while homozygous Hb S has severe manifestation known as sickle cell syndrome. In addition, the connection between heterozygous Hb S with other hemoglobinopathies, especially Hemoglobin C (Hb C) or Hb O-Arab, or heterozygous beta thalassemia can bring a disease as severe as sickle cell syndrome [32]. Although there are some differences between these syndromes, all have similar clinical manifestations, severe anemia. Sickle hemoglobin crystallizes with deoxygenation causing distortion of the erythrocyte and many clinical problems [32]. This single mutation leads to the formation of abnormal hemoglobin, HbS (alpha2betas[s]2), which is much less soluble when deoxygenated than hemoglobin A (HbA) (alpha2beta2) [37]. This insolubility causes aggregates of HbS to form inside sickle erythrocytes as they traverse the circulation [37]. With full deoxygenation, the polymer becomes so extensive that the cells become sickled in shape [37]. Sickling of erythrocytes is facilitated by increased temperature (fever), decreased pH (acidosis), and high mean corpuscular hemoglobin concentration (MCHC) (dehydration) [32]. Powars and Hiti said that the Bs gene cluster haplotypes could be as genetic markers for severe disease expression [38].

Clinical manifestations of sickle cell syndromes include moderate to severe hemolytic anemia, increased severity of certain infections, tissue infarction with organ damage and failure, and recurrent pain episodes [32]. The vaso-occlusive process also seen in the patients with sickle cell disease is complex and is likely to involve interactions between hemoglobin S red blood cells (SS RBCs) and vascular endothelium, as well as between SS RBCs and leukocytes [39]. Rodgers said that, even with high oxygen saturation values, quantities of HbS polymer might be sufficient to alter the rheologic properties of sickle erythrocytes in the absence of morphologic changes, and cells could occlude end arterioles, leading to chronic hemolysis and microinfarction of diverse tissues and this process has led to vaso-occlusive crises and irreversible tissue damage [37]. Rodgers also said that the spectrum of disease severity even among patients with grossly equivalent hematologic indices suggested that many other factors-including genetic, cellular, physiologic, and psychosocial-played a substantial role in determining the course of this disorder [37].

Pathologically, there are two main manifestations of sickle cell anemia: one as hematologic manifestation and the other as non-hematologic manifestation.

Concerning hematologic manifestation, severe normochromic normocytic anemia is mentioned. Lonergan et al. said that rigid deformation of the cell impaired the ability of the cell to pass through small vascular channels; sludging and congestion of vascular beds might result, followed by tissue ischemia and infarction [40]. Similar to the thalassemia, the trapping of a deformed cells by the reticuloendothelial cells, especially in the spleen, can cause hemolysis leading to severe anemia in the patients with sickle cell diseases [40]. However, the hemolytic anemia is generally well tolerated but does lead to premature gallstones in many patients [32]. An unusual but life-threatening complication of sickle cell anemia is sequestration syndrome or splenic sequestration crisis or aplastic crisis, wherein a considerable amount of the intravascular volume is sequestered in an organ, usually the spleen, causing vascular collapse [40]. Juwah et al. recently studied a total of 108 episodes of anemic crises in 108 patients with sickle cell anemia in Nigeria and found that about 4.6% of patients were not jaundiced at presentation even though they were profoundly anemic [41]. They mentioned that malaria appeared to have played a role in precipitating some of the hyper-hemolytic episodes [41].

Concerning non-hematological manifestation, infarction is the common cause leading to the pathology throughout the body in the patient with sickle cell anemia, and it is responsible for the earliest clinical manifestation, the acute pain crisis, which is thought to result from marrow infarction [40]. The pathology can be seen in many organs such as medullary infarcts and epiphyseal osteonecrosis in bone, white matter and gray matter infarcts in brain causing cognitive impairment and functional neurologic deficits and secondary stroke, and also lung infarct [40]. Rarely, pain episodes or splenic infarctions have been seen with extreme lack of oxygen [32]. Sudden death may be slightly more common at the extremes of human endurance [32]. The vaso-occlusive related process is another underlying cause of non-hematologic manifestation of sickle cell anemia [39]. The well-known condition is pulmonary emboli, from marrow infarcts and fat necrosis [40]. Although pulmonary embolism in the patients with sickle cell anemia is not common, it is fatal [41]. Lakkireddy *et al.* noted that it was important for clinicians to be expectant of impending clinical deterioration and likewise be aware that ACS could develop in patients hospitalized for other medical or surgical conditions [42]. In addition, obstruction of retinal vessels may lead to vitreous hemorrhage or retinal detachment with resulting loss of vision [40]. Concerning sickle cell trait, it usually associated with any hematological abnormalities, however, some carriers may have episodes of hematuria and may have more urinary tract infections [32].

Concerning treatment of sickle cell anemia, the general principle of anemia management, an increase in red blood cell production in cases with production defect and a decrease in red blood cell destruction accompanied with red blood cell replacement in cases with increased red blood cell destruction can be applied. Agarwal said that the recent explosion acknowledged in understanding the pathogenesis of this disease had lead to newer dimensions in treatment; some of these included prevention of overwhelming bacterial infection, present indications and controversies regarding blood transfusion, prevention of stroke, acute chest syndrome, hydroxyurea therapy and stem cell transplantation [43]. Concerning the increase in red blood cell production, erythropoietin treatment is used in sickle cell anemia cases, similar to thalasemia [44]. The effective therapeutic result in the pregnant cases was also reported [45]. However, hydroxyurea therapy is another method, more applicable, for increased red blood cell production in the cases with sickle cell anemia. Agarwal said that hydroxyurea therapy probably the best disease modifying agent at the moment [43]. Papassotiriou *et al.* said that administration of hydroxyurea in sickle cell disease was associated with a dramatic increase of HbF along with a significant clinical improvement and, occasionally, increased total hemoglobin levels [46]. They performed a small trial and found that two to three weeks after initiation of treatment, the serum erythropoietin values started to increase and reached levels three to 31 times higher than the baseline two to three weeks later [46]. They concluded that peaks of endogenous erythropoietin might promote proliferation of erythroid precursors, which maintained the capacity to synthesize H bF [46]. The combination of erythropoietin and hydroxyurea therapy has also been tried. Recently, el-Hazmi *et al.* recommended the use of hydroxyurea for the treatment of SCD and a combination therapy using hydroxyurea and erythropoietin for the non-responders [47]. Concerning decreased red blood cell destruction, splenectomy is done for splenic sequestration in older children and with recurrence [40]. However, similar to thalassemia, post-splenectomy cases increase the incidence of sepsis, meningitis, and other serious infections with *Streptococcus pneumoniae*, *Hemophilus influenzae*, *Salmonella* species, and *Mycoplasma pneumoniae* [40]. Concerning the red blood cell replacement, transfusion in sickle cell anemia is also practiced. Al-Saeed and Al-Salem said that regardinhg blood transfusion as therapy and prophylaxis in sickle cell anemia, although advocated as early as the 1940's, there were still debates about its benefits and risks [48]. Danielson said that red blood cell exchange transfusion could, without increasing the whole-blood viscosity, quickly replace abnormal erythrocytes with normal ones and raise the hematocrit resulting in improved delivery of oxygen to hypoxic tissues [49]. In addition, it can prevent stroke [50]. However, transfusion can also be associated with several complications especially blood-borne pathogen transmission. Luckily, secondary hemochromatosis as a post -transfusion complication in sickle cell anemia is not common [51]. Similar to thalassemia, bone marrow transplantation is the new curative therapeutic management of sickle cell anemia. Vermylen said that the disease-free survival (DFS) was good (80-85% in several series), even though many children who received allografts had had already significant sickle-related complications [52]. Vermylen said that the best results were obtained in young children who had HLA-identical sibling donors and are transplanted early in the course of the disease (DFS: 93%) [52]. Vermylen proposed that future directions in the field of stem cell transplantation of sickle cell anemia should include (1) the establishment of new protocols with less toxicity, but still effective, (2) adapted conditioning regimens for adult patients, and (3) new sources of stem cells for broader application: umbilical cord blood and volunteer unrelated donors [52].

Hemoglobin C

Hemoglobin C (Hb C) has a substitution of lysine for glutamic acid in the sixth position of the Beta globin chain [32]. Hb C occurs in higher frequency in individuals with heritage from Western Africa. The Hb C is also prevalent in Italy, Greece, Turkey, and the Middle East [32]. Usanga et al. said that the incidence of Hb C was as high as 6% in western Nigeria [53]. Association of Hb C with the erythrocyte membrane causes red cell dehydration and resulting increase in MCHC [32, 54]. This leads to a shortened red cell survival in Hb C homozygotes and sickling complications in compound heterozygotes for Hb S and Hb C [32]. Similar to other hemoglobinopathies, heterozygote Hb C is mild, usually has target cells on a blood smear and may have a slightly low MCV, while homozygote Hb C is more severe [32, 54]. Individuals with Hb CC disease have a mild hemolytic anemia, microcytosis, and target cell formation. There may be very occasional episodes of joint and abdominal pain, which are attributed to Hb CC disease, and splenomegaly is common. Similar to sickle cell anemia, aplastic crisis and gallstone disease may occur [32, 54]. A combination between heterozygous Hb C and heterozygous Hb S is medically important. These cases have a sickle syndrome which is very similar to sickle cell anemia, however, the hemolysis is usually less severe so the hemoglobin level is higher [32, 55]. Concerning the pathogenesis of the combine Hb S and Hb C disease, it is proposed that HbC enhances, by dehydrating the pathologic red cell, the pathogenic properties of HbS, resulting in a clinically significant disorder, but milder than sickle cell anemia [55]. In addition, retinnitis proliferans, osteonecrosis, and acute chest syndrome have equal or higher incidence in this combined disease, compared to sickle cell anemia: this pathogenic is relating to an increase in the activity of K: Cl cotransport that induces the loss of K(+) and consequently of intracellular water [55]. Since this event creates a sufficient increase of MCHC, so that the lower levels of Hb S found in SC red cells can polymerize rapidly and effectively [55]. The combination between heterozygotes for Hb C and beta thalassemia trait is more complex. If the combination is between Hb C and beta + thalassemia, there is 65 - 70% Hb C, 20 - 30% Hb A, and increased Hb F, but if the combination is between Hb C and beta 0 thalassemia, there is no Hb A and increased Hb F with Hb C [32]. In the first case, the affected patients have a mild anemia, low MCV, and target cells while in the later case, the affected patients have a moderately severe anemia, splenomegaly, and may have bone changes [32]. Fattoum *et al.* studied 11 cases with combination between Hb C and beta thalassemia in Tunisia and found that microcytosis and hypochromia could be detected in every case [56]. In this series, blood transfusions were required in only one patient, who was an infant with HbC/beta + thalassemia [56].

Similar to sickle cell anemia and hemoglobin E disorders, this hemoglobin disorder can be detected by the hemoglobin electrophoresis. However, its motility overlaps with hemoglobin E, therefore, it is sometimes difficult to discriminate between these two disorders. The molecular is still the best definitive diagnostic method, similar to other hemoglobin disorders. Concerning treatment for anemia in hemoglobin C disorders, the principle is similar to those for other hemoglobin disorders. If the heterozygous hemoglobin C presents with mild hemolytic anemia, it is not a problematic case, however, some cases present

with a moderate hemolytic anemia and a massive, painful and even disabling splenomegaly [57]. Splenectomy is an effective method to decrease the pain [57]. However, a postoperative course could be complicated by portal venous thrombosis, which was medically treated [57]. Bruyneel *et al.* said that in only very few cases of hemoglobin C disease, splenectomy, preceded by prophylactic antipneumococcic vaccine, might be indicated from pain and risk of spontaneous splenic rupture [57].

References

[1] Old JM. Screening and genetic diagnosis of haemoglobin disorders. *Blood Rev* 2003;17:43-53.

[2] Fucharoen S, Wanichagoon G. Thalassemia and abnormal hemoglobin. *Int J Hematol* 2002;76 Suppl 2:83-9.

[3] Johnxis JH. Haemoglobinopathies and their occurrence in South East Asia. *Paediatr Indones* 1975;15:112-9.

[4] Fucharoen S, Winichagoon P. Hemoglobinopathies in Southeast Asia. *Hemoglobin* 1987;11:65-88.

[5] Dode C, Berth A, Bourdillon F, Mahe C, Labie D, Rochette J. Haemoglobin disorders among Southeast-Asian refugees in France. *Acta Haematol* 1987;78:135-6.

[6] Rees DC, Styles L, Vichinsky EP, Clegg JB, Weatherall DJ. The hemoglobin E syndromes. *Ann N Y Acad Sci* 1998;850:334-43.

[7] Schrier SL. Pathobiology of thalassemic erythrocytes. *Curr Opin Hematol* 1997;4:75-8.

[8]   Chotivanich K, Udomsangpetch R, Pattanapanyasat K, Chierakul W, Simpson J, Looareesuwan S, White N. Hemoglobin E: a balanced polymorphism protective against high parasitemias and thus severe P falciparum malaria. *Blood* 2002;100:1172-6.

[9]   Tanphaichitr VS, Mahasandana C, Suvatte V, Yodthong S, Pung-amritt P, Seeloem J. Prevalence of hemoglobin E, alpha-thalassemia and glucose-6-phosphate dehydrogenase deficiency in 1,000 cord bloods studied in Bangkok. *Southeast Asian J Trop Med Public Health* 1995;26 Suppl 1:271-4.

[10] Wiwanitkit V, Suwansaksri J, Paritpokee N. Combined one-tube osmotic fragility (OF) test and dichlorophenol-indolphenol (DCIP) test screening for hemoglobin disorders, an experience in 213 Thai pregnant women. *Clin Lab* 2002;48:525-8.

[11] Soograun S, Sirimongkolsakul S, Wiwanitkit V, Mahakitikul B, Pradniwat P, Palasuwan A. Haemoglobinopathy among the medical technologist students, a note from haemoglobin electrophoresis study. *Haema* 2004; 7: 252 – 3.

[12] Brown RG. Determining the cause of anemia. General approach, with emphasis on microcytic hypochromic anemias. *Postgrad Med* 1991;89:161-4.

[13] Marsh WL Jr, Rogers ZR, Nelson DP, Vedvick TS. Hematologic findings in Southeast Asian immigrants with particular reference to hemoglobin E. *Ann Clin Lab Sci* 1983;13:299-306.

[14] Ittarat W, Ongcharoenjai S, Rayatong O, Pirat N. Correlation between some discrimination functions and hemoglobin E. *J Med Assoc Thai* 2000; 83:259-65.

[15] Kulapongs P, Tawarat S, Sanguansermsri T. Dichlorophenolindophenol (DCIP) precipitation test : a simple screening test for hemoglobin E and alpha thalassemia (Thalassemia Conference In Memorial of Dr. Sa-nga Pootrakul At the Mahidol University Faculty of Medicine Siriraj Hospital February 10-11, 1977). *J Med Assoc Thai.* 1978; 61: 62-63.

[16] Wiwanitkit V. Combined osmotic fragility and dichlorophenol-indolphenol test for hemoglobin disorder screening in Thai pregnant subjects: an appraisal. *Lab Hematol* 2004;10:119-20.

[17] Phawaphutanon Na Mahasarakam K, Suksa-ard V, Sanchaisuriya K, Boonfuangfu R, Munkong Y, Fucharoen G, Fucharoen S, Mertz G. Screening for hemoglobin E by the DCIP precipitation test in non anemic people. *Bull Med Tech Phys Ther* 1993; 5: 139-143.

[18] Tunsaringkarn K, Taechachainirun B, Sindhuphak R. Modified DCIP for thalassemia carrier screening for health center in community. *Bull Dept Med Serv* 2002; 27: 103-107

[19] Boonchalermvichian C, Paritpokee N, Bhokaisawan N, Nuchprayoon I, Wiwanitkit V. Marked increase in serum transferrin receptor among Thai children with Hb-E-beta-thalassaemia. *J Paediatr Child Health* 2002;38:601-3.

[20] Paritpokee N, Wiwanitkit V, Bhokaisawan N, Boonchalermvichian C, Preechakas P. Serum erythropoietin levels in pediatric patients with beta-thalassemia/hemoglobin E. *Clin Lab* 2002;48:631-4.

[21] Sanguansermsri T, Matragoon S, Changloah L, Flatz G. Haemoglobin Suan-Dok (alpha 2 109 (G16) Leu replaced by Arg beta 2): an unstable variant associated with alpha-thalassemia. *Haemoglobin* 1979; 3:161-174.

[22] Matragoon S. The hematological studies and structural analysis of haemoglobin Suan-Dok: an alpha chain variant found in association with alpha thalassemia. *Master's thesis (Biochemistry)*, Faculty of Graduate Studies, Mahidol University Thailand, 1978.

[23] Weiss L, Cash FE, Coleman MB, Pressley A, Adams JG, Sanguansermsri T, Liebhaber SA, Steinberg MH. Molecular basis for a thalassaemia associated with the structural mutant haemoglobin Suan–Dok (a2 109 LEU----ARG). *Blood* 1990;76:2630-6.

[24] Suyaphun A, Wiwanitkit V, Suwansaksri J, Nithiuthai S, Sritar S, Suksirisampant W, Fongsungnern A. Malaria among hilltribe communities in northern Thailand: a review of clinical manifestations. *Southeast Asian J Trop Med Public Health.* 2002; 33 Suppl 3: 14-5.

[25] Wiwanitkit V, Suyaphan A. High prevalence of HBsAg seropositivity in Hilltribers in the Mae Jam district in northern Thailand. *MedGenMed* 2002; 4: 26.

[26] Hundrieser J, Sanguansermsri T, Laig M, Pape M, Kuhnau W, Flatz G. Direct demonstration of the HB Suan-Dok mutation in the alpha 2-globin gene by restriction analysis with Sma I. *Haemoglobin* 1990; 14: 69-77.

[27] Sanguansermsri T, Matrakool S, Flatz G. Haemoglobin H-haemoglobin Suan-Dok disease. *Chiangmia Med Bull* 1980; 20: 381 – 91.

[28] Ifediba TC, Stern A, Ibrahim A, Rieder RF. Plasmodium falciparum in vitro: diminished growth in haemoglobin H disease erythrocytes. *Blood* 1985; 65: 452-5.

[29] Laig M, Pape M, Hundrieser J, Flatz G, Sanguansermsri T, Das BM, Deka R, Yongvanit P, Mularlee N. The distribution of the Hb constant spring gene in Southeast Asian populations. *Hum Genet* 1990 ;84:188-90.

[30] Hsia YE, Ford CA, Shapiro LJ, Hunt JA, Ching NS. Molecular screening for haemoglobin constant spring. *Lancet.* 1989;1:988-91.

[31] Viprakasit V, Tanphaichitr VS. Compound heterozygosity for alpha0-thalassemia (-THAI) and Hb constant spring causes severe Hb H disease. *Hemoglobin* 2002;26:155-62.

[32] Eckman   JR.   Hemolgobins–What   the   results   mean.   Available   at *http://www.scinfo.org/hemoglb.htm.*

[33] Joutovsky A, Nardi M. Hemoglobin C and hemoglobin O-Arab variants can be diagnosed using the Bio-Rad Variant II high-performance liquid chromatography system without further confirmatory tests. *Arch Pathol Lab Med* 2004;128:435-9.

[34] Roberts DJ, Williams TN. Haemoglobinopathies and resistance to malaria. *Redox Rep* 2003;8:304-10.

[35] Hebbel RP. Sickle hemoglobin instability: a mechanism for malarial protection. *Redox Rep* 2003;8:238-40

[36] Adewuyi JO, Gwanzura C. Frequency of the sickle haemoglobin gene in Zimbabwe. *East Afr Med J* 1994;71:204-6.

[37] Rodgers GP. Overview of pathophysiology and rationale for treatment of sickle cell anemia. *Semin Hematol* 1997;34(3 Suppl 3):2-7.

[38] Powars D, Hiti A. Sickle cell anemia. Beta s gene cluster haplotypes as genetic markers for severe disease expression. *Am J Dis Child* 1993;147:1197-202

[39] Parise LV, Telen MJ. Erythrocyte adhesion in sickle cell disease. *Curr Hematol R*ep 2003;2:102-8.

[40] Lonergan GJ, Cline DB, Abbondanzo SL. Sickle cell anemia. *Radiographics* 2001;21:971-94

[41] Juwah AI, Nlemadim EU, Kaine W. Types of anaemic crises in paediatric patients with sickle cell anaemia seen in Enugu, Nigeria. *Arch Dis Child* 2004;89:572-6.

[42] Lakkireddy DR, Patel R, Basarakodu K, Vacek J. Fatal pulmonary artery embolism in a sickle cell patient: case report and literature review. *J Thromb Thrombolysis* 2002;14:79-83.

[43] Agarwal MB. Advances in management of sickle cell disease. *Indian J Pediatr* 2003;70:649-54.

[44] Biesma DH. Erythropoietin treatment for non-uremic patients: a personal view. *Neth J Med* 1999;54:10-5.

[45] Bourantas K, Makrydimas G, Georgiou J, Tsiara S, Lolis D. Preliminary results with administration of recombinant human erythropoietin in sickle cell/beta-thalassemia patients during pregnancy. *Eur J Haematol* 1996;56:326-8.

[46] Papassotiriou I, Voskaridou E, Stamoulakatou A, Loukopoulos D. Increased erythropoietin level induced by hydroxyurea treatment of sickle cell patients. *Hematol J* 2000;1:295-300.

[47] el-Hazmi MA, al-Momen A, Kandaswamy S, Huraib S, Harakati M, al-Mohareb F, Warsy AS. On the use of hydroxyurea/erythropoietin combination therapy for sickle cell disease. *Acta Haematol.* 1995;94:128-34.

[48] Al-Saeed HH, Al-Salem AH. Principles of blood transfusion in sickle cell anemia. *Saudi Med J* 2002;23:1443-8.

[49] Danielson CF. The role of red blood cell exchange transfusion in the treatment and prevention of complications of sickle cell disease. *Ther Apher* 2002;6:24-31.

[50] Gebreyohanns M, Adams RJ. Sickle cell disease: primary stroke prevention. *CNS Spectr* 2004;9:445-9.

[51] Flyer MA, Haller JO, Sundaram R. Transfusional hemosiderosis in sickle cell anemia: another cause of an echogenic pancreas. *Pediatr Radiol* 1993;23:140-2.

[52] Vermylen C. Hematopoietic stem cell transplantation in sickle cell disease. *Blood Rev* 2003;17:163-6.

[53] Usanga EA, Andy JJ, Ekanem AD, Udoh EA, Udoh AE. Haemoglobin C gene in south eastern Nigeria. *East Afr Med J* 1996;73:566-7.

[54] Ohba Y, Fujisawa K. Hb, C, D and E hemoglobinopathies. *Nippon Rinsho* 1996;54:2448-53.

[55] Nagel RL, Fabry ME, Steinberg MH. The paradox of hemoglobin SC disease. *Blood Rev* 2003;17:167-78

[56] Fattoum S, Guemira F, Abdennebi M, Ben Abdeladhim A. HbC/beta-thalassemia association. Eleven cases observed in Tunisia. *Ann Pediatr* (Paris). 1993;40:45-8.

[57] M, De Caluwe JP, des Grottes JM, Collart F. Hemoglobinopathy C and splenomegaly in an Ivory Coast patient. Value of splenectomy. *Rev Med Brux* 2003;24:105-7.

Chapter 10

Glucose-6-Phosophate Dehydrogenase Deficiency in Tropical Countries

Introduction to Glucose-6-Phosphase Dehydrogenase Deficiency

Glucose-6-phosphate dehydrogenase (G6PD, EC1.1.1.49) is an enzyme expressed in all tissues, where it catalyses the first step in the pentose phosphate pathway [1 – 3]. This first reaction in the pathway leads to the production of pentose phosphates and reducing power in the form of NADPH for reductive biosynthesis and maintenance of the cellular redox state [1 – 3]. The defect of this enzyme namely G6PD deficiency is the most common sex-linked inherited enzymatic defect, affecting over 400 million persons worldwide [1 – 3]. This disorder can cause hemolytic anemia [1]. The severe hemolysis and hemostatic change is sometimes due to an identifiable chemical trigger, drugs or to infection [1 – 2]. Several widely used drugs in the tropics, especially antimalarial drugs, can induce hemolysis in the patients with G6PD deficiency. G6PD deficiency is prevalent throughout tropical and subtropical regions of the world because of the protection it affords during malaria infection [3]. Ruwende and Hill said that the geographical correlation of its distribution with the historical endemicity of malaria suggested that G6PD deficiency had risen in frequency through natural selection by malaria [4]. This is supported by data from in vitro studies that demonstrate impaired growth of Plasmodium falciparum parasites in G6PD-deficient erythrocytes [4]. Ruwende and Hill noted that recent results from large case control studies conducted in East and West Africa provide strong evidence that the most common African G6PD deficiency variant, G6PD A-, was associated with a significant reduction in the risk of severe malaria for both G6PD female heterozygotes and male hemizygotes [4].

Molecular Basis of Glucose-6-Phosphase Dehydrogenase Deficiency

G6PD plays a key role in the generation of NADPH, which is essential for maintaining glutathione in the reduced state, and in the production of ribose 5-phosphate for the synthesis of nucleotides [1 – 3, 5]. G6PD in its active form is either a dimer or tetramer consisting of identical subunits [1 –3, 5]. It is already known that the cause of G6PD deficiency is the enzymatic defect at the gene level. The glucose-6-phosphate dehydrogenase (G6PD) gene is X-linked. The gene for G6PD is located on the X chromosome [5]. Human red cell G6PD consists of 515 amino acids with a molecular weight of 59,265 daltons [5]. There are numerous mutations that cause a deficiency of this enzyme in erythrocytes [6]. DNA sequence analysis has shown that the vast majority of these are caused by single amino acid substitutions [1 – 3]. Beutler said that different mutations, each characteristic of certain populations, were found, and had been characterized at the deoxyribonucleic acid (DNA) level [6]. Beutler noted that G6PD A-(202A376G) was the most common African mutation while G6PD Mediterranean(563T) was found in Southern Europe, the Middle East and in the Indian subcontinent and several other mutations were common in Asia [6]. Miwa and Fujii said that the mutations responsible for about 78 variants have been determined in G6PD deficiency and some had polymorphic frequencies in different populations [7]. They said that most variants were produced by one or two nucleotide substitutions [7]. Fujii mentioned that except for 7 kinds of variants with small gene deletion, splice site deletion of intron or three nucleotide substitutions, all of those were found to be produced by one or two nucleotide substitutions [5]. They also noted that several molecular studies had disclosed that most of the class 1 G6PD variants associated with chronic hemolysis had the mutations surrounding either the substrate or the NADP binding site [5, 7 - 9]. In addition, the three-dimensional structure of G6PD shows a classical dinucleotide binding domain and a novel beta + alpha domain involved in dimerization [1 –3].

Pathogenesis of Glucose-6-Phosphase Dehydrogenase Deficiency

G6PD deficiency was discovered in the 1950s [10]. This deficiency is an inheritable, X-linked recessive disorder whose primary effect is the reduction of the enzyme G6PD in red blood cells, causing destruction of the cells, called hemolysis [10]. Due to the nature of inheritance, the disease is more common in males. The hemolytic anemia in G6PD deficiency can be divided into either *acute* hemolytic or a *chronic* spherocytic type. The most well known condition is favism. Favism is an acute hemolytic syndrome occurring in G6PD deficient individuals, about 20 %, after the consumption of fava beans [11]. The erythrocytes in affected individuals have insufficient reducing power against toxic peroxydes and free radicals generated during metabolism [12]. Normally, affected individuals are without signs of disease, but under the influence of oxidants severe intravascular hemolysis may occur [12]. One of the most important oxidants is the fava bean which, when ingested, may cause acute favism, a condition which has a 10% mortality if not treated properly [12]. Mareni *et al.* noted that since not all G6PD deficient subjects were sensitive to fava beans, the possibility has been suggested that extra erythrocytic factors might play an important role in the susceptibility to haemolytic favism [13]. They performed a study to test the hypothesis that an autosomal enzyme was involved in the pathogenesis of favism by carrying out a beta-glucosidase assay in small intestine biopsies from normal subjects and G6PD deficient subjects with or without favism [13]. They found that beta-glucosidase might be involved in the absorption and metabolism of fava beans and a quantitative polymorphism could explain the different susceptibility to fava beans of G6PD deficient subjects, however, their observation showed no consistent quantitative polymorphism of beta-glucosidase in the subjects examined [13]. Damonte *et al.* reported that exposure of G6PD-deficient erythrocytes in vitro to autoxidizing divicine, a pyrimidine aglycone strongly implicated in the pathogenesis of favism which leads to late accumulation of intracellular calcium, caused: (i) a marked inactivation of calcium ATPase, without changes in the molecular mass of 134 kD; and (ii) the concomitant loss of spectrin, band 3 and band 4.1, all known substrates of the calcium activated procalpain-calpain proteolytic system, thus, the increased intraerythrocytic calcium apparently results in the degradation of calcium ATPase observed in some favic patients [14]. Damonte *et al.* proposed that both enhanced calcium permeability and a calcium-stimulated degradation of the calcium pump were the mechanisms responsible for the perturbation of erythrocyte calcium homeostasis in favism [14]. However, favism is not common in the tropics. Recently, Kitayaporn *et al.* proposed that G6PD deficiency and fava bean consumption do not produce hemolysis in Thailand [15]. They concluded that this might be due to the presence of different G6PD mutants to those found elsewhere or due to different consumption patterns of fava beans among the Thais compared to people in other areas with high prevalence of G6PD deficiency [15].

The pathogenesis of G6PD in the tropics, especially in Asia, usually relates to drugs or infection. The common problematic drug is the antimalarial drug, which is widely prescribed in the tropic countries where malaria is still endemic. The occurrence of G6PD as well as other inherited hemoglobin disorders in these countries is believed to be due to the natural selection to resist the highly endemicity of malaria. Concerning the malarial parasite, it contains a gene for G6PD and can produce a small quantity of parasite-encoded enzyme, however, it is not clear if the production of this enzyme can be up-regulated in G6PG deficient host red cells [16]. Roth noted that parasitized red cells contained about 10 times more NAD than uninfected red cells, but the NADP(H) content was unchanged [16]. However, the role of NADPH in protecting the parasite-red cell system against oxidative stress, via glutathione reduction, remains controversial [16].

Clinical Manifestations of Glucose-6-Phosphase Dehydrogenase Deficiency

Although most affected individuals are asymptomatic, there is a risk of neonatal jaundice and acute hemolytic anemia, triggered by infection and the ingestion of certain drugs and broad beans (favism) [3]. A rare but more severe form of G6PD deficiency is found throughout the world and is associated with chronic non-spherocytic hemolytic anemia [3]. A common presentation of G6PD deficiency in the tropics is neonatal hyperbilirubinemia [17]. In Asia, neonatal hyperbilirubinemia is a common manifestation of G6PD deficiency [17]. Iranpour et al. studied the prevalence of G6PD deficiency of hyperbilirubinemia in neonates in Iran [18]. They found that only 53 of 705 (7.5%) included cases had G6PD deficiency [18]. In all G6PD deficient neonates no evidence of other factors known to cause hyperbilirubinemia were detected [18]. They concluded that since the prevalence of severe hyperbilirubinemia among our neonates was relatively high and about half of them required exchange transfusion, early detection of this enzymopathy, regardless of sex, and close surveillance of the affected newborns might be important in reducing the risk of severe hyperbilirubinemia and exchange transfusion [18].

In non-pediatric cases, there are some previous studies from tropical countries on the clinical presentations of G6PD deficiency. The common presentation is the hemolytic anemia. The patients usually experience severe fatigue. Bouma et al. studied the prevalence of G6PD deficiency among Pakistani Pathans was 7.0%, and that in Tajik and Turkoman refugees was 2.9% and 2.1% respectively [19]. They found that the type of G-6-PD deficiency in Pathans could cause severe hemolytic crises [19]. They mentioned that the potentially fatal side effects of primaquine treatment in the Pathan communities, and the high risk of re-infection, rendered the anti-relapse treatment policy for Plasmodium vivax obsolete and proposed for the necessary revision of the recommendations for the use of primaquine in the area [19]. It should be noted that the presentation of G6PD deficiency is relating to the triggers. As already described, the triggers are usually drugs and infections. An example of a common problematic drug is primaquine [1 – 3] and of a problematic infection is hepatitis [20 - 21]. If there is no trigger, all cases remain normal. The hemolytic anemia therefore can be seen only in the post – stimulated G6PD deficient cases

Diagnosis of Glucose-6-Phosphase Dehydrogenase Deficiency

Presently, the screening for G-6-PD deficiency is a new screening option for the neonatology unit [17]. The basic hematology and clinical chemistry tests are the choice in screening. Concerning the blood smear interpretation, the hemolytic blood picture can be seen. However, as already mentioned, it can be seen only in the cases with exposure to triggers. In addition, the hemolytic anemia can be seen in many disorders, especially tropical infections, therefore, the usefulness of the blood smear interpretation is limited. The classical qualitative hematology test for G-6-PD deficiency screening is methaemoglobin reduction test (MRT): an examination on color change of deficient red cell [22]. The basis of this in-vitro test is a coloric reaction using sodium nitrite and methylene blue chloride reagent [22]. Color change of blood was assessed qualitatively [22]. Diagnosis of G-6-PD deficiency was made if the sample was too dark brown [22]. The sensitivity of this test from the previous study is 85.7 % [23]. Recently, Sanpawat et al. performed a comparative study between the MRT and the G-6-PD activity assay, a quantitative test using enzymatic principle, and reported a higher sensitivity for G-6-PD activity assay [23]. High specificity (98 - 100 %) of both tests was presented [23]. However, that study did not take into account the cost of the laboratory investigation. Since the tropics presently has an economic crisis, the economic concern in the selection of a screening test is necessary. Owa and osanyintuyi compared the MRT screening to the semiquantitative fluorescent screening method (FSM) and found no significant difference [24]. They concluded that since MHRT could be used at room temperature, and since the materials needed were cheap and easy to get and electricity was not essential, most hospitals should be able to use the MHRT method to screen for G-6-PD deficiency [24].

Concerning the semi-quantitative test, the fluorescent screening method is relatively simple. A widely recommended method is described by Simkins *et al.* [25]. Briefly, a 3mm punch from a dried blood spot sample is placed in a well of a black fluorescent microtiter plate containing calibrators and controls in duplicate [25]. 100 microl of reagent is added and the sample is allowed to react for 30 minutes at ambient temperature after which 200 microl of stop reagent is added [25]. The plate may be read immediately or up to one hour in a fluorescent reader [25]. Of interest, glutathione, ascorbate and bilirubin do not affect the assay while hemoglobin does quench the fluorescence by about 1.1 fluorescence units/g/dHb and this would not cause any false negatives and deficients would not be missed [25]. Another interesting semiquantitative screening method is blue formazan spot test (BFST). Pujades *et al.* noted that the sensitivity of screening by BFST is similar to the reference [26].

Ainoon *et al.* studied the semi-quantitative test for screening of G6PD deficiency and found that that 3.9% of G6PD-deficient neonates were missed by the routine fluorescent spot test and they were found to be exclusively females [28]. This study demonstrates a need to use a method that can correctly classify female heterozygotes with partial G6PD deficiency [28].

Concerning the quantitative test, G6PD activity assay is widely used as the reference in the present day. Echler said that measurement of the enzyme in red cell preparations after buffy coat removal permitted more accurate identification of patients with deficient enzyme activity, especially in the presence of anemia and/or leukocytosis [29]. Presently, there are several test kits for G6PD activity from many manufacturers. These test kits are widely used as the references in diagnosis G6PD in many tropical laboratories. Indeed, the most accurate definitive diagnosis of G-6-PD deficiency requires molecular identification [1 – 3] of the defect gene, however, very few laboratories have the ability to carry it out. Furthermore, they require a high skill medical technologist which is not easily available in developing countries. At present, basic screening tests are still necessary for the diagnosis of G6PD deficiency in the tropics.

Management of Glucose-6-Phosphase Dehydrogenase Deficiency

Since individuals with no exposure develop no pathology, there is no need to treat these cases. However, screening for G6PD deficiency is somewhat useful in the area with high endemicity. Chuu *et al.* recently indicated that severe neonatal jaundice can be effectively prevented by neonatal screening for G-6-PD deficiency [30]. Wiwanitkit also recommended the G6PD screening in combination with ABO blood group and Rh blood group as basic screening tests for the neonates with unexplained pathological hyperbilirubinemia [17]. In the non-pediatric population, there is no recommendation for mass screening of G6PD in the tropics. However, in some risk populations, especially the soldiers in the forest where malaria is endemic, screening might be useful. These soldiers are at risk for malarial infection and subsequent antimalarial – stimulated hemolysis if they have G6PD deficiency [30]. To prevent malarial infection in the cases with G6PD deficiency, doxycycline (100 mg/day), not pyrimethamine, should be given [31]

In the affected cases with post-stimulated hemolysis, the treatment is necessary. The general principles of anemia management, increase red blood cell production, decrease red blood cell destruction and red blood cell replacement are recommended. In the extremely severe cases as those with flavism, prompt treatment is necessary. The unwanted complication, tissue hypoperfusion, which can lead to cellular oxidative and peroxidative damage due to biochemical disorders in the oxygen and substrate metabolism, should be controlled [32]. Corbucci said that reduced glutathione could represent a new and interesting therapeutic approach in marked and acute hypoxic conditions [32]. Transfusion therapy is recommended in cases with severe illness. However, treatment by blood transfusion is usually supportive while effective therapy directed to treat the underlying cause of hemolysis, getting rid of the trigger, is needed [33]. Recently, al-Rimawi *et al.* reported that desferrioxamine in a small dose is effective in the treatment of acute haemolytic crises of G6PD deficiency [34]. They proposed that desferrioxamine could shorten the duration of the crisis and decrease the amount of blood transfusion needed [34]. In the neonatal jaundice cases due to the G6PD deficiency, prompt treatment is also necessary as well, in order to prevent the totally unwanted complication, kernicterus [17]. The phototherapy and possible exchange transfusion in the severe jaundice cases are recommended [17, 35]. Concerning mild hemolytic cases, if the cause is an infection, it should be treated and if the cause is a drug, it should be stopped as well. It should be noted that the best management for the cases with G6PD deficiency is prevention from exposure to the possible triggers.

Summary of Glucose-6-Phosphase Dehydrogenase Deficiency in the Tropics

Glucose-6-Phosphase Dehydrogenase Deficiency in Southeast Asia

The prevalence of G6PD deficiency in Southeast Asia is high. This region is the endemic area of malaria, therefore, there is no doubt for this finding. In this region, the prevalence of G6PD deficiency has been continuously studied. In 1999, Tanphaichitr performed a study in the Thais and found that the prevalence of G6PD deficiency in Thai males ranged from 3-18% depending upon the geographic region and G6PD "Mahidol" (163 Gly --> Ser) was the most common variant found in the Thai population [36]. A similar study was performed in the Thai neonates by Nuchprayoon *et al.* [37]. They found the prevalence of G6PD deficiency as 22.1% in males and 10.1% in females [37]. However, they proposed that G6PD Viangchan (871G>A), not G6PD Mahidol, was the most common deficiency variant in the Thai population [37].

Recently, Iwai *et al.* studied the distribution of G6PD deficiency in Southeast Asia in a total of 4317 participants (2019 males, 2298 females) from 16 ethnic groups in Myanmar, Lao in Laos, and Amboinese in Indonesia who were screened with a single-step screening method [38]. They found the prevalence of G6PD deficient males ranged from 0% (the Akha) to 10.8% (the Shan) [38]. According to this study, 10 different missense mutations were identified in 63 G6PD-deficient individuals (50 hemizygotes, 11 heterozygotes, and 2 homozygotes) from 14 ethnic groups [38]. The 487 G-->A (G6PD Mahidol) mutation was widely seen in Myanmar, 383 T-->C (G6PD Vanua Lava) was specifically found among Amboinese, 871 G-->A (G6PD Viangchan) was observed mainly in Lao, and 592 C-->T (G6PD Coimbra) was found in Malaysian aborigines (Orang Asli) [38].

The special consideration of G6PD deficiency in Thailand is the correlation with malarial infection. The theory of natural selection is widely mentioned. Lederer *et al.* studied 192 male malaria patients, 74 cases with G6PD deficiency and 118 without [39]. In this study, the history of dark urine, and the presence of jaundice, haematocrit, total bilirubin and parasite count on day of admission were not significantly different when comparing both groups, and the number of observed complications did not differ either [39]. Lederer *et al.* reported that G6PD deficient patients had significantly less gastrointestinal disturbances, higher serum glutamic oxalacetic transaminase and significantly lower blood urea nitrogen, when compared with the control group [39]. Lederer *et al.* concluded that G-6-PD deficiency, when the variants were aggregated, in male adult patients has no significant influence on the clinical presentation of malaria [39]. In addition to malaria, the correlation with the other common endemic inherited disease, thalassemia and hemohglobinopathies, is of interest. Insiripong *et al.* studied the prevalence of thalassemia/hemoglobinopathies and G-6-PD deficiency in Thai malarial patients [40]. They found that the numbers of thalassemia/hemoglobinopathies in the malaria group and in the control group were not significantly different and also the occurrence of G-6-PD deficiency in the malaria group was not different from that of the controls [40]. In addition, the clinical manifestations of malaria in any group were quite similar [40]. Insiripong *et al.* concluded that there is no protective effect against malaria in thalassemia/hemoglobinopathies or G-6-PD deficiency [40].

Glucose-6-Phosphase Dehydrogenase Deficiency in South Asia

The prevalence of G6PD deficiency in South Asia is slightly lower than that reported in Southeast Asia. Mohanty *et al.* said that the prevalence varied from 0-27% in different caste, ethnic and linguistic groups [41]. They noted that the major clinical manifestations were drug - induced hemolytic anemia, neonatal jaundice and chronic non-spherocytic hemolytic anemia [41]. Thirteen biochemically characterized variants have been reported from India: G6PD Mediterranean (188 Ser-->Phe) is the most common deficient variant in the caste groups, whereas G6PD Orissa is more prevalent among the tribal of India while the third most common variant is G6PD Kerala-Kalyan [41]. Of interest, G6PD Orissa (44 Ala-->Gly) is a well-known G6PD variant in South Asia [42]. Kaeda *et al.* said that G6PD Orissa was responsible for most of the G6PD deficiency in tribal Indian populations but is not found in urban populations, where most of the G6PD deficiency was due to the G6PD Mediterranean variant [42]. They noted that the KmNADP of G6PD Orissa was fivefold higher than that of the normal enzyme, and this might be due to the fact that the alanine residue that was replaced by glycine was part of a putative coenzyme-binding site [42]. The correlation between the G6PD deficiency and malaria in South Asia has been studied as well. Recently, Kar *et al.* studied G6PD status and hemoglobin E (Hb E) among 708 malarial patients and control groups of Ao Nagas in the extreme northeast of India, next to Southeast Asia, where the malaria is endemic [43]. According to this study, it suggested that malaria was an important ecologic factor in maintaining the high frequency of G6PD deficiency and HbE among the Ao Nagas [43]. Kar *et al.* said that although migrations from adjoining populations that had a high frequency of both these traits could have contributed to the presence of these genes in the Ao Nagas, malaria also could be an essential determinant in maintaining the current high frequency in present-day Ao Nagas [43].

Glucose-6-Phosphase Dehydrogenase Deficiency in West Asia

G6PD deficiency in the West Asia is also mentioned. Usanga and Ameen studied the prevalence of G6PD in some countries in West Asia in 2000 [44]. They studied a total of 3,501 male subjects from six Arab countries living in Kuwait and found that the distribution of G6PD deficiency among the different ethnic groups varied widely, ranging from 1 % for Egyptians to 11.55% for Iranians, however, the activity of the normal enzyme was remarkably similar, with values ranging from 6.1 +/- 0.8 to 6.5 +/- 1.1 IU/g Hb [44]. In this study, a low frequency of the Gd(A) allele was found in two ethnic groups, Egyptians (0.019) and Iranians (0.014). Gd(A-) was present at the very low frequency of 0.006 in another two ethnic groups, Kuwaitis and Jordanians [44]. Of interest, the malaria in this region is not endemic, therefore, the correlation between G6PD and malarial infections in this area is rarely mentioned.

Glucose-6-Phosphase Dehydrogenase Deficiency in Latin America

G6PD deficiency in Latin America can also be seen. In Brazil, Saad *et al.* indicated that G6PD A- with the 202 G-->A mutation was the most frequent G6PD deficiency in the population of southeastern Brazil while the remaining variants had a Mediterranean origin [45]. Of interest, these results are in agreement with the origin of the Brazilian population [45]. Recently Hamel *et al.* performed a similar study in 196 Amazonians in Brazil [46]. According to this study, the most frequent G6PD variant was the widespread and common G6PD A- (202G --> A, 376A --> G) observed in 161 subjects (82.1%). Besides this, Hamel *et al.* found another form of G6PD A- (968T --> C, 376A --> G) in 14 (7.1%) individuals, G6PD Seattle (844G --> C) in 4.6%, G6PD Santamaria (542A --> T, 376A --> G) in 2.5%, and G6PD Tokyo (1246G --> A) in one blood donor [46]. In addition, another 4 novel variants were also identified: G6PD Belem (409C --> T; Pro137His), G6PD Ananindeua (376A --> G, 871G --> A; Asn126Asp, Val291Met), G6PD Crispim with four point mutations (375G --> T, 379G --> T, 383T --> C, and 384C --> T) leading to three amino acid substitutions (Met125Ile, Ala127Ser, and Leu128Pro), and G6PD Amazonia (185C --> A; Pro62His) [46].

Glucose-6-Phosphase Dehydrogenase Deficiency in Africa

Similar to Southeast Asia, this area is another highly endemic area for malaria. The high prevalence of G6PD deficiency can also be seen, similar to Southeast Asia [47]. Ademowo and Falusi studied the prevalence of G6PD deficiency in Nigeria [48]. According to this study, G6PD deficiency was 23.9%, with 4.6% in males and females respectively, and only GdA-1 type was found in subjects with deficient variants [48]. In addition, Ademowo and Falusi found that G6PD activity decreased significantly with age among non-deficient individuals but the range of enzyme activities was wide and overlapping among the different G6PD variants [48].

Similar to Southeast Asia, the correlation between G6PD deficiency and malaria in this region is widely studied. In addition, the correlation between G6PD deficiency and the endemic hemoglobionopathy, hemoglobin S (Hb S), is also widely investigated. Recently, Burchard *et al.* studied the spleen size in the patients with sickle cell anemia, HbAC trait and glucose-6-phosphate-dehydrogenase deficiency in a malaria hyperendemic area of Ghana [49]. According to this study, the spleen rates and sizes did not differ significantly between HbAA-, HbAS- and HbAC-positive individuals [49]. Furthermore, enlargement of spleens was found at similar frequencies in persons with and without glucose-6-phosphate-dehydrogenase (G6PD)-deficiency (G6PD-A(-)) [49]. In 2001, Badens *et al.* reported another interesting study on the molecular basis of hemoglobinopathies and G6PD deficiency in the Comorian population [50]. In this study, the molecular study involved 31 alleles carrying the betaS mutation (Cd 6 [A-->T]), six beta-thalassaemic alleles and 17 G6PD-deficient alleles, selected from a group of carriers or affected subjects [50]. Badens *et al.* found that the allele frequencies were 3% for haemoglobin S, 1% for beta-thalassaemia trait and 9.5% for G6PD deficiency [50]. Molecular analysis had revealed that the African alleles are predominant, being present in almost all the subjects studied. Mediterranean alleles were found for all the beta-thalassaemia mutations and for three G6PD chromosomes out of 17 [50]. Badens *et al.* said that these data were consistent with the mixed Arab and African origin of the population of the Comoro Islands, and were of clinical interest in prenatal and newborn screening plans [50]. Finally, Andoka *et al.* found that G6PD deficiency did exist in the Congolese population and that this enzyme deficiency might be more frequent in the carriers of sickle cell trait [51].

References

[1]   Mehta A, Mason PJ, Vulliamy TJ. Glucose-6-phosphate dehydrogenase deficiency. *Baillieres Best Pract Res Clin Haematol* 2000;13:21-38.

[2]   Kaplan M, Hammerman C. Glucose-6-phosphate dehydrogenase deficiency: a potential source of severe neonatal hyperbilirubinaemia and kernicterus. *Semin Neonatol* 2002;7:121-8.

[3]   Evdokimova AI, Ryneiskaia VA, Plakhuta TG. Hemostatic changes in hereditary hemolytic anemias in children. *Pediatriia.* 1979;8:17-21.

[4]   Ruwende C, Hill A. Glucose-6-phosphate dehydrogenase deficiency and malaria. *J Mol Med* 1998;76:581-8.

[5]   Fujii H. Glucose-6-phosphate dehydrogenase. *Nippon Rinsho* 1995;53:1221-5.

[6]   Beutler E. G6PD: population genetics and clinical manifestations. *Blood Rev* 1996;10:45-52.

[7]   Miwa S, Fujii H. Molecular basis of erythroenzymopathies associated with hereditary hemolytic anemia: tabulation of mutant enzymes. *Am J Hematol* 1996;51:122-32.

[8]   Miwa S, Kanno H, Hirono A, Fujii H. Red cell enzymopathies as a model of inborn errors of metabolism. *Southeast Asian J Trop Med Public Health* 1995;26 Suppl 1:112-9.

[9]   Vulliamy T, Mason P, Luzzatto L. The molecular basis of glucose-6-phosphate dehydrogenase deficiency. *Trends Genet* 1992;8:138-43.

[10] Beutler E. Study of glucose-6-phosphate dehydrogenase: history and molecular biology. *Am J Hematol* 1993;42:53-8.

[11] Oliveira S, Pinheiro S, Gomes P, Horta AB, Castro AS. Favism. *Acta Med Port* 2000l;13:237-40.

[12] Holm B, Jensenius M. Favism. Acute hemolysis after intake of fava beans. *Tidsskr Nor Laegeforen* 1998;118:384-5.

[13] Mareni C, Repetto L, Forteleoni G, Meloni T, Gaetani GF. Favism: looking for an autosomal gene associated with glucose-6-phosphate dehydrogenase deficiency. *J Med Genet* 1984;21:278-80.

[14] Kitayaporn D, Charoenlarp P, Pattaraarechachai J, Pholpoti T. G6PD deficiency and fava bean consumption do not produce hemolysis in Thailand. *Southeast Asian J Trop Med Public Health* 1991;22:176-82.

[15] Damonte G, Guida L, Sdraffa A, Benatti U, Melloni E, Forteleoni G, Meloni T, Carafoli E, De Flora A. Mechanisms of perturbation of erythrocyte calcium homeostasis in favism. *Cell Calcium* 1992;13:649-58.

[16] Roth E Jr. Plasmodium falciparum carbohydrate metabolism: a connection between host cell and parasite. *Blood Cells* 1990;16:453-60.

[17] Wiwanitkit V. Laboratory investigation in neonatal jaundice. *Med J Ubon Hosp* 2001; 22: 231-239.

[18] Iranpour R, Akbar MR, Haghshenas I. Glucose-6-phosphate dehydrogenase deficiency in neonates. *Indian J Pediatr* 2003;70:855-7.

[19] Bouma MJ, Goris M, Akhtar T, Khan N, Khan N, Kita E. Prevalence and clinical presentation of glucose-6-phosphate dehydrogenase deficiency in Pakistani Pathan and Afghan refugee communities in Pakistan; implications for the use of primaquine in regional malaria control programmes. *Trans R Soc Trop Med Hyg* 1995;89:62-4.

[20] Peyramond D, Excler JL. Infectious hepatitis, acute hemolysis and glucose-6-phosphate dehydrogenase deficiency. *Ann Med Interne* (Paris) 1983;134:659-62.

[21] Burka ER. Infectious disease: a cause of hemolytic anemia in glucose-6 phosphate dehydrogenase deficiency. *Ann Intern Med* 1969;70:222-5.

[22] Brewer GJ, Tarlov AR, Alving AS. Methemoglobin reduction test - a new, simple in vitro test for identifying primaquine sensitivity. *Bull World Health Organ* 1960; 22: 633 – 40.

[23] Sanpavat S, Nuchprayoon I, Kittikalayawong A, Ungbumnet W. The value of methemoglobin reduction test as a screening test for neonatal glucose 6-phosphate dehydrogenase deficiency. *J Med Assoc Thai.* 2001; 84 Suppl 1:S91-8.

[24] Owa JA, Osanyintuyi VO. Screening for glucose-6-phosphate dehydrogenase (G-6-PD) deficiency by a simple method. *Afr J Med Med Sci* 1988;17:53-5.

[25] Simkins RA, Culp KM. A simple, rapid fluorometric assay for the determination of glucose 6-phosphate dehydrogenase activity in dried blood spot specimens. *Southeast Asian J Trop Med Public Health* 1999;30 Suppl 2:84-6.

[26] Pujades A, Lewis M, Salvati AM, Miwa S, Fujii H, Zarza R, Alvarez R, Rull E, Corrons JL. Evaluation of the blue formazan spot test for screening glucose 6 phosphate dehydrogenase deficiency. *Int J Hematol* 1999;69:234-6.

[27] Ainoon O, Alawiyah A, Yu YH, Cheong SK, Hamidah NH, Boo NY, Zaleha M. Semiquantitative screening test for G6PD deficiency detects severe deficiency but misses a substantial proportion of partially-deficient females. *Southeast Asian J Trop Med Public Health* 2003;34:405-14.

[28] Echler G. Determination of glucose-6-phosphate dehydrogenase levels in red cell preparations. *Am J Med Technol* 1983;49:259-62.

[29] Chuu WM, Lin DT, Lin KH, Chen BW, Chen RL, Lin KS. Can severe neonatal jaundice be prevented by neonatal screening for glucose-6-phosphate dehydrogenase deficiency?--a review of evidence. *Zhonghua Min Guo Xiao Er Ke Yi Xue Hui Za Zhi* 1996;37:333-41.

[30] Karwacki JJ, Shanks GD, Kummalue T, Watanasook C. Primaquine induced hemolysis in a Thai soldier. *Southeast Asian J Trop Med Public Health* 1989;20:555-6.

[31] Shanks GD, Edstein MD, Suriyamongkol V, Timsaad S, Webster HK. Malaria chemoprophylaxis using proguanil/dapsone combinations on the Thai-Cambodian border. *Am J Trop Med Hyg* 1992; 46:643-8.

[32] Corbucci GG. The role of reduced glutathione during the course of acute haemolysis in glucose-6-phosphate dehydrogenase deficient patients: clinical and pharmacodynamic aspects. *Int J Clin Pharmacol Res* 1990;10:305-10.

[33] Tabbara IA. Hemolytic anemias. Diagnosis and management. *Med Clin North Am* 1992;76:649-68.

[34] al-Rimawi HS, al-Sheyyab M, Batieha A, el-Shanti H, Abuekteish F. Effect of desferrioxamine in acute haemolytic anaemia of glucose-6-phosphate dehydrogenase deficiency. *Acta Haematol* 1999;101:145-8.

[35] Kaplan M, Hammerman C. Severe neonatal hyperbilirubinemia. A potential complication of glucose-6-phosphate dehydrogenase deficiency. *Clin Perinatol* 1998;25:575-90.

[36] Tanphaichitr VS. Glucose-6-phosphate dehydrogenase deficiency in Thailand; its significance in the newborn. *Southeast Asian J Trop Med Public* Health 1999;30 Suppl 2:75-8.

[37] Nuchprayoon I, Sanpavat S, Nuchprayoon S. Glucose-6-phosphate dehydrogenase (G6PD) mutations in Thailand: G6PD Viangchan (871G>A) is the most common deficiency variant in the Thai population. *Hum Mutat* 2002;19:185.

[38] Iwai K, Hirono A, Matsuoka H, Kawamoto F, Horie T, Lin K, Tantular IS, Dachlan YP, Notopuro H, Hidayah NI, Salim AM, Fujii H, Miwa S, Ishii A. Distribution of glucose-6-phosphate dehydrogenase mutations in Southeast Asia. *Hum Genet* 2001 ;108:445-9.

[39] Lederer W, Jongsakul K, Pungpak S, Looareesuwan S, Sathawarawong W, Bunnag D. Glucose-6-phosphate dehydrogenase deficiency in Thailand: the influence on the clinical presentation of malaria in male adult patients. *J Trop Med Hyg* 1988;91:151-6.

[40] Insiripong S, Tulayalak P, Amatachaya C. Prevalences ofthalassemia/hemoglobinopathies and G-6-PD deficiency in malaria patients. *J Med Assoc Thai* 1993 Oct;76:554-8.

[41] Mohanty D, Mukherjee MB, Colah RB. Glucose-6-phosphate dehydrogenase deficiency in India. *Indian J Pediatr* 2004;71:525-9.

[42] Kaeda JS, Chhotray GP, Ranjit MR, Bautista JM, Reddy PH, Stevens D, Naidu JM, Britt RP, Vulliamy TJ, Luzzatto L, et al. A new glucose-6-phosphate dehydrogenase variant, G6PD Orissa (44 Ala-->Gly), is the major polymorphic variant in tribal populations in India. *Am J Hum Genet* 1995;57:1335-41.

[43] Kar S, Seth S, Seth PK. Prevalence of malaria in Ao Nagas and its association with G6PD and HbE. *Hum Biol* 1992;64:187-97.

[44] Usanga EA, Ameen R. Glucose-6-phosphate dehydrogenase deficiency in Kuwait, Syria, Egypt, Iran, Jordan and Lebanon. *Hum Hered* 2000;50:158-61.

[45] Saad ST, Salles TS, Carvalho MH, Costa FF. Molecular characterization of glucose-6-phosphate dehydrogenase deficiency in Brazil. *Hum Hered* 1997;47:17-21.

[46] Hamel AR, Cabral IR, Sales TS, Costa FF, Olalla Saad ST. Molecular heterogeneity of G6PD deficiency in an Amazonian population and description of four new variants. *Blood Cells Mol Dis* 2002;28:399-406.

[47] Verjee ZH. Glucose 6-phosphate dehydrogenase deficiency in Africa--review. *East Afr Med J* 1993;70(4 Suppl):40-7.

[48] Ademowo OG, Falusi AG. Molecular epidemiology and activity of erythrocyte G6PD variants in a homogeneous Nigerian population. *East Afr Med J* 2002;79:42-4.

[49] Burchard GD, Browne EN, Sievertsen J, May J, Meyer CG. Spleen size determined by ultrasound in patients with sickle cell trait, HbAC trait and glucose-6-phosphate-dehydrogenase deficiency in a malaria hyperendemic area (Ashanti Region, Ghana). *Acta Trop* 2001;80:103-9.

[50] Badens C, Martinez di Montemuros F, Thuret I, Michel G, Mattei JF, Cappellini MD, Lena-Russo D. Molecular basis of haemoglobinopathies and G6PD deficiency in the Comorian population. *Hematol J* 2000;1:264-8.

[51] Andoka G, Thiloemba, Moussoki J, Djembo-Taty M, Galacteros F. Evaluation of the incidence of glucose-6-phosphate dehydrogenase deficiency in children with sickle cell anemia in Brazzaville (Congo). *Med Trop* (Mars) 1988;48:249-51.

Chapter 11

Nutritional Anemia in Tropical Countries

Introduction to Nutritional Anemia

Nutrition is necessary for human beings. Nutrition deals with the organic process of nourishing or being nourished, by which an organism assimilates food and uses it for growth and maintenance. Nutrition is the way human bodies take in and use food. Basically, there are five different types of nutrients including carbohydrates, fats, proteins, vitamins and minerals. Nutrients, especially carbohydrates, fats and proteins, are necessary because they are the source of energy for human bodies. Of primary importance in this connection is the bioavailability of carbohydrates and fats as a source of energy so that the muscles can produce ATP [1]. The amount of glycogen in the liver and skeletal muscles and possibly the intramuscular triglyceride levels play a pivotal role in this process [1]. Nutrients also promote growth, help repair body tissues, and regulate body functions [1]. Clinical nutritional support became widely accepted as one of the basic tools of patient care, and knowledge of the metabolism of nutrients has been extended [2]. In particular, the significance of micronutrients in systemic function, importance of gut function on the systemic metabolism and immune system, and involvement of amino acids and fat elements in the development and amelioration of specific disease status such as renal and hepatic failure have been recognized, and specific nutritional support has been created as a treatment strategy [2]. In a healthy person, a state of nutritional balance exists: the amount of food eaten is equal to the amount of nutrients utilized in order to ensure the effective functioning of the body and maintain sufficient reserves [3]. The nutritional balance may be upset under various circumstances: decrease in nutrition, increase in losses, increased needs, decreased absorption, and decreased utilization and when this balance is upset for one or more of the identified reasons, a nutrient deficiency arises [3]. Nutritional deficiency is a major health problem, affecting multiple systems in human bodies including the hematopoietic system [3 – 5].

Concerning hematopoiesis, nutrition plays important roles in the process. Nutrients can be both precursors and regulators in the hematopoiesis process. Among the elements which contribute to the formation and development of red corpuscles and to the synthesis of hemoglobin, the following should be noted: iron; other minerals, i.e., copper, zinc, magnesium, cobalt, molybdenum; vitamins, especially folic acid and vitamin B12; and amino acids [3 – 4]. As already mentioned, nutritional imbalance affects the regular hematopoietic system. The impairment of hematopoietic nutrients, nutrient disorder, can lead to the decreased production of red corpuscles hemoglobin, finally presenting as anemia [3]. Presently, anemia is a major nutritional global problem of public health significance, affecting persons of all ages, sex and economic group [3 - 5]. In medicine, nutritional anemia is the term used for the anemia relating to nutritional defects. Nutritional anemia is a pathologic condition where hemoglobin or hematocrit level becomes abnormally low because of low essential nutrients regardless of the cause of these deficiencies [3 - 5]. Diaz et al. mentioned that micronutrient deficiencies, also known as "hidden hunger", were determining and aggravating factors for health status and quality of life [5]. However, it should be noted that both undernutrition and overnutrition can lead to anemia. In developing countries like those in the tropics, foods are usually insufficient. The nutritional anemia has major consequences not only on the morbidity and mortality in children but also affects growth and intellectual development of these children [3 – 5]. Hercberg and Rouaud said that nutritional anemia could only be overcome if its prevalence, and the respective prevalences of iron, folic acid, and/or vitamin B12 deficiencies, were accurately determined for various population groups through reliable epidemiological studies [3]. They also said that the effective management must cover other factors contributing to the development of nutritional anemia including lack of food, certain customs and habits, and parasitoses [3]. They mentioned that an increase in available foodstuffs, better utilization of resources, and better living conditions led to more balanced nutrition [3].

Anemia and Carbohydrate Malnutrition

Carbohydrate is the major nutrient giving energy or calories to human beings. Pure carbohydrate effects on erythropoiesis are few, however, the compound between carbohydrate and protein, glycoprotein, plays several roles. Human erythropoietin also contains carbohydrate, it is a 30 kDa glycoprotein [6]. It is composed of 165 amino acids and 4 carbohydrate side chains [6]. Erythropoietin maintains red cell production by inhibiting apoptosis of erythrocytic progenitors, and by stimulating their proliferation and differentiation into normoblasts. Lack of erythropoietin results in anemia [6]. Pathologically, a glycolipid namely glycosylphosphatidylinositol (GPI)-anchored molecules is confirmed for its roles in paroxysmal nocturnal hemoglobinuria (PNH) [7 - 8].

Anemia due to carbohydrate malnutrition is also mentioned. In severe protein-calories malnutriton, kwashiorkor, anemia is common [9 - 10]. Glutathione (gamma-glutamyl-cysteinyl-glycine; GSH), the most abundant low-molecular-weight thiol, deficiency is noted for its correspondence to kwashiorkor [11]. In diabetes mellitus, a well-known disorder of carbohydrate metabolism, anemia can be seen. In 2002, Pinero-Pilona et al. said that some patients with new-onset diabetes have a mild normochromic normocytic anemia that was not attributable to usual causes, such as infection, pancreatitis, or blood loss [12]. They proposed that improvement in glycemic control tended to be associated with normalization of hemoglobin levels [12]. They proposed that the cause of such cases of anemia might be either direct "glucose toxicity" to erythrocyte precursors in the bone marrow or perhaps oxidative stress to mature erythrocytes [12]. However, those finding might be only accidental findings. Recently, Soogarun et al. studied the effect of glucose on platelet, another blood cell series, and found a null effect [13].

Anemia and Protein Malnutrition

Several proteins play important roles in the hematopoietic process [14]. Amino acids, the minute compositions of proteins, are important precursors and regulators of erythropoiesis [14]. It is no doubt that protein deficiency can lead to anemia [15].

Nutritional anemia in protein energy malnutrition is an important aspect in clinical nutrition [9 – 10 , 16]. Politt noted that the social environment moderates the effects of an early nutritional insult; it can keep such effect unchanged, or increase or decrease its severity [17]. Vertongen et al. performed a study on the hemolytic anemia observed in protein energy malnutrition in Kivu [18]. They found that the in vitro resistance to oxidative aggressions of the patients' erythrocytes was decreased: when incubated with acetylphenylhydrazine, a higher percentage of the cells showed Heinz bodies, as compared with erythrocytes of local controls [18]. Normal or increased activities were found for certain erythrocyte enzymes involved in the detoxification of activated oxygen: glucose-6-phosphate dehydrogenase, 6-phosphogluconate dehydrogenase and glutathione reductase, however, the level of reduced glutathione was not decreased [18]. In addition, reduced activities were observed for two enzymes containing trace elements: glutathione peroxidase and superoxide dismutase [18]. Vertongen et al. suggested that the shortened erythrocyte lifespan observed in the patients with protein energy malnutrition corresponds to an oxidative process which results from the decrease of both enzyme activities [18]. Mandelbaum et al. also concluded that slight erythrocyte glycolytic abnormalities may occur in the anaemia of Kivu protein energy malnutrition, but that they are not the main cause of the haemolysis observed in this syndrome [19]. In the cases with protein deficiency, Lipschitz and Mitchell noted that hyperalimentation corrected nutritional deficit and returned immune and hematopoietic abnormalities to near normal levels [20].

Anemia and Lipid Malnutrition

Similar to carbohydrate and protein, lipid is also necessary for hematopoeiesis. The adipocyte is the most abundant stromal cell phenotype in adult human bone marrow [21]. Gimble et al. said that adipocytes might share common functions with stromal stem cells, osteoblasts, and hematopoietic supportive cells [21]. Four hypotheses are mentioned: 1) adipocytes may serve a passive role, simply occupying excess space in the bone marrow cavity, 2) they may play an active role in systemic lipid metabolism, 3) adipocytes may provide a localized energy reservoir in the bone marrow and 4) marrow adipocytes may contribute directly to the promotion of hematopoiesis and influence osteogenesis [21]. Defect in lipid can lead to anemia. Congenital Dyserythropoietic anemias (CDAs) is an example of inheried anemia due to lipid defect [22]. In CDA, the red cell membrane is abnormal in at least CDA I and II [22]. Concerning the pathogenesis, a major breakthrough was the identification of the gene, the mutations of which cause CDA I [22]. Delaunay said that the occurrence of lipid rafts in the red cell starts being documented [22]. Delaunay also mentioned that GPI-anchored proteins and a number of minor proteins associated with the rafts allow foreseeing a chapter of great novelty in red cell membrane physiology [22]. PNH is another anemic disease with evidence for lipid defect. This disease is a unique clonal stem cell disorder characterized by intravascular hemolysis, thrombotic events and bone marrow failure [7 – 8, 23]. Meletis and Terpos said that the development of PNH requires not only a somatic mutation of the phospatidylinositol glycan complementation class A (PIG-A) gene, but also a survival advantage of the PNH clone ('dual pathogenesis' theory) [23].

Hypolipidemia is mentioned for its association with anemia [24 – 25]. Noseda said that secondary hypolipidemias were associated with malabsorption, malnutrition and maldigestion including protein-losing gastroenteropathy, with liver diseases, endocrine diseases (hyperthyroidism, hirsutism) and anemia [26]. Yokoyama *et al.* suggested that low serum lipids implied severe bone marrow failure in children with aplastic anemia [27]. Recently, Hartman *et al.* also noted the findings of hypocholesterolemia in the patients with thalassemia, an inherited anemic disorder [28]. Concerning hypertriglyceridemia, a common disorder of lipid metabolism, its correlation to anemia is also documented. Tanzer *et al.* reported that iron deficiency anemia might be linked to the endogenous carnitine synthesis in pediatric age group, and thus hyperlipidemia appeared to be a risk factor for premature cardiovascular diseases [29].

Anemia and Vitamin Malnutrition

Vitamins are important nutrients acting as a regulator in several metabolisms.

In medicine, there are several vitamins, both soluble and non-soluble. Several vitamins are mentioned for their correlation to anemic disorders. Concerning vitamin A, the role of vitamin A deficiency as a contributing factor to anemia has been examined. Vitamin A appears to be involved in the pathogenesis of anemia through diverse biological mechanisms, such as the enhancement of growth and differentiation of erythrocyte progenitor cells, potentiation of immunity to infection and reduction of the anemia of infection, and mobilization of iron stores from tissues [30]. Vitamin A can improve hematological indicators and enhance the efficacy of iron supplementation [31]. Xerophthalmia is now recognized as a late manifestation of severe deficiency [32]. Milder deficiency increases the severity of infectious morbidity, exacerbates iron deficiency anemia, retards growth, and is responsible for one to three million childhood deaths each year [32]. Epidemiological surveys show that the prevalence of anemia is high in populations affected by vitamin A deficiency in developing tropical countries [30]. Semba RD, Bloem said that improvement of vitamin A status had generally been shown to reduce anemia [30]. Control of vitamin A deficiency is now a major health challenge and goal of both UNICEF and the World Health Organization (WHO) [32].

Concerning vitamin B1 or thiamine, it is required for all tissues and is found in high concentrations in skeletal muscle, heart, liver, kidneys and brain [33]. Thiamine diphosphate is the active form of thiamine, and it serves as a cofactor for several enzymes involved primarily in carbohydrate catabolism and the enzymes are important in the biosynthesis of a number of cell constituents, including neurotransmitters, and for the production of reducing equivalents used in oxidant stress defenses and in biosyntheses and for synthesis of pentoses used as nucleic acid precursors [33]. Thiamine uptake by the small intestines and by cells within various organs is mediated by a saturable, high affinity transport system [33]. Alcohol affects thiamine uptake and other aspects of thiamine utilization, and these effects may contribute to the prevalence of thiamine deficiency in alcoholics [33]. The major manifestations of thiamine deficiency in humans involve the cardiovascular (wet beriberi) and nervous (dry beriberi, or neuropathy and/or Wernicke-Korsakoff syndrome) systems [33]. Singleton and Martin noted that a number of inborn errors of metabolism had been described in which clinical improvements can be documented following administration of pharmacological doses of thiamine, such as thiamine-responsive megaloblastic anemia (TRMA) [33]. TRMA is an autosomal recessive disorder with features that include megaloblastic anemia, mild thrombocytopenia and leukopenia, sensorineural deafness and diabetes mellitus [34]. Genetically, the disease is caused by mutations in the SLC19A2 gene encoding a high-affinity thiamine transporter [34]. Blood transfusion is useless for correction of anemia in TRMA [35]. Treatment with pharmacological doses of thiamine ameliorates the megaloblastic anemia and diabetes mellitus [34].

Concerning vitamin B2 or riboflavin, it is unique among the water-soluble vitamins in that milk and dairy products make the greatest contribution to its intake in Western diets [36]. Meat and fish are also good sources of riboflavin, and certain fruit and vegetables, especially dark-green vegetables, contain reasonably high concentrations [36]. Riboflavin enhances the hematological response to iron, and its deficiency may account for a significant proportion of anemia in many populations [31]. Powers said that poor riboflavin status interfered with iron handling and contributes to the etiology of anemia when iron intakes are low, however, various mechanisms for this have been proposed, including effects on the gastrointestinal tract that might compromise the handling of other nutrients [36]. Riboflavin deficiency might exert some of its effects by reducing the metabolism of other B vitamins, notably folate and vitamin B 6 [36 - 37].

Concerning vitamin B6 or pyroxidine, it is also described for its association with anemia [38]. Sideroblastic anemia is the most common anemia mentioned for the correlation to vitamin B 6 [38]. Fishman et al. mentioned that vitamin B6 effectively treats sideroblastic anemia [31]. In the patients with sideroblastic anemia, hypochromic microcytic red cell appearance can be seen. Bone marrow smear always shows a normocellular marrow with augmented severely dysplastic erythropoesis and Prussian-blue staining revealed an increased number of ring sideroblasts [39 - 40]. Pyridoxine-responsive, X-linked sideroblastic anaemia (XLSA) has been shown to be caused by missense mutations in the erythroid-specific ALA synthase gene, ALAS2 [39 - 40]. A loose correlation has been found between the in vitro kinetics and stability of the catalytic activity of the recombinant variant enzymes and the in vivo severity and pyridoxine-responsiveness of the anemia [39]. Enhanced instability in the absence of pyridoxal phosphate (PLP) or decreased PLP and substrate binding have been noted [39]. Mutations in the same gene which affect mitochondrial processing, terminate translation prematurely, or are thought to abolish function altogether causing an XLSA[39]. A major complication of this disorder is its accompanying increased iron absorption and iron overload which occurs in patients and female heterozygotes [39]. Concerning treatment, this type of anemia is responding well to pyridoxine treatment [39 – 40].

Concerning vitamin B 12, there are numerous evidences that the deficiency of vitamin B12 can lead to megaloblastic anemia. An association between neuropsychiatric disorders and vitamin B12 deficiency has been recognized since 1849 when pernicious anemia was first described [41]. It has been suggested that deficiency of vitamin B12 might contribute to age-associated cognitive impairment [42]. Malouf et al. said that low serum vitamin B12 concentrations were found in more than 10% of older people. They also noted that a high prevalence of low serum vitamin B12 levels, and other indicators of vitamin B12 deficiency, had been reported among people with Alzheimer's disease [42]. Although readily treatable with vitamin B12, pernicious anemia continues to captivate investigative endeavors of those interested in the pathophysiology and pathogenesis of this disorder [41]. Notable advances have been made in understanding properties of intrinsic factor, vitamin B12-binding proteins, structure and de novo synthesis of vitamin B12, mechanism of action of vitamin B12-dependent enzymes in man, and metabolic consequences of reduced activities of these enzymes in pernicious anemia [41]. Both cellular and humoral factors may contribute to immune-mediated processes in pernicious anemia, although as yet, it has not been established with certainty that pernicious anemia is an autoimmune disorder [41]. Apart from the pernicious anemia, vitamin B 12 deficiency induced anemia can be seen in the patients with alcoholism. It can also be seen in vegans. Concerning the laboratory investigations relating to diagnosis of vitamin B 12 deficiency are macrocytic isocytic red blood cell in peripheral blood smear, hypersegmented neutrophil in peripheral blood smear and increase mean corpuscular volume (MCV). However, the best confirmation test is the determination of blood vitamin B 12 level. In cases that the blood vitamin B 12 is less than < 100 pg/ml, the definitive diagnosis is mage. Since the determination of vitamin B12 level required a complicated analyzer, there is also the application of the mathematical model for determination of blood vitamin B 12 [43]. However, Oh and Brown recently noted that diagnosis of vitamin B12 deficiency was typically based on measurement of serum vitamin B12 levels; however, about 50 percent of patients with subclinical disease have normal B12 levels [44]. They proposed a more sensitive method of screening for vitamin B12 deficiency as measurement of serum methylmalonic acid and homocysteine levels, which were increased early in vitamin B12 deficiency [44].

Similar evidences are documented for the megaloblastic anemia due to folate or vitamin F deficiency. Both folate and vitamin B12 can cure and prevent megaloblastic anemia [31]. Li et al. said that the vitamin that is most commonly deficient in the American diet was folate [45]. Severe folate deficiency in humans is known to cause megaloblastic anemia and developmental defects, especially neural tube defect, and is associated with an increased incidence of several forms of human cancer [45]. Li et al. said that although the exact mechanisms by which this vitamin deficiency might cause these diseases were not known at the present time, recent work had shown that folate deficiency also causes genomic instability and programmed cell death or apoptosis [45]. It is known that the DNA mismatch repair pathway mediates folate deficiency-induced apoptosis [45]. Similar to vitamin B 12 deficiency, alcoholism and vegetarianism can be the contributing factor to folate deficiency. The laboratory investigations relating to diagnosis of folate deficiency is similar to vitamin B 12 deficiency. Methionine metabolism is regulated by folate, and both folate deficiency and abnormal hepatic methionine metabolism are recognized features of alcoholic liver disease (ALD) and abnormal methionine metabolism and hepatocellular apoptosis develop in the cases with ALD [46]. Halsted et al. said that folate deficiency promoted and folate sufficiency protected against the early onset of methionine cycle-mediated ALD [46]. The determination of blood folate level is still the definitive diagnostic tool and the mathematical model is also developed to simplify the determination [44].

Concerning vitamin C, it enhances the absorption of dietary iron, although population-based data showing its efficacy in reducing anemia or iron deficiency are lacking [31]. Vitamin C deficiency or scurvy is a common nutritional disorder in the rural areas of the tropics. Unlike most animals, which form ascorbic acid by metabolizing glucose, humans require an exogenous source [47]. Vitamin C occurs primarily in fruits and vegetables, and scurvy develops from inadequate consumption of these sources, usually because of ignorance about proper nutrition, psychiatric disorders, alcoholism, or social isolation [47]. The earliest symptom of scurvy, occurring only after many weeks of deficient intake, is fatigue while the most common cutaneous findings are follicular hyperkeratosis, perifollicular hemorrhages, ecchymoses, xerosis, leg edema, poor wound healing, and bent or coiled body hairs [47]. Gum abnormalities, which occur only in patients with teeth, include gingival swelling, purplish discoloration, and hemorrhages [47]. Anemia is frequent, leukopenia occasional [47]. Hirschmann and Raugi said that treatment with vitamin C results in rapid, often dramatic, improvement [47].

Concerning vitamin D, it should be noted that the anemia and thrombocytopenia were the results of myelofibrosis, which was secondary to vitamin D deficiency [48]. Refractory anemias and the myelodysplastic syndromes are a group of hematopoietic stem cell disorders characterized by ineffective and dysplastic hematopoiesis, leading to persistent peripheral cytopenias [49]. Since defective cellular maturation is the central pathogenetic feature, improved differentiation may result in correction of neutropenia and thrombocytopenia [49]. However, al-Eissa and al-Mashhadani noted that clinical trials using retinoic acid and vitamin D3 analogues are not satisfactory and only small numbers of patients may benefit from receiving them [49].

Concerning vitamin E or alpha-tocopherol, there is now convincing evidence that vitamin E is a specific erythropoietic factor for nonhuman primates and swine, however, there is no evidence that vitamin E is normally required as an erythropoietic factor for humans and many species of animals [50]. Drake and Fitch proposed that the lack of a requirement for vitamin E in erythropoiesis in humans is due to a metabolic adaptation that circumvents the need for the role that the vitamin otherwise would serve and there was reason to believe that this metabolic adaptation is deranged in patients with protein calorie malnutrition [50]. They noted that the patients with protein calorie malnutrition responded with reticulocytosis and a limited increase in hemoglobin concentration when vitamin E was given before their metabolic derangement is reversed by correcting their other nutritional deficiencies [50]. In addition, some proposed that vitamin E relates to anemia of prematurity. . It has been thought that deficiency of vitamin E is at least partly responsible for the anemia which often occurs 4 to 6 wk after premature birth, and routine dietary supplementation with vitamin E is frequently recommended [51]. However, Fishman et al. mentioned that vitamin E supplementation given to preterm infants had not reduced the severity of the anemia of prematurity [31].

Concerning vitamin K, many disorders due to deficiency of the vitamin K-dependent clotting factors are described [52]. Vitamin K deficiency can occur in the newborn, or at later stages in life when there is intestinal malabsorption [52]. The anemia due to the hemorrhagic episodes in vitamin K deficiency can be expected [53].

In addition, it is noted that hemolytic uremic syndrome accompanied with vitamin K deficiency can make it more easy to bleed [54].

Anemia and Mineral Malnutrition

Several minerals are mentioned for the correlation to anemia. Many biometals play important roles in the erythropoietic processes. The main biometals relating to anemia include iron, copper, zinc, selenenium and cobalt [55]. It is well documented that iron deficiency can lead to hypochromic microcytic anemia. This anemia is the most common type of anemia in all age groups all over the world. The details of the iron deficiency anemia will be presented in another chapter. Concerning copper, copper deficiency is usually the consequence of decreased copper stores at birth, inadequate dietary copper intake, poor absorption, elevated requirements induced by rapid growth, or increased copper losses [56]. The most frequent clinical manifestations of copper deficiency are anemia, neutropenia, and bone abnormalities [56]. Other, less frequent manifestations are hypopigmentation of the hair, hypotonia, impaired growth, increased incidence of infections, alterations of phagocytic capacity of the neutrophils, abnormalities of cholesterol and glucose metabolism, and cardiovascular alterations [57]. Measurements of serum copper and ceruloplasmin concentrations are currently used to evaluate copper status [57]. Wilson's disease is an inherited disorder of copper transport in the organism, transmitted in autosomal recessive fashion [58]. It is caused by dysfunction in homologous copper-transporting adenosine triphosphatases [58]. Grudeva-Popova et al. noted that hemolytic anemia was a recognized but rare (10-15%) complication of the disease [58]. They noted that most often Coombs' negative acute intravascular hemolysis occurred as a consequence of oxidative damage to the erythrocytes by the higher copper concentration [58]. However, it should be noted that hemolytic anemia as the other complication of Wilson's disease can be the result of other etiology such as hepatitis viral coinfection [59].

Concerning zinc, zinc takes part in the catalytic function of many metalloenzymes: it plays a role in conformational stability [60]. Of the intracellular zinc, only a small part is bound to metalloenzymes, most being coordinated to binding sites of nonspecific proteins [60]. It is noted that a syndrome of zinc deficiency associated with anaemia, hepatosplenomegaly, dwarfism, and hypogonadism is known [60 - 62]. Concerning selenium,

selenium deficiency has been associated with cases of congestive cardiomyopathy, skeletal myopathy, anemia, enhanced cancer risk, elevated incidence of cardiovascular disease, immune system alterations, hair and nail changes, and abnormalities in thyroid hormone metabolism [63]. Of interest, Bonomini and Albertazzi said that these symptoms are frequently present in chronic uremic patients and supposed pathogenetic mechanisms of selenium disturbance in uremia, and the possible role of selenium deficiency on some uremic abnormalities [63]. Concerning cobalt, cobalt is an unique trace element for man as it can only reveal its essential properties if provided directly as its biological active form, cobalamin or vitamin B12, the daily requirement of which is 1 to 2 micrograms in adults [64]. Since cobalt is an important composition of vitamin B 12, therefore, the correlation between cobalt and anemia is not in doubt.

Summary of Nutritional Anemia in the Tropics

Nutritional anemia, the most widespread nutritional disorder in the world, affects mainly developing countries and to a lesser extent developed nations [3]. It is estimated that 500 million to 1 billion individuals in the world are affected by nutritional anemia [3]. Unavailability of foods remains the main public health problem in the tropics. Besides deficiencies of food-specific nutrients like iron, folic acid, B12 protein, vitamin C, vitamin E, trace elements are common in those developing countries [3 – 5]. In addition, poor health facilities, poor socioeconomic status, faulty dietary patterns, the degree of urbanization, ethnic background, prevalence of hook worm and other worm infestations, repeated bacterial infections also influence the incidence of nutritional anemia particularly in children [3 – 5]. Here, the summary of nutritional anemia in different areas in the tropics is presented.

Nutritional Anemia in Tropical Asia

South Asia is always mentioned for nutritional health problems.
Concerning nutritional anemia, there are several interesting reports from South Asia.
It should be noted that anemia is the most common nutritional problem in India affecting more than half of the total population, particularly in children and pregnant women. Available studies on the prevalence of nutritional anemia in India show that 65% infant and toddlers, 60% 1-6 years of age, 88% adolescent girls (3.3% had hemoglobin < 7.0 g/dl; severe anemia) and 85% pregnant women (9.9% having severe anemia) were anemic [65]. Kapur *et al.* said that the prevalence of anemia was marginally higher in lactating women as compared to pregnant women and the commonest was iron deficiency anemia [65]. A national program to combat nutritional anemia in India has been launched [66]. The program solicits the support of various departments in implementing dietary modification and supplementation measures: 1) pregnant women are recommended to have one big tablet per day for 100 days after the first trimester of pregnancy; a similar dose applies to lactating women and IUD acceptors, 2) preschool children (ages 1-5 years) are recommended to take

one small tablet per day for 100 days every year and 3) for treatment of severe anemia, women in the reproductive age group are recommended to take three adult tablets per day for a minimum of 100 days [66]. Kapur *et al.* said that national programmes to control and prevent anemia have not been successful [65]. They proposed that nutrition education to improve dietary intakes in families for receiving needed macro/micro nutrients as protein, iron and vitamins like folic acid, B12, A and C for hemoglobin synthesis was important and medicinal iron was necessary to control anemia [65]. They also noted that addition of folate with iron controlled anemia and was neuroprotective [65].

Of interest, there are nutritional anemic cases due to the local belief in South Asia. Megaloblastic anaemia in the vegetarian Hindu communities are mentioned [66].

The nutritional problem in Southeast Asia still exists, especially in the rural community settings. Recently Wiwanitkti and Sodsri performed a study in a rural area near the Thai-Cambodia border and found that being underweight is still the problem of the children there [66]. Iron deficiency anemia is the most common nutritional anemic problem in Southeast Asia [68]. Luckily, Gopalan said that food production in the countries of South and South-East Asia has shown a general upward trend during the last decade despite the considerable increase in population in many of these countries: the increase being specially marked in such countries as Vietnam, Cambodia, Indonesia, and Malaysia [69]. A correlation between nutritional anemia and other tropical anemias, especially hemoglobinopathies and malarial infection, are also considerable problem in Southeast Asia [70]. Similar to South Asia, megaloblastic anemia due to vegetarianism in some Buddhism groups can be seen. The nutritional anemia can be seen in West Asia as well. Iron deficiency anemia is also the most common type of nutritional anemia. However, the data on the nutritional anemia in West Asia is not as much as those of Southeast Asia and South Asia [70].

Nutritional Anemia in Tropical Africa

Concerning Africa, it is the most problematic area of the world for the nutritional health problem. Numerous nutritional surveillances in the African population have been continuously performed. Masawe noted that nutritional anemia, including iron-deficiency anaemia, megaloblastic anaemia due to folate deficiency or vitamin B12 deficiency, or both, and protein deficiency-anemia was widespread throughout Africa and it was particularly common in growing children, women of child-bearing age, pregnant women and lactating mothers [71]. Masawe said that the anemia was also especially common during the second half of the dry season and the first half of the wet season, when food supplies were limited. Masawe indicated that in all cases, the anemia was caused either by limited dietary intake, excessive loss of nutrients or excessive utilization [71]. Masawe also mentioned that the evidence in favor of increased susceptibility to infections in megaloblastic anemia and protein-deficiency anemia was overwhelming, but in iron-deficiency anemia the available information argues in favor of reduced susceptibility to infections, except after initiation of iron therapy [71]. Masawe proposed that the treatment of nutritional anemia should include replacement of the deficient nutrients and blood transfusion in severe cases, prevention of further nutrient losses and treatment of associated complications [71]. Similar to Southeast

Asia, a correlation between nutritional anemia and other tropical anemias, especially hemoglobinopathies and malarial infection, should also be considered [71].

References

[1]   Saris WH, van Loon LJ. Nutrition and health--nutrition and performance in sports. *Ned Tijdschr Geneeskd* 2004;148:708-12.

[2]   Iwasaki T, Ohyanagi H. Advance and perspective of clinical nutrition. *Nippon Geka Gakkai Zasshi.* 2004;105:196-9.

[3]   Hercberg S, Rouaud C. Nutritional anaemia. *Child Trop* 1981;(133):1-36.

[4]   Campbell K. Anaemia: causes and treatment. *Nurs Times* 2003;99:30-3.

[5]   Diaz JR, de las Cagigas A, Rodriguez R. Micronutrient deficiencies in developing and affluent countries. *Eur J Clin Nutr* 2003;57 Suppl 1:S70-2.

[6]   Jelkmann W, Metzen E. Erythropoietin in the control of red cell production. *Anat Anz* 1996;178:391-403.

[7]   Shichishima T, Noji H. A new aspect of the molecular pathogenesis of paroxysmal nocturnal hemoglobinuria. *Hematology* 2002;7:211-27.

[8]   Hall C, Richards SJ, Hillmen P. The glycosylphosphatidylinositol anchor and paroxysmal nocturnal haemoglobinuria/aplasia model. *Acta Haematol* 2002;108:219-30.

[9]   Pereira SM, Begum A. The manifestations and management of severe protein-calorie malnutrition (kwashiorkor). *World Rev Nutr Diet* 1974;19:1-50.

[10]   The anemia of Kwashiorkor. *Nutr Rev* 1968;26:273-5.

[11]   Wu G, Fang YZ, Yang S, Lupton JR, Turner ND. Glutathione metabolism and its implications for health. *J Nutr* 2004;134:489-92.

[12]   Pinero-Pilona A, Litonjua P, Devaraj S, Aviles-Santa L, Raskin P. Anemia associated with new-onset diabetes: improvement with blood glucose control. *Endocr Pract* 2002;8:276-81.

[13]   Soogarun S, Wiwanitkit V, Suwansaksri J. Platelet count neither decreases nor relates to blood glucose level. *Clin Appl Thromb Hemost* 2004;10:187-8.

[14]   Motoyoshi K. Molecular mechanism of hematopoiesis and its clinical presentation. *Nippon Naika Gakkai Zasshi* 2004;93 Suppl:52-6.

[15]   Adams EB. Anemia associated with protein deficiency. *Semin Hematol* 1970;7:55-66

[16]   Desai N, Choudhry VP. Nutritional anemia in protein energy malnutrition. *Indian Pediatr* 1993;30:1471-83.

[17]   Pollitt E. Developmental sequel from early nutritional deficiencies: conclusive and probability judgements. *J Nutr* 2000;130(2S Suppl):350S-353S.

[18]   Vertongen F, Heyder-Bruckner C, Fondu P, Mandelbaum I. Oxidative haemolysis in protein malnutrition. *Clin Chim Acta* 1981;116:217-22.

[19]   Mandelbaum IM, Mozes N, Fondu P. Erythrocyte glycolysis in protein-energy malnutrition. *Clin Chim Acta* 1982;124:263-75.

[20] Lipschitz DA, Mitchell CO. The correctability of the nutritional, immune, and hematopoietic manifestations of protein calorie malnutrition in the elderly. *J Am Coll Nutr* 1982;1:17-25.

[21] Gimble JM, Robinson CE, Wu X, Kelly KA. The function of adipocytes in the bone marrow stroma: an update. *Bone* 1996;19:421-8.

[22] Delaunay J. Red cell membrane and erythropoiesis genetic defects. *Hematol J* 2003;4:225-32.

[23] Meletis J, Terpos E. Recent insights into the pathophysiology of paroxysmal nocturnal hemoglobinuria. *Med Sci Monit* 2003;9:RA161-72.

[24] Rifkind B, Gale M. Hypolipidemia in anemia. *Am Heart J* 1968;76:849-50.

[25] Hashima JA, Afroz N. Hypolipidemia in anemia. *Am Heart* J 1969;78:840.

[26] 26. Noseda G. Hypolipidemias. *Schweiz Med Wochenschr* 1975;105:1233-7.

[27] Yokoyama M, Suto Y, Sato H, Arai K, Waga S, Kitazawa J, Maruyama H, Ito E. Low serum lipids suggest severe bone marrow failure in children with aplastic anemia. *Pediatr Int* 2000;42:613-9.

[28] Hartman C, Tamary H, Tamir A, Shabad E, Levine C, Koren A, Shamir R. Hypocholesterolemia in children and adolescents with beta-thalassemia intermedia. *J Pediatr* 2002;141:543-7.

[29] Tanzer F, Hizel S, Cetinkaya O, Sekreter E. Serum free carnitine and total triglycerid levels in children with iron deficiency anemia. *Int J Vitam Nutr Res* 2001;71:66-9.

[30] Semba RD, Bloem MW. The anemia of vitamin A deficiency: epidemiology and pathogenesis. *Eur J Clin Nutr* 2002;56:271-81.

[31] Fishman SM, Christian P, West KP. The role of vitamins in the prevention and control of anaemia. *Public Health Nutr* 2000;3:125-50.

[32] Sommer A. Xerophthalmia and vitamin A status. *Prog Retin Eye Res* 1998;17:9-31.

[33] Singleton CK, Martin PR. Molecular mechanisms of thiamine utilization. *Curr Mol Med* 2001;1:197-207.

[34] Ozdemir MA, Akcakus M, Kurtoglu S, Gunes T, Torun YA. TRMA syndrome (thiamine-responsive megaloblastic anemia): a case report and review of the literature. *Pediatr Diabetes* 2002;3:205-9.

[35] Rosskamp R, Zigrahn W, Burmeister W. Thiamine-dependent anemia and thrombocytopenia, insulin-dependent diabetes mellitus and sensorineural deafness--case report and review. *Klin Padiatr* 1985;197:315-7.

[36] Powers HJ. Riboflavin (vitamin B-2) and health. *Am J Clin Nutr* 2003;77:1352-60.

[37] Cherstvova LG. Biological role of vitamin B2 in iron deficiency anemia. *Gematol Transfuziol* 1984;29:47-50.

[38] Vitamin B6 (pyridoxine and pyridoxal 5'-phosphate) - monograph. *Altern Med Rev* 2001;6:87-92.

[39] May A, Bishop DF. The molecular biology and pyridoxine responsiveness of X-linked sideroblastic anaemia. *Haematologica* 1998;83:56-70.

[40] Heller T, Hochstetter V, Basler M, Borck V. Vitamin B6-sensitive hereditary sideroblastic anemia. *Dtsch Med Wochenschr* 2004;129:141-4.

[41] Kass L. Newer aspects of pernicious anemia. CRC Crit Rev Clin Lab Sci 1978;9:1-47

[42] Malouf R, Areosa Sastre A. Vitamin B12 for cognition. *Cochrane Database Syst Rev* 2003;(3):CD004326

[43] Wiwanitkit V. Mathematical model for vitamin B12 and folate from RIA correlation curve, a short report. *Asean J Radiol* 2002;8:163-165.

[44] Oh R, Brown DL. Vitamin B12 deficiency. *Am Fam Physician* 2003;67:979-86.

[45] Li GM, Presnell SR, Gu L. Folate deficiency, mismatch repair-dependent apoptosis, and human disease. *J Nutr Biochem* 2003;14:568-75.

[46] Halsted CH, Villanueva JA, Devlin AM. Folate deficiency, methionine metabolism, and alcoholic liver disease. *Alcohol* 2002;27:169-72.

[47] Hirschmann JV, Raugi GJ. Adult scurvy. *J Am Acad Dermatol* 1999;41:895-906.

[48] Gruner BA, DeNapoli TS, Elshihabi S, Britton HA, Langevin AM, Thomas PJ, Weitman SD. Anemia and hepatosplenomegaly as presenting features in a child with rickets and secondary myelofibrosis. *J Pediatr Hematol Oncol* 2003;25:813-5.

[49] al-Eissa YA, al-Mashhadani SA. Myelofibrosis in severe combined immunodeficiency due to vitamin D deficiency rickets. *Acta Haematol.* 1994;92:160-3.

[50] Drake JR, Fitch CD. Status of vitamin E as an erythropoietic factor. *Am J Clin Nutr* 1980;33:2386-93.

[51] Bell EF, Filer LJ Jr. The role of vitamin E in the nutrition of premature infants. *Am J Clin Nutr* 1981;34:414-22.

[52] Prentice CR. Acquired coagulation disorders. *Clin Haematol* 1985;14:413-42.

[53] Nishio T, Nohara R, Aoki S, Sai HS, Izumi H, Miyoshi K, Morikawa Y, Mizuta R. Intracranial hemorrhage in infancy due to vitamin K deficiency: report of a case with multiple intracerebral hematomas with ring-like high density figures. *No To Shinkei* 1987;39:65-70.

[54] Silliman CC, Ford DM, Lane PA. Hemolytic uremic syndrome complicated by vitamin K deficiency. *Am J Pediatr Hematol Oncol* 1991;13:176-8.

[55] Hercberg S, Rouaud C. Nutritional anaemia. *Child Trop* 1981;(133):1-36.

[56] Uauy R, Olivares M, Gonzalez M. Essentiality of copper in humans. *Am J Clin Nutr* 1998;67(5 Suppl):952S-959S.

[57] Olivares M, Uauy R. Copper as an essential nutrient. *Am J Clin Nutr* 1996;63:791S-6S.

[58] Grudeva-Popova JG, Spasova MI, Chepileva KG, Zaprianov ZH. Acute hemolytic anemia as an initial clinical manifestation of Wilson's disease. Folia Med (Plovdiv) 2000;42:42-6

[59] Wiwanitkit V. Wilson's disease with hepatitis C infection. *Chula Med J* 2002; 46: 747 – 51.

[60] Seeling W, Ahnefeld FW, Dick W, Fodor L. The biological significance of zinc (author's transl). *Anaesthesist* 1975;24:329-42.

[61] Haeger K. Zinc and zinc deficiency--a clinical review. *Lakartidningen* 1973;70:3243-6.

[62] Prasad AS. Discovery of human zinc deficiency: impact on human health. *Nutrition* 2001;17:685-7.

[63] Bonomini M, Albertazzi A. Selenium in uremia. *Artif Organs* 1995;19:443-8.

[64] Kapur D, Agarwal KN, Agarwal DK. Nutritional anemia and its control. *Indian J Pediatr* 2002;69:607-16.

[65] Kumar A. National nutritional anaemia control programme in India. *Indian J Public Health* 1999;43:3-5.

[66] Chanarin I, Malkowska V, O'Hea AM, Rinsler MG, Price AB. Megaloblastic anaemia in a vegetarian Hindu community. *Lancet* 1985;2:1168-72.

[67] Wiwanitkit V, Sodsri P. Underweight schoolchildren in a rural school near the Thai-Cambodian border. *Southeast Asian J Trop Med Public Health* 2003;34:458-61.

[68] Khor GL. Update on the prevalence of malnutrition among children in Asia. *Nepal Med Coll J* 2003;5:113-22.

[69] Gopalan C. Current food and nutrition situation in south Asian and south-east Asian countries. *Biomed Environ Sci* 1996;9:102-16.

[70] Baker SJ. Nutritional anaemias. Part 2: *Tropical Asia. Clin Haematol* 1981;10:843-71.

[71] Masawe AE. Nutritional anaemias. Part 1: *Tropical Africa. Clin Haematol* 1981;10:815-42.

Chapter 12

Iron Deficiency in the Tropics

Introduction to Iron Deficiency Anemia

Iron deficiency anemia (IDA) is the most common anemia that can be seen in both sexes of all age groups in any region of the world. Iron is the basic mineral nutrient required for the erythropoietic process. The iron in the heme form is the main composition of hemoglobin in the red blood cell. However, human bodies cannot auto-generate iron for usage, therefore, the source of iron is totally intake. In addition, some part of iron can be derived from the turnover of the red blood cells in human bodies. Any conditions that affect the regular process of iron intake can lead to the deficiency of iron. Generally, ingestion is the main method of iron intake into human bodies. Daily iron losses in males are about 1 mg (14 micrograms kg-1), while the average additional requirements incurred in women include menstruation (0.6 mg), pregnancy (2.7 mg) and lactation (less than 0.3 mg) [1]. Requirements during pregnancy are not evenly distributed and increase to between 5-6 mg in the last trimester of pregnancy, which is more than can be absorbed from even an optimal diet [1]. The recommended food sources of easily absorbed iron are animal products, which contain heme iron. Iron sources that have high iron availability include liver, red beef, tuna, liver, oyster and egg yolk. Non-heme iron can be derived from grains, wheat, millet, oat, vegetable (broccoli, spinach, collards and asparagus) and fruit (prune and raisin). It should be noted that the dietary intake of iron in underdeveloped countries is based mainly on non-heme iron which is absorbed to a lesser degree that heme iron and is subjected to many interferences from inhibitors generally present in the diets, such as phenols, phytates, fibers, etc [2]. About one-quarter of the iron in heme proteins is absorbed regardless of the other components in the diet, while non-heme iron absorption is subject to the interplay of promoting and inhibiting substances in the diet [1]. In addition, *vitamin C* also increases iron absorption. Unluckily, vitamin C deficiency is always common in the area where iron deficiency is endemic. Thus diets rich in enhancers of non-heme iron absorption, chiefly meat and/or ascorbic acid, have high iron bioavailability (about 3 mg per day) while diets in which inhibitors, such as polyphenols and phytates, predominate are poor sources of iron (less than 1 mg per day) [1]. In addition, undernutrition is still the problem of those tropical developing countries, therefore, it is no doubt that iron deficiency anemia is common in the tropics [3]. In human bodies, iron distributes into several sites and performs an important function in normal processes (Table 12.1). In human bodies, iron can be found in hemoglobin, myoglobin and etc. Concerning iron loss, there are several ways that iron can be lost from human bodies including in urine (about 0.1 mg/day), feces (about 0.6 mg/day), cutaneous cell, perspiration (about 0.1mg/day) and menstruation (about 25-30 mg/day in female). Excessive loss of iron via these ways can also bring iron deficiency anemia.

Table 12.1. Sites of iron distribution in human bodies

Sites	Brief description
Large metabolic pool	o This site including those irons found in hemoglobin, myoglobin, cytochrome, other ferroprotiens and other ferroenzymes. All of irons in metabolic iron cycle will pass the life cycle of red blood cell, erythropoiesis, circulating with carriage by red blood cell and reabsorption.
Storage pool	o This site appears in the form known as "ferritin." The main sources of ferritin in human bodies are hepatocytes in liver and macrophages.
Transit pool	o This site appears bound to transferrin, circulating in plasma.

Concerning hematopoiesis, iron and erythropoiesis are inextricably linked [4].

Generally, erythropoiesis is a dynamic process that requires 30-40 mg of iron per day[4]. The erytropoiesis is also under the effect of a hormone, secreted from renals, namely erythropoietin. In normal circumstances, this is met from red cell destruction but in anemia this will not be the case [4]. Reduced iron stores will limit iron supply to erythroblasts but normal or raised iron stores may not be able to supply iron fast enough [4]. While hemoglobin and serum ferritin concentrations reflect the major iron pools, iron supply to erythroid cells can only be assessed by measuring effective hemoglobinization through the percentage of hypochromic red cells in the circulation [4]. Food fortification with iron is considered to be the best and cheapest long-term approach for correcting the deficiency [3]. The iron source selected for this purpose has to be soluble, and of high bioavailability, even in a diet rich in inhibitors [3].

Molecular and Genetic Basis of Iron Deficiency Anemia

Human and animal studies have shown that amino acids and peptides influence iron absorption from the intestinal lumen [5]. A newly identified iron regulator, hepcidin, appears to communicate body iron status and demand for erythropoiesis to the intestine, and in turn, modulates intestinal iron absorption [6]. Concerning hepcidin, it was first purified from human blood and urine as an antimicrobial peptide and was found to be predominantly expressed in the liver [6]. Leong and Lonnerdal said that a lack of hepcidin expression had been associated with iron overload, and overexpression of hepcidin results in iron-deficiency anemia in mice [6]. They said that hepcidin expression was also affected by hypoxia and inflammation and was decreased in hemochromatosis patients, thus, the relationship between body iron status and hepcidin was altered in hemochromatosis patients. They also noted that transcription factors, such as C/EBPalpha, were also suggested to be involved in the regulation of hepcidin gene expression [6]. Brittenham noted that a nuclear DNA-binding protein, NF-E2, might be involved in the regulation of both hemoglobin synthesis in erythroid cells and of iron absorption in the intestine [7]. Hephaestin is another membrane-bound multicopper ferroxidase necessary for iron egress from intestinal enterocytes into the circulation [8]. Ireg1, SLC11A3, also known as Ferroportin1 or Mtp1, is the putative intestinal basolateral iron transporter [8]. Recently, Chen et al. compared iron levels and expression of genes involved in iron uptake and storage in sla mice and C57BL/6J mice fed iron-deficient, iron-overload, or control diets [8]. They found that both iron-deficient wild-type mice and sla mice showed increased expression of Heph and Ireg1 mRNA, compared to controls, whereas only iron-deficient wild-type mice had increased expression of the brush border transporter Dmt1 and unlike iron-deficient mice, sla mouse enterocytes accumulated nonheme iron and ferritin [8]. They indicated that Dmt1 could be modulated by the enterocyte iron level, whereas hephaestin and Ireg1 expression respond to systemic rather than local signals of iron status, thus, the basolateral transport step appeared to be the primary site at which the small intestine responded to alterations in body iron requirements [8].

Inter-organ transport and uptake of nonheme iron is largely performed by the complex transferring-transferring receptor system [5]. Cytoplasmic iron regulatory proteins (IRPs) and the iron responsive elements (IREs) to which they bind allow mammals to make use of the essential properties of iron while reducing its potentially toxic effect [5]. Composed mainly of monocytes and tissue macrophages, the reticuloendothelial system (RES) plays two major roles in iron metabolism: it recycles iron from senescent red blood cells and it serves as a large storage depot for excess iron [9]. Knutson and Wessling-Resnick said that several studies characterizing the function and regulation of Nramp1, DMT1, HFE, FPN1, CD163, and hepcidin were rapidly expanding our knowledge of the molecular aspects of RE iron handling [9].

Brittenham said that molecular mechanisms for the cellular uptake, storage, and utilization of iron were clarified in investigations of the structure and functions of transferrin, transferrin receptor, ferritin, erythroid delta-aminolevulinic acid synthase, and the RNA-binding protein termed the IREs [7]. Transferrin receptor is a protein widely studied for the correlation to the iron deficiency anemia at present. Transferrin receptor 1 and putative Stimulator of Fe Transport (SFT) represent two different proteins involved in iron metabolism in mammalian cells [10]. The expression of TfR1 in the duodenum of subjects with normal body iron stores has been mainly localized in the basolateral portion of the cytoplasm of crypt cells, supporting the idea that this molecule may be involved in the sensing of body iron stores [10]. Barisani and Conte said that TfR1 expression demonstrated an inverse relationship with body iron stores as assessed by immunohistochemistry with anti-TfR1 antibodies in iron deficiency anemia [10].

Concerning genetic polymorphism, there are several polymorphisms mentioned for their correlation to iron deficiency anemia. A functional consequence, G-->A mutation at cDNA nucleotide 829 (G277S) was associated with a reduction in total iron binding capacity (TIBC) [11]. Lee *et al.* said that the G277S genotype was a risk factor for iron deficiency anemia in menstruating white women [11]. They mentioned that iron deficiency anemia was present in 27% of homozygous G277S/G277S women, 10% of G277G/G277S heterozygous women and 5% of homozygous wild-type G277G/G277G women [11]. Recently, Jackson *et al.* studied the influence of HFE genotype on iron status in 10,556 blood donors [12]. They found that mean values increased for transferrin saturation (TS) and serum ferritin (sFn), and decreased for unsaturated iron binding capacity (UIBC) in the order: donors lacking the mutations, H63D heterozygotes, C282Y heterozygotes, H63D homozygotes, compound heterozygotes and C282Y homozygotes, but serum ferritin (sFn) concentrations were no higher in H63D heterozygotes and C282Y heterozygous women than in donors lacking mutations [12]. However, the percentage of donors failing the screening test for anaemia or of those with sFn < 15 microg/l did not differ among the genotype groups [12].

The genetic basics in many infections related to iron deficiency anemia have also been studied for their clinical importance. Concerning the hookworm infestation, a most well-known tropical parasitic infestation relating to iron deficiency anemia, Harrison *et al.* identified the major anticoagulant inhibitor of coagulation factor Xa from the hookworm parasite *Ancylostoma ceylanicum* using reverse transcription PCR and 3'-rapid amplification of cDNA ends [13]. They noted that despite approximately 50% amino acid similarity, A. ceylanicum anticoagulant peptide 1 (AceAP1) was both immunologically and mechanistically distinct from AcAP5, its homologue isolated from the dog hookworm Ancylostoma caninum [13]. They suggested that factor Xa inhibitory activity was predictive of hookworm bloodfeeding capabilities in vivo [13]. *Helicobacter pylori* is another gastrointestinal infection relating to iron deficiency anemia, which is widely studied for the effect of its genetic polymorphism. *H. pylori* infection is thought to contribute to iron-deficiency anemia, especially during puberty [14]. Generally, the ferritin protein Pfr of H. pylori is homologous to eukaryotic and prokaryotic ferritins [14]. Recently, Choe *et al.* performed a study to analyze the H. pylori pfr status in gastric biopsy specimens according to clinical data, including antral gastritis with or without iron-deficiency anemia [14]. According to this study, the Ser39Ala mutation was found in 100% (26/26), Gly111Asn in 26.9% (7/26), and Gly82Ser in 11.5% (3/26) and there were no significant differences in the mutations of the pfr regions between the iron deficiency anemia positive and negative groups [14]. Choe *et al.* concluded the mutation in the pfr gene did not relate with the clinical phenotype, iron deficiency anemia [14]. Jeon *et al.* said that the *H. pylori* feoB gene product, a high-affinity ferrous iron transporter, might play a central role in iron acquisition and virulence [15]. They undertook a study in 14 Korean patients to analyze H. pylori feoB status according to clinical data, including antral gastritis with or without IDA [14]. They noted that although statistically significant differences were observed at four sites (K127T, A273S/P, I438V and I441T) between IDA positive and negative, the number of specimens was too low to assess the significance of the differences. They concluded that the four polymorphisms of the feoB gene observed appeared to be related to the clinical phenotype of IDA, but the relation was unclear because of the small number of strains studied [15].

Pathogenesis of Iron Deficiency Anemia

Any disorder thst disturbs the normal regulation process of iron metabolism in human bodies can cause iron disorders [16]. Such disorders can lead to the iron decreasing.

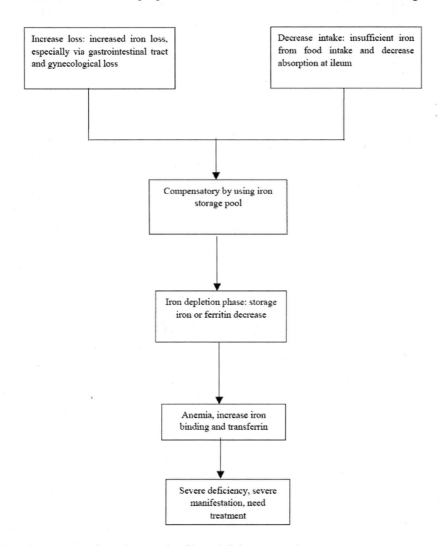

Figure 12.1. Summary on the pathogenesis of iron deficiency anemia

Concerning the phase of iron decreasing, there are three main phases: iron depletion, early iron deficiency and late iron deficiency. Concerning iron depletion, it is the first phase. In this phase, the iron stores in the body decrease but do not cause an overt effect. Although there is no clinical manifestation, the laboratory investigations can show low serum ferritin levels and decreased hemoglobin levels [17]. Concerning the early iron deficiency phase, more laboratory aberrations including low levels of serum ferritin, transferrin saturation, and increased levels of erythropoiesis protoporphyrin can be seen [17]. Clinical manifestation can be detected. Concerning the late iron deficiency, gross specific clinical manifestation such as koilonychia can often be detected. Decreased mean corpuscular volume of red blood cells is common. The iron deposit in bone marrow can be rarely demonstrated.

As previously mentioned the clinical manifestation of iron decreasing starts when there is iron deficiency. The common sign and symptoms of anemia can be seen in any case with iron deficiency anemia. In addition to the usual clinical symptoms of anemia, there may also be symptoms affecting the skin, mucosa, and appendages of the skin [18]. The clinical manifestations of iron deficiency anemia can be subtle, but irreversible delayed psychomotor development may occur if the anemia is severe and prolonged [19 – 20].

Diagnosis of Iron Deficiency Anemia

Iron deficiency anemia is one of the most common diseases worldwide [19 – 20]. In the majority of cases, the presence of hypochromic microcytic anemia and biochemical evidence for depletion of body iron stores makes the diagnosis relatively straightforward [19 – 20]. Based on medicine, diagnosis of iron deficiency anemia must be based on the history taking, physical examination and laboratory investigation. Before a diagnosis of iron deficiency anemia, the diagnosis of anemia is required.

The diagnosis of anemia and consequent classification as hypochromic microcytic type led to the suspicious case of iron deficiency anemia. Concerning history taking, some histories are clues for further diagnosis of iron deficiency anemia including chronic peptic ulcer, history of hypermenorrhea and history of insufficient food intake. Concerning physical examination, some signs including koilonychia are hallmarks for diagnosis of iron deficiency anemia. From the basic data from history taking and physical examination, additional laboratory investigations are required for confirmation of a diagnosis. However, in several clinical conditions, classic biochemical indices such as serum iron, transferrin saturation, and ferritin may not be informative or may not change rapidly enough to reflect transient iron-deficient states, functional iron deficiency, such as the ones that develop during recombinant human erythropoietin (r-HuEPO) therapy [19 – 20].

Concerning laboratory investigations, the basic investigation such as blood smear examination is still a useful tool in a setting with limited resources. However, this method has poor diagnostic property. It is difficult to discriminate between iron deficiency anemia and the other common hypochromic microcytic anemia in the tropics, hemoglobinopathies. Although the poikilocytosis with anisocytosis can be used for discrimination between iron deficiency anemia and thalassemia, the trait form of hemoglobinopathies can be very similar to iron deficiency anemia. It should also be noted that the low MCV and MCH results from automated hematology analyzer can be seen in both iron deficiency anemia and trait form of thalassemia and hemoglobinopathy [21]. The additional modification of automated hematology analyzer, using the mathematical model (Table 12.2) based on the automated hematology analyzer is another useful application in discrimination between iron deficiency anemia and thalassemia [22 – 24]. However, the application of these basic principles should be done carefully. In tropical countries, the co-occurrence of both thalassemia and iron deficiency anemia can be seen. Another limitation of these basic principles is the case of iron deficiency anemia after iron treatment. The identification and treatment of iron deficiency in settings such as r-HuEPO therapy, anemia of chronic disease, and iron deficiency of early childhood may be improved by the use of red cell and reticulocyte cellular indices, which reflect in almost real time the development of iron deficiency and the response to iron therapy [19 – 20].

Table 12.2. Some mathematical models for discrimination between iron deficiency anemia and thalassemia.

Authors	Models
Shine and Lai [22]	$0.01 \times MCH \times (MCV)^2$
Green and King [23]	$RDW \times MCH \times (MCV)^2 / Hb \times 100$
Mentzer [24]	MCV/RBC

Concerning the biochemistry tests, there are several tests for diagnosis of iron deficiency anemia. The determination of serum iron is difficult, and therefore is not recommended as a diagnostic tool. Suwansaksri *et al.* performed a comparative study on different methods for determination of serum iron [25]. The recommended diagnostic test for the diagnosis of iron deficiency anemia is ferritin. The ferritin level reflects the storage pool of iron in human bodies. It is useful in the diagnosis of phases of decreasing iron. However, Wiwanitkit and Preechakas recently proposed that the serum ferritin level might not be useful in the setting where the prevalence of thalassemia is high such as in Thailand [26]. In the thalassemia cases, the serum ferritin is high and if the thalassemia combines with iron deficiency, the serum ferritin level is hard to predict [26]. The new diagnostic tool is the serum transferrin receptor. Beguin concluded that soluble TfR represented a valuable quantitative assay of marrow erythropoietic activity as well as a marker of tissue iron deficiency [27]. The soluble transferrin receptor (sTfR) has been introduced as a sensitive, early and highly quantitative new marker of iron depletion, increasing in proportion to tissue iron deficit [28]. Unlike conventional laboratory tests, the sTfR is not an acute phase reactant and remains normal in patients with chronic disease [28]. Baillie *et al.* found that the sTfR concentration was shown to be the most efficient test in predicting bone marrow iron stores in 20 patients with anemia of chronic disease (75% efficiency) and in 18 patients with rheumatoid arthritis (RA) (94% efficiency) [28]. They noted that measurement of sTfR might be a useful addition in the differential diagnosis of anemia of chronic disease and iron deficiency anemia [28]. The ratio of serum transferrin receptor (sTfR) to serum ferritin (R/F ratio) has been shown to have excellent performance in estimating body iron stores, but it cannot be used widely because of the lack of standardization for sTfR assays [19 – 20]. The combination of hematologic markers such as reticulocyte hemoglobin content, which decreases with iron deficiency, and R/F ratio may allow for a more precise classification of anemias [19 – 20]. However, the most reliable diagnostic test but invasive test is the bone marrow examination. The absence of iron stores in the bone marrow remains the most definitive test for differentiating iron deficiency from the other microcytic states, anemia of chronic disease, thalassemia, and sideroblastic anemia [29]. However, Massey noted that measurement of serum ferritin, iron concentration, transferrin saturation and iron-binding capacity, and, more recently, serum transferrin receptors may obviate proceeding to bone marrow evaluation [29]. However, all biochemistry tests are expensive and seem not available in the rural communities where the prevalence of iron deficiency anemia is high. Diagnosis by the iron treatment trial is recommended. Recently, Nuchprayoon *et al.* noted that therapeutic trial of iron is useful as a diagnostic test in anemic females except those with high RBC (> 4.4 x 10(6)/microl) and very low MCV (< 69 fl), a subgroup which most likely has thalassemia and are least likely to benefit from iron treatment [30]. In addition to the laboratory investigations for diagnosis of iron deficiency anemia, the investigations for diagnosis of the underlying causes of iron deficiency anemia is also needed. These tests include the stool examination for parasite and occult blood.

Treatment of Iron Deficiency Anemia

To treat iron deficiency anemia, one can apply to the basic principle of the treatment of anemia. The easiest method for the treatment of iron deficiency anemia is iron treatment. Iron treatment is a direct method to increase red blood cell production. Oral iron sulfate, 120 mg elemental iron per day for at least 2 months, is recommended [30]. However, since the co-occurrence between iron deficiency anemia and hemoglobinopathy can be seen in the tropics, the decision to prescribe iron treatment must be carefully considered since in the cases with hemoglobinopathy the iron treatment is useful and sometimes harmful. The iron supplementation is not only a method for treatment but also a method for diagnosis, as previously mentioned [30]. In addition, iron supplementation can be a good preventive tool, especially in high-risk populations, such as in the tropics. Iron fortification of food has been proposed as a strategy to reduce the high prevalence of iron deficiency [31]. However, poor consumer acceptance, unacceptable taste, and discoloration of the iron-fortified foods have been frequently listed as causes of unsuccessful iron fortification programs [31].

Bovell-Benjamin and Guinard noted that an excellent prospect for improving consumer acceptance of iron-fortified foods is the incorporation of a thorough, organized, and unified approach to sensory evaluation practices of iron fortification programs for product optimization [31]. Baynes and Cook said that the intermittent administration of iron supplements once or twice weekly rather than daily had been advocated by international health agencies in recent years [32]. Indeed, iron supplementation is recommended for the pregnant in the highly endemic area of iron deficiency anemia [33]. However, Favier *et al.* said that a selective supplementation reserved to anemic women must be preferred to a systematic supplementation, which improves biological parameters of mothers but has no effect on newborns [34]. They said that iron was a potentially toxic element and an unjustified supplementation could expose individulas to high iron levels and lead to an oxidative stress, which is also observed in pregnancy pathologies including pre-eclampsia and gestational diabetes [34]. They noted that as a precaution, iron supplementation may be reserved to anemic women or those with high anemia risk, while for others, nutritional advice must permit them to reach their iron recommendation [34].

Although the treatment of choice is oral iron therapy, several factors limit its efficacy, such as requirement of long-term treatment and intolerance to gastrointestinal side effects of oral iron administration. Concerning other treatments for iron deficiency anemia, there are some documents on those methods. Blood transfusion is rarely recommended in the severely ill. In 2002, Sandoval *et al.* retrospectively studied 42 children with severe iron deficient anemia [35]. In this study, 29 received oral iron and 13 required parked red blood cell transfusions because of co-morbid cardiorespiratory distress [35]. Similar to blood transfusion, parenteral iron infusion is recommended in severe iron deficiency anemia. It also is recommended in the cases where individuals cannot tolerate the oral iron treatment [36 – 37]. In 2002, Reynoso-Gomez *et al.* carried out a prospective, longitudinal, uncontrolled clinical trial to evaluate the safety and efficacy of total-dose intravenous iron infusion in the treatment of iron deficiency anemia in adult, non-pregnant patients [36]. They confirmed that total-dose iron infusion was a safe and effective method to treat iron deficiency anemia that might be used in patients with an intolerance or unresponsiveness to oral iron or in patients with who did not benefit from other iron schedules, as well as initial therapy in selected cases [36]. They also noted that it provided a swift correction of hematocrit allowing, in some cases, elective surgery without the need of a blood transfusion [36]. There are now three parenteral iron products available: iron dextran, ferric gluconate, and iron sucrose [37]. In addition to the treatment of anemia, the treatment for the underlying cause of iron deficiency anemia, such as antihelminthic drug for hookworm infestation and antacid for peptic ulcer, is recommended.

Summary of Iron Deficiency Anemia in the Tropics

Iron deficiency anemia can be seen all over the world. In the tropics, the prevalence of iron deficiency anemia is very high. Anemia is still the present health problem of many developing tropical countries. In Asia, the high prevalence of iron deficiency anemia is due to malnutrition and parasitic infestations. Khor said that besides protein-energy malnutrition, Asian children also suffered from micronutrient deficiency [38]. Khor noted that iron deficiency anaemia affects 40-50% of preschool and primary school children [38]. Concerning West Asia, Musaiger explored the magnitude of the problem and factors that contribute to the high prevalence of anemia in Arab Gulf countries [39]. According to this study, the prevalence of iron deficiency anemia among preschool children ranged from 20% to 67%, while that among school children ranged from 12.6% to 50% and the percentage of pregnant women who suffered from this anemia ranged from 22.7% to 54% [39]. Musaiger mentioned that infant feeding practices, food habits, parasitic infection, parity, early age at marriage, and geographical location were among the most important factors associated with iron deficiency anemia in this region [39]. Musaiger noted that programs to prevent and control this anemia, are urgently needed [39]. Concerning South Asia, the iron deficiency anemia is an important public health problem. Recently, Kumar mentioned the strategies of the National Nutritional Anemia Control Program (NNACP) in India [40]. This program focuses on three vital strategies: promotion of regular consumption of foods rich in iron, provisions of iron and folate supplements in the form of tablets to the high risk groups, and identification and treatment of severely anemic cases [40]. The malnutrition is mentioned as the most important factor leading to iron deficiency anemia in South Asia [38, 40].Concerning Southeast Asia, iron deficiency anemia is also an important tropical anemia. As already mentioned, the difficulty in diagnosis of iron deficiency anemia in this region is mainly due to the high prevalence of hemoglobin E trait. Because these two disorders have high prevalence in Southeast Asia, the co-occurrence can be seen. The discriminative diagnosis on these two conditions is necessary and can be performed based on therapeutic iron trial [30]. The medical importance of hookworm infestation as a contributing factor to iron deficiency anemia for the population in Southeast Asia should also be mentioned. Charoenlarp *et al.* mentioned that a combined program, possibly including parasite control and food fortification, should be considered [41]. In Africa, the high prevalence of iron deficiency anemia can be seen as well.

Both malnutrition and infection are important factors for iron deficiency anemia in this region. Indeed, malnutrition-related disorders are common in Africa. It has been noted that nutritional anemia, including iron-deficiency anemia, megaloblastic anaemia due to folate deficiency or vitamin B12 deficiency, and protein deficiency-anaemia was widespread throughout Africa [42]. These disorders are particularly common in growing children, women of child-bearing age, pregnant women and lactating mothers [42]. Masawe noted that the anemia in Africa was especially common during the second half of the dry season and the first half of the wet season, when food supplies were limited [42]. The high prevalence of hookworm-infestation induced iron deficiency anemia can be seen. Bhargava performed a study in Tanzania and found that treatment of the hookworm infestation also improved anemia in the cases with iron deficiency anemia [43]. In addition, Oppenheimer said that iron treatment has been associated with acute exacerbations of infection, in particular malaria [44]. Oppenheimer noted that several subsequent studies in Africa using oral iron showed deleterious effects [44]. Oppenheimer said that knowledge of malarial endemicity, immunity with respect to age and the prevalence of haemoglobinopathies was important in planning interventions for iron supplementation in this area [44].

Concerning Latin America, iron deficiency anemia is also the public anemic health problem [45]. Similar to other tropical regions of the world, the Pan American Health Organization of the World Health Organization (PAHO/WHO) proposed several strategies to combat iron deficiency anemia in this area [46]. Similar to other tropical areas, iron fortification is recommended [46]. Recently, Borigato and Martinez performed an interesting experiment in Brazil. They performed a study to determine the efficacy of cooking food in iron pots to prevent anemia in premature infants. They found that the iron added to food cooked in iron pots was bioavailable, however, this increased iron availability was insufficient to satisfy the high iron requirements of the group of preterm infants [47]. Concerning Polynesia, the iron deficiency anemia is also documented. A hookworm disease is also prevalent in Polynesia as well as in the tropical regions of Africa, Southern Asia, and Latin America [48].

References

[1]   Bothwell TH, Baynes RD, MacFarlane BJ, MacPhail AP. Nutritional iron requirements and food iron absorption. *J Intern Med* 1989;226:357-65.

[2]   Cavill I. Erythropoiesis and iron. *Best Pract Res Clin Haematol* 2002;15:399-409.

[3]   Fleming AF. Iron deficiency in the tropics. *Clin Haematol* 1982;11:365-88.

[4]   MacPhail AP. Iron deficiency and the developing world. *Arch Latinoam Nutr* 2001 ;51:2-6.

[5]   Tapiero H, Gate L, Tew KD. Iron: deficiencies and requirements. *Biomed Pharmacother* 2001;55:324-32.

[6]   Leong WI, Lonnerdal B. Hepcidin, the recently identified peptide that appears to regulate iron absorption. *J Nutr* 2004;134:1-4.

[7]   Brittenham GM. New advances in iron metabolism, iron deficiency, and iron overload. *Curr Opin Hematol* 1994;1:101-6.

[8]   Chen H, Su T, Attieh ZK, Fox TC, McKie AT, Anderson GJ, Vulpe CD. Systemic regulation of Hephaestin and Ireg1 revealed in studies of genetic and nutritional iron deficiency. *Blood* 2003 1;102:1893-9.

[9]   Knutson M, Wessling-Resnick M. Iron metabolism in the reticuloendothelial system. *Crit Rev Biochem Mol Biol* 2003;38:61-88.

[10] Barisani D, Conte D. Transferrin receptor 1 (TfR1) and putative stimulator of Fe transport (SFT) expression in iron deficiency and overload: an overview. *Blood Cells Mol Dis* 2002;29:498-505.

[11] Lee PL, Halloran C, Trevino R, Felitti V, Beutler E. Human transferrin G277S mutation: a risk factor for iron deficiency anaemia. *Br J Haematol* 2001 ;115:329-33.

[12] Jackson HA, Carter K, Darke C, Guttridge MG, Ravine D, Hutton RD, Napier JA, Worwood M. HFE mutations, iron deficiency and overload in 10,500 blood donors. *Br J Haematol* 2001;114:474-84.

[13] Harrison LM, Nerlinger A, Bungiro RD, Cordova JL, Kuzmic P, Cappello M. Molecular characterization of Ancylostoma inhibitors of coagulation factor Xa. Hookworm anticoagulant activity in vitro predicts parasite bloodfeeding in vivo. *J Biol Chem* 2002;277:6223-9.

[14] Choe YH, Hwang TS, Kim HJ, Shin SH, Song SU, Choi MS. A possible relation of the Helicobacter pylori pfr gene to iron deficiency anemia? *Helicobacter* 2001;6:55-9.

[15] Jeon BH, Oh YJ, Lee NG, Choe YH. Polymorphism of the Helicobacter pylori feoB Gene in Korea: a Possible Relation with Iron-Deficiency Anemia? *Helicobacter* 2004;9:330-4.

[16] Nimeh N, Bishop RC. Disorders of iron metabolism. *Med Clin North Am* 1980;64:631-45.

[17] Brugnara C. Iron deficiency and erythropoiesis: new diagnostic approaches. *Clin Chem* 2003;49:1573-8.

[18] Weissinger F. Basic principles and clinical significance of iron deficiency. *Fortschr Med* 1997;115:35-8.

[19] Jaeger M, Schneider W. Manifestation of iron deficiency. *Med Klin* (Munich) 1996; 91:580-8.

[20] Leung AK, Chan KW. Iron deficiency anemia. *Adv Pediatr.* 2001;48:385-408.

[21] Richter S. Erroneous diagnosis of iron deficiency anemia. *Folia Haematol Int Mag Klin Morphol Blutforsch* 1989;116:781-3.

[22] Shine I, Lai S. A strategy to detect α-thalassemia minor. *Lancet* 1977 1: 692 – 694.

[23] Green R, King R. A new red cell discriminant incorporating volume dispersion for differentiating iron deficiency anemia from thalassemia minor. *Blood Cells* 1989 15: 481-491.

[24] Mentzer W. Differentiation of iron deficiency from thalassemia. *Lancet* 1973 1: 449 – 452.

[25] Suwansaksri J, Sookarun S, Wiwanitkit V, Boonchalermvichian C, Nuchprayoon I. Comparative study on serum iron determination by different methods. *Lab Hematol* 2003;9:234-6.

[26] Wiwanitkit V, Preechakas P, Paritpokee N, Boonchalermvichian C. Serum ferritin level by RIA among anemic and non anemic pediatric subjects. *Asean J Radiol* 2002; 2: 167-170.

[27] Beguin Y. Soluble transferrin receptor for the evaluation of erythropoiesis and iron status. *Clin Chim Acta* 2003 ;329:9-22.

[28] Baillie FJ, Morrison AE, Fergus I. Soluble transferrin receptor: a discriminating assay for iron deficiency. *Clin Lab Haematol* 2003;25:353-7.

[29] Massey AC. Microcytic anemia. Differential diagnosis and management of iron deficiency anemia. *Med Clin North Am* 1992;76:549-66.

[30] Nuchprayoon I, Sukthawee B, Nuchprayoon T. Red cell indices and therapeutic trial of iron in diagnostic work-up for anemic Thai females. *J Med Assoc Thai* 2003;86 Suppl 2:S160-9.

[31] Bovell-Benjamin AC, Guinard JX. Novel approaches and application of contemporary sensory evaluation practices in iron fortification programs. *Crit Rev Food Sci Nutr* 2003;43:379-400.

[32] Baynes RD, Cook JD. Current issues in iron deficiency. *Curr Opin Hematol* 1996;3:145-9

[33] Grischke EM. Nutrition during pregnancy--current aspects. *MMW Fortschr Med* 2004;146:29-30.

[34] Favier M, Hininger-Favier I. Is systematic iron supplementation justified during pregnancy? *Gynecol Obstet Fertil* 2004;32:245-50.

[35] Sandoval C, Berger E, Ozkaynak MF, Tugal O, Jayabose S. Severe iron deficiency anemia in 42 pediatric patients. *Pediatr Hematol Oncol* 2002;19:157-61.

[36] Reynoso-Gomez E, Salinas-Rojas V, Lazo-Langner A. Safety and efficacy of total dose intravenous iron infusion in the treatment of iron-deficiency anemia in adult non-pregnant patients. *Rev Invest Clin* 2002;54:12-20.

[37] Silverstein SB, Rodgers GM. Parenteral iron therapy options. *Am J Hematol* 2004;76:74-8.

[38] Khor GL. Update on the prevalence of malnutrition among children in Asia. *Nepal Med Coll J* 2003;5:113-22.

[39] Musaiger AO. Iron deficiency anaemia among children and pregnant women in the Arab Gulf countries: the need for action. *Nutr Health* 2002;16:161-71.

[40] Kumar A. National nutritional anaemia control programme in India. *Indian J Public Health* 1999;43:3-5.

[41] Charoenlarp P, Dhanamitta S, Kaewvichit R, Silprasert A, Suwanaradd C, Na-Nakorn S, Prawatmuang P, Vatanavicharn S, Nutcharas U, Pootrakul P, et al. A WHO collaborative study on iron supplementation in Burma and in Thailand. *Am J Clin Nutr* 1988;47:280-97.

[42] Masawe AE. Nutritional anaemias. Part 1: *Tropical Africa. Clin Ha*ematol 1981;10:815-42.

[43] Bhargava A, Jukes M, Lambo J, Kihamia CM, Lorri W, Nokes C, Drake L, Bundy D. Anthelmintic treatment improves the hemoglobin and serum ferritin concentrations of Tanzanian schoolchildren. *Food Nutr Bull* 2003;24:332-42.

[44] Oppenheimer SJ. Iron and infection in the tropics: paediatric clinical correlates. *Ann Trop Paediatr* 1998;18 Suppl:S81-7.

[45] Gandra VR. Iron deficiency anemia in Latin America and the Caribbean. *Bol Oficina Sanit Panam* 1970 ;68:375-87.

[46] Freire WB. Strategies of the Pan American Health Organization/World Health Organization for the control of iron deficiency in Latin America. *Nutr Rev* 1997;55:183-8.

[47] Borigato EV, Martinez FE. Iron nutritional status is improved in Brazilian preterm infants fed food cooked in iron pots. *J Nutr* 1998;128:855-9.

[48] Georgiev VS. Parasitic infections. Treatment and developmental therapeutics. 1. Necatoriasis. *Curr Pharm Des* 1999;5:545-54.

Chapter 13

Tropical Sprue and Anemia

Introduction to Tropical Sprue

Tropical sprue is a malabsorption syndrome of unknown cause that is prevalent in the tropics and subtropics. Although the true etiology of tropical sprue is still unknown at present, infection is believed to cause tropical sprue. Indeed, tropical malabsorption remains an important clinical problem for both the indigenous population of tropical countries and for short-term visitors and longer-term residents from the industrialized world [1]. In young children, persistent diarrhea and malabsorption can result in severe retardation of growth and development [1]. The most common cause of tropical malabsorption is an intestinal infection, notably the small intestinal protozoa, including Giardia intestinalis, Cryptosporidium parvum, Isospora belli, Cyclospora cayetanensis, and the microsporidia [1]. However, it should also be noted that these parasitic infestations are not common in the immunocompetent hosts but in immunodeficient hosts [2]. However, the cryptosporidium can be the exception, which can be seen in the immunocompetent hosts in a poor sanitation setting such as an orphanage center [3]. Also noted are tropical sprue, which still remain an important diagnostic option, but much less common than it was 20 to 30 years ago [3]. The fact that tropical sprue are usually diagnosed after ruling out other possible causes, the decreased incidence of tropical sprue can be due to the development of diagnostic technology for many infectious agents at present.

Medically, tropical sprue is a disease of the small intestine characterized by a malabsorption syndrome with a subtotal or partial mucosal atrophy [4]. It is observed in Asia and Central America, however, it appears to be rare in Africa. Its real frequency is unknown since small bowel biopsys were not routinely done [4]. Gras *et al.* said that the disease beginning as chronic diarrhea was later on characterized by an aphtoid stomatitis and a macrocytic anemia [4]. They also said that bacterial overgrowth as well as giardiasis might be trigger factors of the disease, the pathogenesis of which was still incompletely understood [4].

Molecular and Genetic Basis of Tropical Sprue

Haghighi and Wolf said that aside from infectious intestinal diseases with known etiology, there is a group of gastrointestinal disorders mainly affecting the small intestine of individuals predominantly living in, but also visiting or returning from the Third World, usually the tropics. These disorders range from asymptomatic structural and/or functional abnormalities of the gastrointestinal mucosa, subclinical enteropathy (SE) to a fully symptomatic condition highlighted by malabsorption of nutrients with associated nutritional deficiencies responsive to folate and broad spectrum antibiotic treatment namely tropical sprue [5]. They said that mounting evidence supported an infectious cause in many instances, however, the exact nature of the infection, whether initiated and/or perpetuated by enterotoxigenic coliform bacteria, virus or a combination of these, was unclear [5]. Therefore, further studies, including those using molecular techniques, are needed in order to clarify this problem [5]. Presently, there are several attempts to find the true etiologies of tropical sprue using the molecular biology investigative tools. However, the non-infectious disorders are also investigated. Ghatei *et al.* said that chromatography of plasmas from healthy subjects and patients with dumping syndrome, active celiac disease, and tropical sprue showed that only the second major peak of R59 immunoreactivity reflected the basal or postnutrient increases in the plasma enteroglucagon concentration [6]. They also noted that in the patients with exaggerated enteroglucagon release, the rise was again found to be entirely due to an increase in this peak of immunoreactivity [6]. Jejunal brush-border folate hydrolase, an enzyme essential and rate-limiting in folate absorption, is also mentioned for its correlation to tropical sprue [7]. Halsted noted that brush-border folate hydrolase activity and pteroylpolyglutamate hydrolysis were inhibited in disease and conditions associated with folate deficiency, including celiac and tropical sprue, the use of sulfasalazine to treat inflammatory bowel disease, and chronic alcoholism [7]. Basically, brush-border folate hydrolase is an exopeptidase located on the jejunal brush-border surface that liberates hydrolytic products of pteroylpolyglutamates in a progressive fashion, with a final release of pteroylglutamate [7]. Halsted proposed that regulating the synthesis and expression of brush-border folate hydrolase might be critical to the availability of dietary folate [7].

Concerning the genetic basics of tropical sprue, there are some documents on this topic. The pathogenesis of nontropical sprue is determined by both genetic factors, demonstrated with a strong association with certain HLA haplotypes (B8, DR3, DR7 and DC3) and presumably also environmental events including virus infection, which render the mucosa susceptible to gluten [8]. However, the association of HLA haplotyes to tropical sprue is rarely mentioned [8]. Menendez-Corrada *et al.* studied 27 Puerto Rican patients with tropical sprue proven by intestinal biopsy and clinical response to folic acid [9]. In this study, HLA type of all cases was determined with a microcytotoxicity assay [9]. According to this study, 25 of all patients had at least one antigen of the Aw-19 series and the strongest association was with Aw-31, for which the relative risk was 10.6 [9]. Menendez-Corrada *et al.* noted that the absence of a B-locus or haplotype effect suggested a marker association only, rather than an immune association [9].

Pathogenesis of Tropical Sprue

As already mentioned, the true pathogenesis of tropical sprue is still unknown. However, the pathogenetic insult in tropical sprue appears to be a persistent overgrowth of the small intestine by enteric pathogens after a bout of turista [8].

In 2003, Ghoshal et al. noted that response to antibiotics in tropical sprue might suggest a role for bacterial contamination of the small bowel, which was known in diseases with prolonged orocecal transit time (OCTT) [10]. Ghoshal et al. studied 13 patients with tropical sprue for frequency, nature and degree of bacterial contamination of the small bowel by quantitative culture of jejunal aspirate, glucose hydrogen breath test (GHBT), and OCTT by lactulose hydrogen breath test before and after treatment [10]. They found that 10 of 13 patients with tropical sprue had bacterial contamination compared with 3/12 of the controls (cases with irritable bowel syndrome: IBS) [10]. In this study, median colony count in tropical sprue was higher than IBSP and gram-negative aerobic bacilli were commonly isolated in tropical sprue but not in IBS [10]. In addition, median OCTT was longer in tropical sprue than IBS and healthy subjects [10]. Ghoshal et al. concluded that aerobic bacterial contamination of the small bowel was common in the patients with tropical sprue. They also noted that prolonged OCTT in tropical sprue correlated with fecal fat and normalized in a subset of patients after treatment [10].

Concerning malnutrition in tropical sprue, the cause of the malabsorption syndrome is multifactorial and results from both intraluminal and cellular events [8]. Westergaard noted that the digestion of proteins, carbohydrates, and lipids in the patients with tropical sprue was compromised due to decreased pancreatic and biliary secretion [8]. Westergaard also mentioned that the absorption of the digestive products was also severely affected due to decreased activity of microvillus enzymes, dipeptidases and disaccharidases, and a presumed reduction in the number of transport carriers [8]. Indeed, recent cell kinetic studies of the turnover of the intestinal epithelium in sprue have convincingly demonstrated that the flat mucosa is caused by increased efflux, cell death, with compensatory crypt hyperplasia [8]. Malik et al. recently studied 10 with tropical sprue and 10 with IBS as controls to characterize the immunocytes in the jejunal mucosa [11]. They found that no correlation was evident between the different immunocytes (IgA, IgG, and IgM) and the duration of illness, serum albumin, and tests for absorption of fat, B-12, and D-xylose [11]. In addition, although many previous studies indicated that many patients with tropical sprue in southern India have triglyceride accumulation within the cells of the intestinal mucosa, Tiruppathi et al. noted that the degree of essential fatty acid depletion observed is unlikely to be the cause of the mucosal accumulation of triglyceride in tropical sprue [12].

Concerning anemia in the tropical sprue, the common type is megaloblastic anemia. The megaloblastic anemia in the tropical sprue is believed to be due to the malabsorption. Lucas and Mathan noted that, as in coeliac disease, mucosal surface pH in the jejunum was elevated above normal in tropical sprue and might reflect the extent to which normal ion transport processes were affected [13]. They noted that mucosal surface pH correlated directly with 3 day-mean fecal fat excretion and inversely with xylose and vitamin B12 absorption values but not with the nutritional indicators serum albumen, folate or blood hemoglobin levels [13]. Kapadia et al. studied the intraluminal fate of orally administered radioactive vitamin B12 in control subjects with normal vitamin B12 absorption and those with vitamin B12 malabsorption due to tropical sprue [14]. According to this study, in control subjects, 1 to 21% of the dose was bound to sedimentable material and 37 to 75% was bound to immunoreactive intrinsic factor. However, in subjects with vitamin B12 malabsorption due to tropical sprue, the results were identical with the control subjects [14]. Bacteriological studies showed a statistically significant correlation between both the number of flora in the jejunum and the number of bacteroides in both the jejunum and ileum and vitamin B12 malabsorption [14]. In addition, in patients with tropical sprue who have normal intrinsic factor secretion, the vitamin B12 absorptive defect was not due to binding of the vitamin to bacteria or to alteration to the intrinsic factor vitamin B12 complex in the intestinal lumen [14]. Kapadia *et al.* said that the lesion appeared to be one of the mucosal cell receptors or of the cells themselves, possibly caused by bacterial toxins [14].

Concerning weight loss in tropical sprue, the respective roles of reduced dietary intake and malabsorption in the pathogenesis of weight loss in persons with chronic tropical sprue have been evaluated by Klipstein and Corcino [15]. According to their study, dietary intake was found to be significantly less in a group of 45 patients with tropical sprue, all of whom had anorexia due to deficiency of folate and/or vitamin B12, than in a group of 51 healthy controls [15]. They noted that weight loss was equally prominent in those patients with tropical sprue who had normal absorption of fat and protein as in those who had excessive fecal loss and reduced absorption of these nutrients [15]. They also noted that treatment of five sprue patients with folic acid or vitamin B12 for 2 weeks resulted in improved appetite and increased dietary intake with weight gain in the absence of significant improvement in intestinal absorption. However, treatment with oral tetracycline for a similar period of time in five other patients was not associated with vitamin repletion, return of appetite, or weight gain [15]. Klipstein and Corcino proposed that reduced dietary intake resulting from anorexia caused by vitamin deficiency was significant, and sometimes the most important factor in the pathogenesis of weight loss in persons with chronic tropical sprue [15].

Clinical Presentation of Tropical Sprue

The sprue syndromes, tropical and nontropical sprue, were both described as disease entities in the 1880s and share similar morphological features with varying degrees of villus atrophy of the small intestinal mucosa, and both were presented clinically with malabsorption [8]. The clinical presentation is identical between tropical and non-tropical sprue [8]. The distinction between tropical and nontropical sprue is based on the history, especially exposure to a tropical environment, and the response to treatment [8]. Khokhar and Gill recently performed a study in Pakistan to review the experience of patients presenting with clinical manifestations of tropical sprue and assess their diagnosis and management, response to treatment and follow up [16]. In this study, a total of 42 patients were investigated. All patients presented with diarrhea, weight loss, anorexia and had megaloblastic anemia and in all patients, a distal duodenal biopsy showed partial villous atrophy [16]. They concluded that tropical sprue presented with diarrhea, anorexia, weight loss, and megaloblastic anemia and the partial villous atrophy had been a constant finding [16]. Kirchgatterer *et al.* also noted that chronic diarrhea, anorexia and anemia could be seen in the patients with tropical sprue [17]. They noted that tropical sprue predominantly occurred during or after a longer stay in endemic areas, however, if chronic diarrhea and signs of malabsorption develop after a short journey to India, South-East Asia and parts of the Caribbean, tropical sprue has to be considered [17]. Kirchgatterer *et al.* said that differential diagnosis in any patient who recently returned from the tropics might be a challenge [17].

Lim said that a diagnosis of tropical sprue, an infrequent affliction of inhabitants and travelers in tropical regions, should be considered in the patients with a compatible history, malabsorption, and chronic diarrhea [18]. They noted that tropical sprue could occur in either endemic or epidemic form and could be preceded by acute gastroenteritis [18]. To diagnose anemia relating to tropical sprue, the diagnosis of anemia due to the standard definition and the diagnosis of tropical anemia must be derived. Concerning the laboratory diagnosis for anemia relating to tropical sprue, laboratory tests showed megaloblastic anemia, folate deficiency and steatorrhea [19]. Stool specimens for bacterial pathogens and parasites were negative [19]. Endoscopy and biopsy from the distal portion of the duodenum revealed a broadening and shortening of the villi and an increased infiltration of the lamina propria by chronic inflammatory cells, plasma cells and lymphocytes [19]. Gras *et al.* noted that treatment of tropical sprue with antibiotics and folic acid is efficient and has a diagnostic value [4]. Effective therapeutic results can be derived from this treatment trail [4]. However, they also noted that the use of pediatric endoscope would assist in the incidences of tropical sprue and asymptomatic tropical sprue in Africa South of the Sahara, where the endoscope is usually not available [4]. They noted that peroral biopsie of the small intestine should be requested, in any intestinal syndrome, observed in tropical areas without an ascertained etiologic diagnosis [4].

Treatment of Anemia Due to Tropical Sprue

Treatment of tropical sprue is indicated in many cases since there are effective therapeutic methods. Tropical sprue is cured by treatment with tetracycline and folic acid, whereas nontropical sprue responds to a gluten-free diet [8]. Kapadia *et al.* reported their experience in using tetracycline 1 g per day and folic acid 5 mg per day for treatment of tropical sprue [14]. They found that all patients responded to treatment within 4 weeks [14]. According to their study, total treatment lasted 3 months and resulted in complete resolution of symptoms and weight gain, and the follow up lasted for a mean of 5 years and no relapses were noted [14]. They concluded that the response to treatment with tetracycline and folic acid had been uniformly successful [14]. First, sulfonamided was recommended for treatment of tropical sprue, however, it had been substituted by tetracycline [20]. Westergaard said that the recommended length of treatment with tetracycline was 6 months and it should be given in combination with folate [20]. Westergaard noted that this treatment had been shown to normalize mucosal structure in the small intestine and resolve malabsorption in most patients with tropical sprue, however, there was a substantial relapse rate in treated patients who return to, or remain in, endemic areas in the tropics [20].

Concerning treatment of anemia due to tropical sprue, Westergaard said that it was necessary to treat anemia in any cases with tropical sprue because the patients with tropical sprue are typically also with macrocytic anemia due to malabsorption of folate and/or vitamin B12 [20]. Westergaard mentioned that treatment of tropical sprue with folic acid replacement was introduced more than 50 years ago and had become standard medical treatment [20]. Although the combination between tetracycline and folic acid is the standard recommendation for treatment of tropical sprue, if treatment is started late, vitamin B12 is also then necessary [14]. Vitamin B 12 replacement is usually added if there is evidence of B12 deficiency or malabsorption [20]. Westergaard said that treatment of tropical sprue with folate and B12 cured the macrocytic anemia and the accompanying glossitis, and often resulted in increased appetite and weight gain [20]. However, Westergaard noted that even prolonged treatment with these vitamins failed to restore villus atrophy, and malabsorption usually persisted [20]. Concerning other methods for treatment of anemia, transfusion and erythropoietin therapy has never been recommended in tropical sprue.

Summary of Anemia Due to Tropical Sprue in the Tropics

As already mentioned, tropical sprue can be seen in the tropics and can lead to tropical anemia [21]. The high prevalence of tropical sprue is mentioned in South Asia. Mathan stated that tropical sprue could be frequently seem in the southern part of India [22]. Mathan said that the stomach, the small intestine and colon were affected and malabsorption resulted in nutrient deficiency in these cases [22]. Mathan noted that enterocyte damage, the primary lesion in southern Indian tropical sprue, was the result of a persistent lesion of the stem cell compartment and that this lesion occurred on a background of tropical enteropathy and the available evidence suggested that an immunity-conferring agent might be responsible for initiating the damage [22]. The high prevalence in Latin America was also noted. Concerning other tropical areas of the world, the high prevalence of tropical sprue is also expected, however, it might be underdiagnosed [1].

Surprisingly, most case reports of tropical sprue are not documented from the endemic area. These cases usually were reported in travelers who visited the tropics. Klipstein believes that the change in the world political situation, the rapidity of transportation, and the availability of effective therapy have altered the pattern of sprue in persons going to the tropics [23]. The importance of traveling medicine can be confirmed by this situation [24]. Indeed, Wiwanitkit said that the gastrointestinal disorders following traveling in the tropics is an important problem in present traveling medicine [24]. Gone are the days when expatriates lived for years in tropical areas, progressed into the full-blown pattern of thedebilitating disease when they acquired sprue, and then were never totally cured either by their return home or by the then-available forms of therapy [23]. Klipstein noted that today, visitors to the tropics usually return home by jet aircraft within weeks or months after acquiring the disease, and thus they are presented with just manifestations of small bowel disease in the absence of nutritional deficiencies [23]. Klipstein noted that the differential diagnosis usually fell between sprue and giardiasis in this circumstance [23]. In addition, Klipstein mentioned that sprue among the indigenous population of the tropics remains largely unchanged: a chronic debilitating disorder that represents a significant contributory factor to the pathogenesis of morbidity and malnutrition in some areas, in contrast to the situation in travelers [23].

References

[1]   Farthing MJ. Tropical malabsorption. *Semin Gastrointest Dis* 2002;13:221-31.
[2]   Wiwanitkit V. Intestinal parasitic infections in Thai HIV-infected patients with different immunity status. *BMC Gastroenterol* 2001;1:3.
[3]   Saksirisampant W, Nuchprayoon S, Wiwanitkit V, Yenthakam S, Ampavasiri A. Intestinal parasitic infestations among children in an orphanage in Pathum Thani province. *J Med Assoc Thai* 2003;86 Suppl 2:S263-70.
[4]   Gras C, Chapoy P, Aubry P. Tropical sprue (author's transl). *Med Trop* (Mars) 1981;41:449-54.
[5]   Haghighi P, Wolf PL. Tropical sprue and subclinical enteropathy: a vision for the nineties. *Crit Rev Clin Lab Sci* 1997;34:313-41.
[6]   Ghatei MA, Uttenthal LO, Christofides ND, Bryant MG, Bloom SR. Molecular forms of human enteroglucagon in tissue and plasma: plasma responses to nutrient stimuli in health and in disorders of the upper gastrointestinal tract. *J Clin Endocrinol Metab* 1983; 57:488-95.
[7]   Halsted CH. Jejunal brush-border folate hydrolase. A novel enzyme. *West J Med* 1991;155:605-9.
[8]   Westergaard H. The sprue syndromes. *Am J Med Sci* 1985;290:249-62.
[9]   Menendez-Corrada R, Nettleship E, Santiago-Delpin EA. HLA and tropical sprue. *Lancet* 1986;2:1183-5.
[10]   Ghoshal UC, Ghoshal U, Ayyagari A, Ranjan P, Krishnani N, Misra A, Aggarwal R, Naik S, Naik SR. Tropical sprue is associated with contamination of small bowel with aerobic bacteria and reversible prolongation of orocecal transit time. *J Gastroenterol Hepatol* 2003;18:540-7.
[11]   Malik AK, Mehta SK, Chandrashekhar Y, Mahajan A, Nanda V, Kochhar R. Quantitation of immunoglobulin-containing cells in the jejunal lamina propria in tropical sprue. *J Clin Gastroenterol* 1992;14:163-6.
[12]   Tiruppathi C, Hill PG, Mathan VI. Plasma lipids in tropical sprue. *Am J Clin Nutr* 1981;34:1117-20.
[13]   Lucas ML, Mathan VI. Jejunal surface pH measurements in tropical sprue. *Trans R Soc Trop Med Hyg* 1989;83:138-42.
[14]   Kapadia CR, Bhat P, Jacob E, Baker SJ. Vitamin B12 absorption--a study of intraluminal events in control subjects and patients with tropical sprue. *Gut* 1975;16:988-93.
[15]   Klipstein FA, Corcino JJ. Factors responsible for weight loss in tropical sprue. *Am J Clin Nutr* 1977;30:1703-8.
[16]   Khokhar N, Gill ML. Tropical sprue: revisited. *J Pak Med Assoc* 2004;54:133-4.

[17] Kirchgatterer A, Allinger S, Balon R, Tuppy H, Knoflach P. Tropical sprue as the cause of chronic diarrhea after travel to Southeast Asia. *Z Gastroenterol* 1998;36:897-900.

[18] Lim ML. A perspective on tropical sprue. *Curr Gastroenterol Rep* 2001;3:322-7.

[19] Santini R, Horta E, Millan S, Fradera J, Maldonado N. Laboratory tests to use in the diagnosis of tropical sprue in Puerto Rico. *Bol Asoc Med P R* 1971;63:223-7.

[20] Westergaard H. Tropical Sprue. *Curr Treat Options Gastroenterol* 2004;7:7-11.

[21] Baker SJ. Nutritional anaemias. Part 2: *Tropical Asia. Clin Haematol* 1981;10:843-71.

[22] Mathan VI. Tropical sprue in southern India. *Trans R Soc Trop Med Hyg* 1988;82:10-4.

[23] Klipstein FA. Tropical sprue in travelers and expatriates living abroad. *Gastroenterology* 1981 ;80:590-600.

[24] Wiwanitkit V. Amazing Thailand Year 1998-1999 Tourist's health concepts. *Chula Med J* 1998; 42: 975 – 84.

Chapter 14

Anemia and Tropical Toxin

Introduction to Tropical Toxin

According to the definition provided in Webster's 1913 Dictionary, toxin is a poisonous product formed by an organism, such as a pathogenic bacterium, a plant or an animal, usually having a high molecular weight, often a protein or a polysaccharide, but occasionally a low-molecular weight agent such as tetrodotoxin [1]. Several toxins are documented at present. Toxin insult is an important disorder in medicine. In tropical areas, there are several toxins. These toxins can be dangerous to human beings in contact with them. Thus, these tropical toxins are a very important topical medicine. There are several methods for insults of tropical toxin. The common methods are ingestion and being hurt by envenomous living things. Each toxin poses its poisonous effect to individual specific organs.

Clinical toxinology encompasses a broad range of medical conditions resulting from envenomation by venomous terrestrial and marine organisms, and also poisoning from ingestion of animal and plant toxins [2]. According to White *et al.,* toxin-related diseases were largely a cause of morbidity and mortality worldwide, particularly in the tropical and subtropical areas [2]. Management of toxin-related disease was often difficult, and in many cases, meticulous supportive care was all that was available [2]. In the specialty area of venomology, emergency physicians were traditionally most interested in the description of a variety of envenomation syndromes and, subsequent to this, the most appropriate investigative and therapeutic strategies to employ when envenomation was necessary [3]. Presently, the mainstream treatment is the use of antivenoms for many envenomations and poisoning, although these do not exist for all dangerous organisms [2]. Unfortunately, antivenoms are not an economically viable product, so development and manufacture of these agents have been limited [2]. According to White *et al.,* there was a need for improvement in the prevention and management of toxin-related diseases, and this will require well-designed studies to define the extent of the problem, initiatives to improve the prevention and management of these conditions, and development of new, as well as continuation of current, and antivenom supplies [2].

Anemia Relating to Important Tropical Toxin

Anemia relating to tropical toxin can be seen. Some important tropical toxins and clinical correlation to anemia are hereby presented.

1. Venomous Snake Toxin and Anemia

Snake bite is the single most important toxin-related disease, causing substantial mortality in many parts of Africa, Asia, and the Americas [2]. The most vital snake families are Viperidae and Elapidae, causing a range of clinical effects including local necrosis, neurotoxicity, coagulopathy and hemorrhage, myotoxicity and renal toxicity [2]. These effects vary according to geography and type of snake [2]. In the tropical areas, venomous snakes are common and therefore envenomations from snakebites are also common. Snakes of the families Viperidae and Elapidae were responsible for the high incidence of morbidity and mortality after snake bites in the countries of West Africa, the Indian subcontinent, South-East Asia, New Guinea and Latin America [4].

Concerning several snakes, the hematological toxic snakes are the group mentioned for the clinical correlation to the blood cell. Generally, hemotoxic snakes are represented by the family Viperidae, and subfamilies Viperinae and Crotalinae [5]. The important members of hematological toxic snakes in the tropics are green pit viper, Malayan's pit viper and Russell's viper [5]. Concerning the green pit viper (*Trimeresurus albolabris*, *Trimeresurus purpureomaculatus* and *Trimeresurus macrops*), there are several reports concerning its toxin effect on the coagulation and red blood cell [6]. After a green pit viper bites, thrombocytopenia and increased fibrinolytic activity were observed in addition to defibrination [6]. Hypofibrinogenemia with normal levels of the other clotting factors was observed [6]. In addition, thrombocytopenia, which resulted from platelet aggregating activity of the venom, has been described [6]. These pathological effects act synergistically to cause bleeding in the victims, and clinical features of these venomous snakebites vary from asymptomatic to fatal bleeding [6]. Recently, Wiwanitkit and Suwansaksri said that the green pit viper toxin could induce the red blood cell morphology change, and decrease the mean corpuscular volume (MCV) [7]. Hemorrhagin is an important component of green pit viper toxin. Both hemorrhagic and proteolytic activities are inhibited by EDTA, suggesting that the hemorrhagin is a metalloprotease [8]. The hemorrhagin hydrolyzed all gelatin preparations derived from types I, II, III and IV collagen, whereas it hydrolyzed only type IV native collagen [8]. Tan *et al.* studied the proteolytic specificity of rhodostoxin, the major hemorrhagin from Malayan's pit viper venom using oxidized B-chain of bovine insulin as substrate and found that 6 peptide bonds were cleaved: Ser9-His10, His10-Leu11, Ala14-Leu15, Tyr16-Leu17, Gly20-Glu21 and Phe24-Phe25 [9]. Concerning Russell's viper, not only hemorrhagic but also nephrotoxic effects of its venom were documented. The coagulation abnormalities following Russell's viper bite were compatible with disseminated intravascular coagulopathy [10]. The hemolytic activity of Russel's viper venom is mentioned since 1970 [11]. Recently, a potent toxin with phospholipase A2 (PLA2) and hemolytic activity in vitro was purified from the Russell's viper venom [12]. Chakraborty *et al.* said that the purified protein (RVV-PFIIc') of 15.3 kDa molecular weight, and a lethal toxicity dose (LD50i.p.) of 0.1 mg/kg body weight, was the most toxic PLA2 so far reported from the Indian subcontinent. The material also possessed anticoagulant activity as it enhanced the prothrombin induced plasma clotting time in vitro [12]. Although the bleeding is common in the three previously described viper snakes, the anemia due to their biting are not widely mentioned. Concerning the other viper toxins, toxin of Gaboon viper (*Bitis gabonica*) is proved to be a hemorrhagic toxin [13]. Marsh performed an animal study and found that there was a slight reduction in total red cell numbers and hemoglobin concentration as a result of the mild internal hemorrhage induced by the venom [13]. Marsh concluded that Gaboon viper venom produced a marked disturbance of iron handling by the liver without an associated change in erythropoiesis [13]. However, the mild hemorrhage was insufficient to produce a microcytic hypochromic anemia [13]. In 1994, Gillissen *et al.* reported a case presenting with neurotoxicity, hemostatic disturbances and hemolytic anemia after a bite by a Tunisian saw-scaled or carpet viper (Echis 'pyramidum'-complex) [14]. In addition, Benbassat and Shalev said that envenomation by the snake *Echis coloratus* caused a local swelling and hemostatic failure. They said that most cases recover uneventfully, however, about one-third of the victims bleed or develop anemia. One known death due to renal failure has been reported [15]

In addition to the viper snakes, other snakes are also mentioned for their clinical correlation to anemia. Jibly *et al.* reported that laboratory tests and clinical exams could show a Coombs positive hemolytic anemia without significant signs of coagulopathy in a case following envenomation by a North American crotalid [16].

Conclusively, the anemia relating to snake bite is usually the hemolytic anemia and associated with hemostatic disorders [17 – 18]. Concerning treatment of hematological toxic snakebite, specific hyperimmune serum or antivenom is the mainstay of medical treatment for severe envenoming. In cases with mild symptoms, close follow up is recommended since the application of antivenom also poses high risk for anaphylaxis [4]. Ancillary treatments such as assisted ventilation, repletion of circulating volume, renal dialysis and surgical debridement of necrotic tissues are needed in some critically severe cases [4].

2. Marine Envenomation and Anemia

Marine-related envenomations are common, but severe effects are less so [2]. Anemia due to marine envenomation is seldom reported. However, the hemolytic effect due to toxins from some jellyfish is medically important. *Cyanea capillata* is an example of jellyfish containing hemorrhagic toxin [19]. However, the most well known jellyfish containing hemolytic toxin is box jellyfish or sea wasp (*Chironex fleckeri*) [20]. Comis *et al.* studied the stability of both the lethal and hemolytic activities of box jellyfish tentacle extract and found that both activities were higher when no buffers or water were used during the initial extraction [21]. Also, when the extract was first filtered through a Sep-pak C18 cartridge, the residual lethal titre, after incubation for 24 hr at room temperature was increased 16-fold and hemolysis was increased 2.6-fold [21]. In this study, evidence for proteolytic activity in the extract was also obtained and monitored by size exclusion HPLC [21]. Generally the deadly box jellyfish is distributed widely in the tropical Pacific region and known as Habu-kurage [21].

3. Arthropod Sting and Anemia

Arachnid envenomation results mainly in morbidity, particularly scorpion stings which can cause severe systemic envenomation [2]. Scorpion stings are a common medical problem in middle and southern America, North Africa and the Middle East [4]. Warrell said that vasodilator drugs were important to counter the effects of massive catecholamine release [4]. Spider bite is far less of a problem, and the majority of medically important cases can be attributed to widow spiders (*Latrodectus* spp.) and recluse spiders (*Loxosceles* spp.) [2]. Warrell noted that bites by spiders and stings by hymenoptera were responsible for deaths and morbidity in some tropical countries [4].

Concerning spider, the toxic spider bite varies in intensity, causing reactions ranging from an area of severe necrosis to a mild cutaneous reaction [22]. *Loxosceles reclusa* or brown recluse spider is a well known toxic spider found in America and causes necrotic arachnidism [22 - 23]. Hemolytic anemia is mentioned following this spider bite [24]. Loxoscelism, or envenomation by the brown recluse spider, may result in necrotic lesions and systemic reactions [22 – 23]. Eichner said that the patients usually had brisk intravascular hemolysis with direct Coombs' tests positive for complement and with peripheral blood smears showing spherocytosis, erythrophagocytosis, and leukoerythroblastosis [25]. Eichner suggested that the hemolytic anemia that can follow the bite of the brown recluse spider could be confused with autoimmune hemolytic anemia [25]. Eichner said that the patients usually had brisk intravascular hemolysis with direct Coombs' tests positive for complement and with peripheral blood smears showing spherocytosis, erythrophagocytosis, and leukoerythro-blastosis [25]. Eichner suggested that the hemolytic anemia that can follow the bite of the brown recluse spider could be confused with autoimmune hemolytic anemia [25]. Histologically, the skin lesion resembles a cutaneous Arthus reaction [26]. The reaction mechanism involves interactions between complement, neutrophils, and the clotting system [26]. Wright *et al.* studied 111 patients with suspected brown recluse spider bites and found that mild hemolytic anemia developed in one patient and another had mild hemolysis and a mild coagulopathy [27]. Majeski and Durst said that treatment was unsatisfactory, and no antivenom was currently available and even though a specific test was available for loxoscelism, diagnosis remained difficult [22]. However, Willie and Morrow said that dapsone is used in the management of local reactions to the bite of the brown recluse spider [28]. Futrell said that it was best treated with analgesics, avoidance of early surgical debridement, and oral dapsone [26].

Concerning scorpion its sting can bring toxin to the stung person. The main effect of scorpion sting is the anaphylactoid and anaphylactic reactions. The main treatment for scorpion sting is control of allergic reaction and pain. In severe cases, renal failure can be seen due to scorpion sting [29]. Hemolytic-uremic syndrome (HUS) following a scorpion sting is also mentioned [30]. Recently, Bahloul et al. reported two cases were reported with HUS due to scorpion stings [31]. These two cases were marked with acute anemia without bleeding, requiring blood transfusion, acute renal failure, low platelets and signs of hemolysis [31].

Concerning the hymenoptera sting, bee and wasp stings are common. They can lead to allergic reaction, with severe anaphylaxis in some cases. In severe cases of hymenoptera stings, the toxic reaction can be manifested by shock, acute renal failure, tissue damage of the skin, muscles and liver and hemolysis which can result in the patients' death [32]. These symptoms occurred as a result of the cytotoxic effects of bee venom components such as melittin, phospholipase and kinins [32]. They noted that the course of the disease was the initial phase mimicking an anaphylactic shock, hemolysis and rhabdomyolysis, which led to acute renal failure with tubular necrosis [32]. Bee envenomation can lead to hemolytic anemia although that is not as often as wasp envenomation. Thrombotic thrombocytopenic purpura (TTP) characterized by the pentad of microangiopathic hemolytic anemia, thrombocytopenia, neurologic symptoms, renal insufficiency, and fever was also reported due to bee sting [33].

Wasp envenomation can induce intravascular hemolysis, which causes acute renal failure, volume overload, hypertension, anemia, hyponatremia, hyperkalemia, and metabolic acidosis. Vachvanichsanong et al. noted that peritoneal dialysis was required for short periods in the cases with severe or multiple wasp envenomation [34].

4. Bacterial Toxin and Anemia

Several tropical bacterial toxins are well documented as the important causes of anemia. As mentioned in the previous chapter, shiga toxin is the bacterial toxin leading to severe hemolysis [35]. This toxin becomes an important problem relating to food sanitation in the tropics [33]. Another tropical bacterial toxin that can cause hemolysis is mycoplasma toxin. Mycoplasma pneumoniae is reported as a bacterial agent leading to paroxysmal noctural hemoglobinuria [36]. In those cases, transitory paroxysmal cold hemoglobinuria is usually associated with anti-P specificity of biphasic hemolysin: the Donath-Landsteiner-antibody exhibited anti-P specificity; hemolytic activity was partially inhibited against papainized erythrocytes at $0 \, C°$ incubation temperature and increased to $8 \, C°$ [36].

In addition, Streptococcus pneumoniae can also cause HUS. Special attention must be given in order to avoid giving plasma to patients with S. pneumoniae-associated HUS [37].

In addition to toxin, toxoid can also induce anemia. Presently, tetatus toxoid is widely used as a prophylactic agent for tetanus. It has been recommended as both post-exposure and standard childhood vaccination programs in the tropics. The hemolytic anemias after DPT immunization has also been mentioned [38 – 39]. In severe cases, HUS was also reported [38].

5. Fungal Toxin and Anemia

Several fungal toxins can be seen in the tropics. One of the most common fungal toxins is aflatoxin. In the tropics, Aflatoxin contamination can be detected in many food products, such as grains, animal tissue and fluids, milk, spices, fermented food and beverages, which have been carried out for a long time [40]. Aflatoxin contamination in all of the above can be determined based on fundamental techniques, thin-layer chromatography (TLC), high pressure liquid chromatography (HPLC), gas chromatography-mass spectrometry (GC-MS), enzyme-link immunosorbent assay (ELISA), monoclonal antibody affinity chromatography, photoacoustic spectrometry and fluorescence technology [40]. Since aflatoxin contamination of food and feed have gained global significance due to its deleterious effect on human and animal health and its importance in international trade, continued detection should be performed by a simple-to-operate, rapid, reliable, and cost-effective method, particularly in developing countries [40]. Hematologically, aflatoxin is mentioned for its correlation to anemia. In 1975, Tung *et al.* studied the effects of graded doses of dietary aflatoxin (0, 0.625, 1.25, 2.5, 5.0, and 10.0 mug./g.) on hemoglobin, packed blood cell volume, erythrocyte count, leucocyte counts, bone marrow lipid, and bone marrow nucleic acids of chickens [41]. According to their study, the hemoglobin, packed cell volume, and erythrocyte count were reduced significantly to about the same extent by any given dose. Microscopic examination of stained smears of the bone marrow revealed a hyperplastic response including the granulocytic elements. Chemical analyses of the marrow revealed decreased lipid content and an increased content of ribonucleic acid and deoxyribonucleic acid [41]. Concerning complete blood count, total leucocytes increased by about threefold by aflatoxin (10 mug/g). Differential leucocyte counts revealed that the heterophils increased while the eosinophils were unaffected and the basophils, lymphocytes, and monocytes were decreased [41]. According to this data, Tung *et al.* suggested that aflatoxin caused a hemolytic anemia in chickens, that aflatoxin, by itself, was not involved in the hemorrhagic anemia syndrome of chickens [41]. In 1986, Liggett *et al.* said that preliminary laboratory examinations in dogs with aflatoxicosis revealed toxic hepatitis, bilirubinuria and anemia [42]. Dietert *et al.* performed another study in a chicken model and found that while the number of peripheral erythrocytes was reduced following exposure to AF-B1, the differentiation status of erythrocytes was apparently unaltered [43]. According to their study, mean cell volume, percentage of circulating reticulocytes, and incidence of an erythroid differentiation marker and chicken fetal antigen were parameters in which no treatment effects were observed [43].

6. Mushroom Toxin and Anemia

Mushroom poisoning can occurs in most parts of the world, but the types and methods of poisoning vary considerably between continents [2]. Toxic mushrooms are usually accidentally ingested due to misunderstanding of the local population.

The anemia due to mushroom toxin is also mentioned [44]. *Gyromitra esculenta* (Persoon ex Fries) mushrooms have been responsible for severe intoxications and even deaths [45]. Clinical data are characterized primarily by vomiting and diarrhea, and, afterward, by jaundice, convulsions and coma [45]. Michelot and Toth observed that frequent consumption can cause hepatitis and neurological diseases [46]. The species of concern are mainly *G. esculenta*, *G. fastigiata and G. gigas*; nevertheless, recent advances in chromatography, biochemistry and toxicology have established that other species within the Ascomycetes may also prove to be toxic [45]. This mushroom, contains gyromitrin (N-methyl-N-formyl-N-acetyl-hydrazone), a toxic compound that is converted to hydrazines in the stomach [47]. It is mainly neurotoxic, but it may also induce moderate hepatic damage and hemolysis [47]. Michelot stated that the toxins gyromitrin and its higher homologues are converted in vivo into MFH (N-methyl-N-formyl-hydrazine) then into MMH (N-Methylhydrazine) [45]. The toxicity of these latter chemicals, which are chiefly hepatotoxic and even carcinogenic, has been established through in vivo, and in vitro experiments with monocelled cultures and biochemical systems [45]. Gamier et al. noted that the intoxication due to gyromitrin was most frequent in Eastern Europe [48]. They noted that the clinical picture associating cytolytic hepatitis, seizures, and hemolysis reminded the physicians of intoxication by hydrazine and therefore, awareness of gyromitrin intoxication was necessary [48].

Another mushroom mentioned for the association with hemolysis is *Amanita phalloides* [49 – 50]. The molecular weight of phallolysin, the toxic haemolysin from this mushroom, was established by gel chromatography to be 30000 daltons [49 – 50]. Basically, many of the physical properties of phallolysin are strikingly similar to those of staphylococcal alpha-toxin: molecular weight, existence of multiple forms, pI values, amino acid composition, and thermolability (60 degrees C) [49 – 50]. Studies by Faulstich et al. on the mechanism of cytolytic activity, enabled them to distinguish at least three sequential events: binding of the toxin to human erythrocytes, K+ release, and membrane rupture and subsequently hemoglobulin release [50]. They said that these steps could be characterized by different kinetics as well as by different temperature dependencies [50].

Additionally, primary hemolysis is well documented as immunohemolysis after repeated ingestion of involute paxillus or Brown Roll-Rim (*Paxillus involutus*) [51]. Brown Roll-Rim is a dangerous poisonous mushroom with symptoms of poisoning that occur a few hours after consumption [52]. Olesen said that repeated consumption may cause sensitization to a heat-stable toxin, resulting in hemolysis, which might be of all degrees [52]. Thus, severe gastrointestinal symptoms might be due to a heat-instable toxin [52]. Olesen noted that the treatment consists of corticosteroid and possibly plasmapheresis and symptomatic therapy in cases with immune hemolysis [52].

In summary, Flammer and Gallen concluded that primary hemolysis induced by antigens and toxins of mushrooms must be distinguished from hemolysis secondary to shock and disseminated intravascular coagulation with disruption of erythrocytes caused by severe poisoning with many mushroom species [51].

They said that direct hemolysis was reported after eating raw mushrooms with a high content of hemolysins and that hemolysis was only speculative in monomethylhydrazine poisoning by false morels (*G. esculenta*) [51]. They also mentioned that secondary hemolysis due to shock was not uncommon [51].

7. Phytotoxin and Anemia

Similar to mushroom poisoning, plant poisoning can occurs in most parts of the world, but the types and methods of poisoning vary considerably between continents [2]. Plants that may intoxicate animals include sorghum, greasewood, halogeton, water hemlock, Japanese yew, larkspur, lupine, milk-weed, philodendron, oleander, castor bean and precatory bean [52]. The hematological aberration, including anemia, due to plant is mentioned in medicine. However, most of the anemias due to plants are due to the sensitization of hemolytic process in glucose-6-phosphate dehydrogenase deficient subjects. Direct plant toxin leading to anemia is less common. There are some reports of the effects of phytotoxins in an animal model.

Adam *et al.* reported that *Chrozophora obliqua* was related to macrocytic hypochromic anemia and leucopenia in the rats [55]. Bracken fern (*Pteridium aquilinum*) was another plant mentioned for anemia due to its toxicity [56]. Marrero *et al.* reported that sick animals showed anemia, leukopenia and urine that turned from pink to intense red color with the presence of blood clots [56]. Red maple (*Acer rubrum*) is also mentioned as the etiological agent for hemolytic anemia in zebras [57].

However, there is still a lack of information about phytotoxin and anemia in human beings.

References

[1]   Definition of Toxin. Available at http://www.webster-dictionary.org/definition/toxin

[2]   White J, Warrell D, Eddleston M, Currie BJ, Whyte IM, Isbister GK. Clinical toxinology--where are we now? *J Toxicol Clin Toxicol* 2003;41:263-76.

[3]   Bailey P, Wilce J. Venom as a source of useful biologically active molecules. *Emerg Med* (Fremantle) 2001;13:28-36.

[4]   Warrell DA. Venomous bites and stings in the tropical world. *Med J Aust* 1993;159:773-9.

[5]   Chanhome L, Cox MJ, Wilde H, Jintakoon P, Chaiyabutr N, Sitprija V. Venomous snakebite in Thailand. I: Medically important snakes. *Mil Med* 1998;163:310-7.

[6]   Wiwanitkit V. A Review of the Hematologic Effects of Green Pit Viper Venom. *Toxin Reviews* 2004; 23: 105 – 10.

[7]   Wiwanitkit V, Suwansaksri J. Effect of green pit viper toxin on red blood cell index (an interim analysis). *Toxicology* 2001; 164: 178 – 9.

[8]   Khow O, Chanhome L, Omori-Satoh T, Puempunpanich S, Sitprija V. A hemorrhagin as a metalloprotease in the venom of Trimeresurus purpureomaculatus: purification and characterization. *Toxicon* 2002;40:455-61.

[9]   Tan NH, Ponnudurai G, Chung MC Proteolytic specificity of rhodostoxin, the major hemorrhagin of Calloselasma rhodostoma (Malayan pit viper) venom. *Toxicon* 1997;35:979-84.

[10]   Mahasandana S, Rungruxsirivorn Y, Chantarangkul V. Clinical manifestations of bleeding following Russell's viper and Green pit viper bites in adults. *Southeast Asian J Trop Med Public Health* 1980;11:285-93.

[11]   Dass B, Chatterjee SC, Devi P. Haemolytic activity of Russell's viper venom. *Indian J Med Res* 1970;58:399-408.

[12] Chakraborty AK, Hall RH, Ghose AC. Purification and characterization of a potent hemolytic toxin with phospholipase A2 activity from the venom of Indian Russell's viper. *Mol Cell Biochem* 2002;237:95-102.

[13] Marsh NA. The effect of Gaboon viper venom on iron exchange in the rat. *Br J Exp Pathol* 1979;60:395-9.

[14] Gillissen A, Theakston RD, Barth J, May B, Krieg M, Warrell DA. Neurotoxicity, haemostatic disturbances and haemolytic anaemia after a bite by a Tunisian saw-scaled or carpet viper (Echis 'pyramidum'-complex): failure of antivenom treatment. *Toxicon* 1994;32:937-44.

[15] Benbassat J, Shalev O. Envenomation by Echis coloratus (Mid-East saw-scaled viper): a review of the literature and indications for treatment. *Isr J Med Sci* 1993;29:239-50.

[16] Gibly RL, Walter FG, Nowlin SW, Berg RA. Intravascular hemolysis associated with North American crotalid envenomation. *J Toxicol Clin Toxicol* 1998;36:337-43.

[17] Sipahioglu H. Explanation of the anemias seen in snake bite, scorpion stings, and arachnidism with enzyme blockage. *Turk Tip Cemiy Mecm* 1968;34:87-100.

[18] Sipahioglu H. A search for glucose-6-phosphate dehydrogenase deficiency, among Toros Seljouck Turks, in both normal and pathological conditions. The explanation of hemolytic anemias seen, in snake bite and poisonous insect bites cases. Three cases of favism and hemolytic syndrome. *Turk Tip Cemiy Mecm* 1968;34:101-15.

[19] Walker MJ. Pharmacological and biochemical properties of a toxin containing material from the jellyfish, Cyanea capillata. *Toxicon* 1977;15:3-14.

[20] Comis A, Hartwick RF, Howden ME. Stabilization of lethal and hemolytic activities of box jellyfish (Chironex fleckeri) venom. *Toxicon* 1989;27:439-47.

[21] Nagai H, Takuwa-Kuroda K, Nakao M, Oshiro N, Iwanaga S, Nakajima T. A novel protein toxin from the deadly box jellyfish (Sea Wasp, Habu-kurage) Chiropsalmus quadrigatus. *Biosci Biotechnol Biochem* 2002;66:97-102.

[22] Majeski JA, Durst GG Sr. Necrotic arachnidism. *South Med J* 1976;69:887-91.

[23] Foil LD, Norment BR. Envenomation by Loxosceles reclusa. *J Med Entomol* 1979;16:18-25.

[24] Chu JY, Rush CT, O'Connor DM. Hemolytic anemia following brown spider (Loxosceles reclusa) bite. *Clin Toxicol* 1978;12:531-4.

[25] Eichner ER. Spider bite hemolytic anemia: positive Coombs' test, erythrophagocytosis, and leukoerythroblastic smear. *Am J Clin Pathol* 1984;81:683-7.

[26] Futrell JM. Loxoscelism. *Am J Med Sci* 1992;304:261-7.

[27] Wright SW, Wrenn KD, Murray L, Seger D. Clinical presentation and outcome of brown recluse spider bite. *Ann Emerg Med* 1997;30:28-32.

[28] Wille RC, Morrow JD. Case report: dapsone hypersensitivity syndrome associated with treatment of the bite of a brown recluse spider. *Am J Med Sci* 1988;296:270-1.

[29] Malhotra KK, Mirdehghan CM, Tandon HD. Acute renal failure following scorpion sting. *Am J Trop Med Hyg* 1978;27:623-6.

[30] Mocan H, Mocan MZ, Kaynar K. Haemolytic-uraemic syndrome following a scorpion sting. *Nephrol Dial Transplant* 1998;13:2639-40.

[31] Bahloul M, Ben Hmida M, Belhoul W, Ksibi H, Kallel H, Ben Hamida C, Chaari A, Chelly H, Rekik N, Bouaziz M. Hemolytic-uremic syndrome secondary to scorpion envenomation (apropos of 2 cases). *Nephrologie* 2004;25:49-51.

[32] Nittner-Marszalska M, Malolepszy J, Mlynarczewski A, Niedziolka A. Toxic reaction induced by Hymenoptera stings. *Pol Arch Med Wewn* 1998;100:252-6.

[33] Ashley JR, Otero H, Aboulafia DM. Bee envenomation: a rare cause of thrombotic thrombocytopenic purpura. *South Med J* 2003;96:588-91.

[34] Vachvanichsanong P, Dissaneewate P, Mitarnun W. Non-fatal acute renal failure due to wasp stings in children. *Pediatr Nephrol* 1997;11:734-6.

[35]   Cherla RP, Lee SY, Tesh VL. Shiga toxins and apoptosis. *FEMS Microbiol Lett.* 2003;228:159-66.

[36] Boccardi V, D'Annibali S, Di Natale G, Girelli G, Summonti D. Mycoplasma pneumoniae infection complicated by paroxysmal cold hemoglobinuria with anti-P specificity of biphasic hemolysin. *Blut* 1977;34:211-4.

[37] Kaplan BS, Cleary TG, Obrig TG. Recent advances in understanding the pathogenesis of the hemolytic uremic syndromes. *Pediatr Nephrol* 1990;4:276-83.

[38] Guerra Au, Lorenzoydeibarreta J, Temesio N. Hemolytic-uremic syndromes following triple vaccination (diptheria-pertussis-tetanus) *Arch Pediatr Urug.*1965 ;36:26-38.

[39] Downes KA, Domen RE, McCarron KF, Bringelsen KA. Acute autoimmune hemolytic anemia following DTP vaccination: report of a fatal case and review of the literature. *Clin Pediatr* (Phila) 2001;40:355-8.

[40] Waenlor W. The contamination of aflatoxin in food products. *Chula Med J* 2002; 46: 843 –9.

[41] Tung HT, Cook FW, Wyatt RD, Hamilton PB. The anemia caused by aflatoxin. *Poult Sci* 1975 ;54:1962-9.

[42] Liggett AD, Colvin BM, Beaver RW, Wilson DM. Canine aflatoxicosis: a continuing problem. *Vet Hum Toxicol* 1986;28:428-30.

[43] Dietert RR, Bloom SE, Qureshi MA, Nanna UC. Hematological toxicology following embryonic exposure to aflatoxin-B1. *Proc Soc Exp Biol Med* 1983;173:481-5.

[44] Louria DB, Smith JK, Finkel GC. Mycotoxins other than aflatoxins: tumor-producing potential and possible relation to human disease. *Ann N Y Acad Sci* 1970;174:583-91.

[45] Michelot D. Poisoning by Geromitra esculenta. *J Toxicol Clin Exp* 1989;9:83-99.

[46] Michelot D, Toth B. Poisoning by Gyromitra esculenta--a review. *J Appl Toxicol* 1991;11:235-43.

[47] Karlson-Stiber C, Persson H. Cytotoxic fungi--an overview. *Toxicon* 2003;42:339-49.

[48] Garnier R, Conso F, Efthymiou ML, Riboulet G, Gaultier M. Acute poisoning by Gyromitra esculenta (author's transl). *Toxicol Eur Res* 1978;1:359-64.

[49] Seeger R. Some physico-chemical *properties of phallolysin obtained from Amanita phalloides. Naunyn* Schmiedebergs Arch Pharmacol 1975;288:155-62.

[50] Faulstich H, Buhring HJ, Seitz J. Physical properties and function of phallolysin. *Biochemistry* 1983;22:4574-80.

[51] Flammer R, Gallen S. Hemolysis in mushroom poisoning: facts and hypotheses. *Schweiz Med Wochenschr* 1983;113:1555-61.

[52] Olesen LL. Poisoning with the brown roll-rim mushroom, Paxillus involutus. *Ugeskr Laeger* 1991;153:445.

[53] Jakobsen PH, Bate CA, Taverne J, Playfair JH. Malaria: toxins, cytokines and disease. *Parasite Immunol* 1995;17:223-31.

[54] Mount ME, Feldman BF. Practical toxicologic diagnosis. *Mod Vet Pract* 1984;65:589-95.

[55] Adam SE, Al-Redhaiman KN, Al-Qarawi AA. Toxicity of Chrozophora obliqua in rats. *Phytother Res.* 1999;13:630-2.

[56] Marrero E, Bulnes C, Sanchez LM, Palenzuela I, Stuart R, Jacobs F, Romero J. Pteridium aquilinum (bracken fern) toxicity in cattle in the humid Chaco of Tarija, Bolivia. *Vet Hum Toxicol* 2001;43:156-8.

[57] Weber M, Miller RE. Presum*ptive red maple (Acer rubrum) toxicosis in Grevy's zebra (Equus grevyi). J Zoo Wildl Med* 1997;28:105-8.

Chapter 15

Occupational Induced Anemia in the Tropics

Occupation and Anemia

One cannot deny that the general population has to spend most of their daily lives working. Their health is therefore related to their working activities. At present, the concept of occupational medicine should be applied. To take care of their health a person should focus not only on the biopsychological aspects but also the social aspect. Individual genetic makeup is the basic component determining the response of each person, while environmental factors act as a superimposition factor aggravating manifestation of disorder in each individual [1].

Several factors in daily work can lead to the development of hematological disorders including anemia. Exposure to biological, physical and chemical insults during work can be the underlying etiologies for anemia.

The intensity, duration and prevention of exposure also modifies the expression of the anemic manifestation. The knowledge of occupational anemia is therefore an important concept for general practitioners at present. This chapter summarizes some important anemic disorders in some occupational groups in the tropics.

Anemia in Agricultural Occupations

Agricultural occupations are the basic occupational group of most of the people living in developing countries in the tropics. Fleming mentioned that the humans evolved as hunter-gatherers, and the invention and spread of agriculture had been followed by changes in diet. The environment and population densities resulted in a globally high prevalence of anemias due to nutritional deficiencies of iron, folate and (locally) vitamin B12, to infestations by hookworm and schistosomes, to malaria, and to the natural selection for the genes for sickle-cell diseases, beta-thalassaemias, alpha-thalassaemias, glucose-6-phosphate dehydrogenase deficiency, ovalocytosis and possibly (locally) elliptocytosis [2]. Fleming also noted that the recent explosion of population was driving an expansion of agriculture, especially the cultivation of rice, and this has often led to disastrous increases of transmission of malaria, schistosomiasis and other diseases, to widespread chemical pollution, and to degradation of the environment [2]. Although food production appears to have kept pace with population growth in macro statistics, 35% of the population in sub-Saharan Africa, 22% of the Asian population, and 22% of developing market economies were estimated to be malnourished in the mid-1980s [3]. Graber *et al.* posited that farming methods and activities were both affected by and had an impact on local and global environmental ecosystems [3]. The urgent need for increased food production is matched by the urgent need for assessment and control of the health impact of agricultural development [2].

Anemia, as the commonest manifestation of human disease, is a frequent consequence [2]. The agricultural–related occupations are mentioned for their correlation with anemia, as previously stated. Presently, the high prevalence of anemia in the primitive agricultural communities in the tropics are still reported. Suyaphan and Wiwanitkit recently reported a high prevalence of anemia among the hilltribers in agricultural communities in Thailand [4]. Igbedioh also indicated the high prevalence of anemia and mulnutrition in the rural agricultural communities in Nigeria [5]. Igbedioh proposed remedial programs, including increased support for the rural farmers, strengthening of the rural credit schemes that were specifically targeted at the poor, distribution of vitamin A and iron supplements in rural health centres, encouraging production of low cost weaning diets and integrating nutrition education in primary health care schemes and in educational curricula [5]. Recently, Gilgen *et al.* conducted a randomized clinical intervention trial over 24 weeks on a tea estate in north-east Bangladesh to investigate the effect of iron supplementation and anthelmintic treatment on the labor productivity of adult female tea pluckers [6].

They found that there was a negative association between the intensity of helminth infections (eggs/g faeces) and all measures of labor productivity for all three detected worms; *Ascaris lumbricoides*, *Trichuris trichiura* and hookworms [6]. In addition, lower hemoglobin values and anemia were both associated with lower labour productivity and more days sick and absent [6].

Concerning the population of agricultural occupations, their underlying risks for anemia are different. Concerning the farmer who worked bare-footed, the high prevalence of hookworm infestation and anemia can be seen. Since they practiced the risky behavior, not wearing shoes during daily work, they had a greater chance contacting the hookworm contamination in the soil. Carr-harris said that personal hygiene was always affected by inadequate supplies in the rural agricultural communities [7]. They also noted that another hazard was waste disposal which, if improperly managed, resulted in hookworm and ascarias infestations. As previously mentioned, Carr-harris noted that barefoot people are particularly affected [7]. In 1989, Chandiwana *et al.* performed an examination of 1635 fecal samples from rural farm workers with poor living conditions in Zimbabwe and found that hookworms were the commonest helminths (61.7%) in these populations [8]. They noted that age-prevalence and age-intensity profiles for hookworms showed that infection increased with age, with a peak in the adult age groups [8]. Recently, Wiwanitkit *et al.* also reported a high prevalence of parasitic contamination in the soil samples collected from agricultural communities in northern Thailand [9]. The high prevalence of hookworm infestation as well as the high rate of parasitic contamination in the agricultural communities in tropical countries can warrant the high prevalence of hookworm-induced anemia in these settings [2].

Concerning the forester who worked in the tropical monsoon forests in the tropics, they had a high risk of malarial infection. Kimerling *et al.* performed a study among the forest workers in Cambodia [10]. According to the KAP assessment, they identified that the young, male forest worker was the highest risk group [10]. In their study, the primary reason found for patient delay in seeking hospital care was self-treatment at home with drugs purchased through private sellers [10]. Indeed, the anemia in the forestry area of tropical countries is mentioned for its strong correlation to the malarial infection [11 – 12]. In addition to the forester, the gardener who performed their garden activities in the area near the forest also had a high risk of getting malaria and subsequently an anemic complication [12]. Another problem for the gardener in the tropics is the poor control of pesticide usage in their gardens. Recently, Soogarun *et al* noted for the low level of serum cholinesterase in the Thai gardeners indicating high exposure to the pesticide [13 – 14]. The accumulation of the pesticide can also lead to anemia. Aplastic anemia is accepted as the complication of chronic intoxication of pesticide. Rugman and Cosstick said that the temporal association between chemical exposure and the onset of first symptoms of anemia was strongly supportive [15]. Muir *et al.* also identified significant risks for aplastic anemia associated with self-reported exposure to solvents, radiation and pesticides in the workplace [16].

Concerning fisherman, the risk for anemia due to their daily work is less than other previously mentioned agricultural occupations. However, due to modern technology, using the machinery on fishing ships, the risk for accumulated exposure to fuel, which can subsequently lead to aplastic anemia, is also mentioned [17]. Conclusively, since agricultural occupations are the main occupations in the tropics, tropical anemia as a subsequent result should be a concern.

Anemia in Industrial Occupations

Generally, three factors, population, consumption levels per person, and technology, have an impact on environmental damage [18]. Harrion said that reduction of 125 million hectares in forests was observed in developing countries between 1971-1986 [18]. Harrison noted that the increase in farmland was responsible for 80% of the deforestation [18]. Population growth related to about 80% of the increased farmland; thus, 64% of deforestation was contributed by the population factor [18]. A main problem leading to the deforestation is industrialization. Harrion concluded that the cities mainly invaded into the forests [18]. At present, industrialization invades into many tropical countries. countries can face environmental problems if there is no good practi several industrial occupations have replaced the old agricultural o Several problems in occupational medicine including anemia a industrial workers in the developing tropical countries.

The industrial-related anemia is usually due to the effect of toxic pollutants from industries can lead to the anemia (Table 15.1) [19 toxic pollutants noted for their correlation to anemia include manganese, arsenic, benzene, toluene and styrene. Concerning lead, it has a wide range of applications, and its production and use result in contamination of the environment, including food and drinking water [20]. Naturally, lead is found naturally in earth and present in almost all parts of the environment, such as food, air, water, dust, soil, paint, and tissues of living organisms including humans [21]. Grandjean said that geochemical studies indicated that the majority of lead in ecosystems originated from industrial operations, and that human lead intake has increased 100-fold above the "natural" level [21]. Grandjean said that biochemical interference with heme biosynthesis could be detected as a result of current lead exposures, inhibition of aminolevulinate dehydratase and accumulation of zinc protoporphyrin in erythrocytes being the earliest effects [20]. Grandjean said that anemia was uncommon except for cases of lead poisoning, but even slightly increased lead absorption results in a decrease in hemoglobin concentrations [20]. Lead has been known to be toxic to most living things at high doses [21]. This metal is being used in various aspects including the manufacturing of storage batteries, production of chemicals, paints and gasoline additives, and it is also used to make various metal products including sheet lead, solder, and pipes [21]. Grandjean also noted that modern neurobehavioral test methods have disclosed an increased prevalence of psychological dysfunction associated with augmented lead absorption [21]. The well-known and excessive environmental exposures are from the air of industrial and heavy traffic areas [21]. The high level of blood lead implying the high exposure of the industrial workers in the tropics is reported. Recently, Suwansaksri et al. reported the high level of blood lead among the garage workers in Bangkok [22]. In addition, Suwansaksri and Wiwanitkit also reported similar results among the mechanics as well [23]. As previously mentioned, chronic exposure to lead can lead to anemia. Grandjean noted that biochemical and behavioral changes could occur below the recommended limit for blood lead concentrations of 60 micrograms/100 ml [20]. The well-known anemic disorder, sideroblastic anemia, is described due to lead poisoning. Lead intoxication results in a disturbance of heme biosynthesis, its degree depending on the severity and duration of exposure to lead [24]. A mild secondary, sideroblastic anemia is common; basophilic stippling may occur, especially in severe lead poisoning [24]. Increased excretion in the urine of delta-aminolevulinic acid and coproporphyrin III may occur; porphobilinogen excretion is not usually increased while delta-aminolevulinate dehydratase, coproporphyrin oxidase, and ferrochelatase activities are reduced; delta-aminolevulinate synthetase activity is increased [24]. In addition, erythrocyte protoporphyrin (FEP and ZPP) is increased [24]. Therefore, monitoring for the exposure to lead among the risk exposed workers is necessary [22 – 23]. Presently, several diagnostic tests for lead toxicity are available [20]. Of those tests, the protoporphyrin concentration in the blood seems to be the best risk indicator [20]. However, Porphyrinurias as well as porphyrias can be observed after exposure to hexachlorobenzene, chlorinated dibenzodioxins, polychlorinated biphenyls, polybrominated biphenyls and vinyl chloride [19].

Concerning mercury, the hemolytic anemia due to chronic exposure is reported. Rothstein said that mercury influenced a large number of protein-mediated functions in red ll membranes including transport phenomena, related enzyme activities and sructural s such as deformability and phospholipid asymmetry [25]. They noted that the l groups that were the targets for mercurials were found in different locations in the the outer surface, internal compartments, or cytoplasmic surface [25]. In addition to mercury, lead and cadmium are two other metallic pollutants mentioned as underlying corresponding agents for hemolytic anemia. Concerning copper, aplastic anemia is mentioned for the cases with chronic exposure [19]. However, arsenic is more widely mentioned for the correlation to aplastic anemia. Hall said that symptomatic arsenic poisoning was not often seen in occupational exposure settings, however, long-term exposure could result in chronic toxicity [26]. Benramdane *et al.* noted that although acute intoxication had become rare, arsenic was still a dangerous pollution agent for industrial workers and people living in the vicinity of emission sources [27]. Concerning arsenic toxicity, skin pigmentation changes, palmar and plantar hyperkeratoses, gastrointestinal symptoms, anemia, and liver disease are common [26]. In addition, noncirrhotic portal hypertension with bleeding esophageal varices, splenomegaly, and hypersplenism may occur [26]. Concerning the hematotoxic effect of arsenic, not only anemia but also bone marrow depression can be seen [26]. Hall said that workplace exposure or chronic ingestion of arsenic-contaminated water or arsenical medications was associated with development of skin, lung, and other cancers [26]. Therefore, it is necessary to monitor the aresenic exposure among workers at risk. The analysis of urine, blood, fingernails and hair has been used to monitor occupational exposure to arsenic. Concerning treatment, Hall suggested the use of chelating agents such as dimercaprol (BAL), dimercaptosuccinic acid (DMSA), and dimercaptopanesulfonic acid (DMPS) [26].

Table 15.1. Anemia due to toxic effects of some common industrial pollutants [19]

Types of anemia	Examples of industrial pollutants
1. Aplastic anemia	o benzene, pesticides, arsenic, cadmium and copper
2. Megaloblastic anemia	o arsenic, chlordane, benzene and nitrous oxide
3. Hemolytic anemia	o arsenic, methyl chloride, naphthalene, lead, cadmium and mercury

Concerning cadmium, it is a heavy metal that is found as an important pollutant from many industries. Chronic exposure to cadmium in industry gives rise to a proteinuria which may be tubular, glomerular or mixed in character [28]. This proteinuria may be accompanied or preceded by a variety of other renal effects [28]. Bernard *et al.* said that three main groups of thresholds for urinary cadmium have been identified for the induction of these effects with corresponding thresholds in the renal cortex in active male workers [28]. Bernard *et al* suggested that subclinical changes in tubular function may occur in the general population above a threshold of urinary cadmium as low as 2 micrograms/24h [28]. Of interest, the contamination of cadmium from industry to the environment is widely mentioned at present. Recently, Parkpian *et al.* reported an interesting finding in Thailand that improvements in farm management significantly reduced elevated levels of lead and cadmium in soil and plants [29]. The toxicity of cadmium is therefore an interesting topic in tropical medicine at present. Although less common than nephrotoxicity, the hematotoxicity of cadmium is also mentioned [19]. The hematologic effect of cadmium includes anemia [19]. Aplastic anemia is the most common anemic disorder resulting from chronic cadmium exposure [19]. In 1985, Hays and Margaretten performed an animal experiment in CBA/H mice that drank water containing 300 mg/L cadmium chloride for 12 months [30]. According to this study, the animals reflected the marrow alterations by demonstrating an anemia with reticulocytopenia and neutropenia [30]. The mice did not show increased mortality or increased susceptibility to infections; however, their body weight was significantly reduced [30]. In addition, iron deficiency was demonstrated in the cadmium-treated mice and the animals had a hypochromia of the peripheral red cells and diminished marrow iron stores [30]. Hays and Margaretten concluded that the anemia of cadmium toxicity was probably the combined result of bone marrow hypoplasia and iron deficiency [30].

In addition to the metallic pollutant, volatile hydrocarbon compound is another group of industrial pollutant that relates to anemia. Of several volatile hydrocarbons, benzene is the most widely mentioned compound for its correlation to anemia.

Benzene is a colorless poisonous liquid with a sweet - odor [31]. Breathing extremely high levels of benzene can result in death while exposure to high levels can cause drowsiness, dizziness, rapid heart rate, headaches, tremors, confusion, and unconsciousness [31]. Long-term benzene exposure is hematotoxic, genotoxic, genetoxic and immunotoxic. Concerning the hematological effect of benzene, all three blood cell series can be insulted. The recent data suggested that benzene activate peripheral lymphocytes, and cause changes in the incidence of CD25+/CD4+ T lymphocytes that may represent a distinct subset of immune-regulatory T cells [32].

In 2004, Wiwanitkit et al. reported the effect of benzene exposure on platelets [33]. According to this study, they found that although there was no statistical significance, the platelet count and PCT decreased while the urine benzene biomarker increased [33]. In addition, using the upper normal limit biomarker level as the cutoff level, the statistically significant lower platelet count and PCT was observed in the subjects with urine biomarkers higher than the upper normal limit [33]. Concerning the effect on red blood cells, Bogadi-Sare et al. recently said that the results confirm that benzene exposure below 15 ppm might produce qualitative abnormalities, particularly macroerythrocytosis and increased red cell glycerol resistance, in the absence of an overt quantitative decrease in circulating blood cells [34]. They said increased resistance to the hemolytic action of glycerol was a potentially useful biological monitoring procedure in medical surveillance of benzene exposed workers [34]. Bogadi-Sare et al. also suggested that potential threshold concentration for hematologic effects of benzene was lower than 15 ppm [34]. Presently, it is accepted that benzene exposure is an important risk for aplastic anemia. In addition, low levels and long term exposure to benzene is associated with hematotoxicity including aplastic anemia, acute myelogenous leukemia, and lymphoma [35]. Concerning the underlying genetic factor for those hematological complications due to benzene exposure, Chen et al. said that genetic polymorphism of I metabolic enzymes(CYP2E1, NQO1, MPO) and II metabolic enzymes (GST, PST) involved benzene metabolite and interindividual variation in their genetic susceptibility to hematotoxicity from benzene exposure [36]. At present, work with benzene is subject to the Control of Substances Hazardous to Health (COSHH) Regulations 1999. Hence, benzene exposure is of particular concern because of ongoing exposure to thousands of workers in industrial plants. As indicated, benzene exposure becomes the present problem in the industrial-workers in developing countries. For example, Suwansaksri and Wiwanitkit recently reported the high exposure to benzene among a sample of mechanics in Bangkok, Thailand [37].

Monitoring for benzene exposure among the at-risk workers is recommended. Current biomonitoring methods such as urinary phenol, S-phenylmercapturic acid, and trans-trans muconic acid were found to be unreliable as analytical methods to detect benzene exposure. Of several biomarkers, urine ttMA determination is a helpful test for monitoring [38 – 39]. Recently, Joo et al. noted that TCR beta levels in plasma could be used as a new biomarker and a possible therapeutic target for benzene exposure [35].

Concerning toluene, although there are fewer evidences on its hematoxic effect, it is mentioned for the correlation to anemia. Toluene is an important toxic volatile agent found in many modern industrial processes [40]. Toluene exposure is of particular concern because of the ongoing exposure of thousands of workers in industrial plants and recent research has indicated that toluene exposure can result in chronic toxicity [40]. Its effects are central nervous system excitation followed by central nervous system depression, at times accompanied by seizures. Acute exposure to very high doses of toluene may cause sudden death as a result of ventricular arrhythmias, reflex vagal inhibition, respiratory depression, and anoxia. Chronic toxicity may involve the nervous system, heart, kidney, and liver. As previously mentioned, the hematotoxic effect of toluene is not common. However, hemolytic anemia as well as aplastic anemia due to trinitrotoluene intoxication has been continuously reported [41 – 43]. Similar to benzene exposure, the toluene exposure becomes the present problem in industrial-workers in the developing countries. For example, Wiwanitkit et al recently reported the high exposure to benzene among a sample of press workers in Bangkok, Thailand [40]. Urine hippuric acid determination is helpful for monitoring a group of workers at risk for exposure to toluene. This biomarker can be determined by simple urine colorimetric method, which is feasible for the developing countries with limited resources in the tropics. In 2002, Wiwanitkit et al. indicated that smoking did not influence the urinary hippuric acid levels and therefore it was recommended as a biomarker for toluene exposure [44]. The other biomarker for monitoring of toluene exposure is o-cresol [45]. However, this test is more complicated than urine hippuric acid determination and therefore not recommended. Recently, urinary benzylmercapturic acid (or N-acetyl-S-benzyl cysteine, BMA), a mercapturate metabolite of toluene is available. Ioue et al. noted that BMA is superior to hippuric acid and o-cresol as a marker of occupational exposure to toluene [46]. However, BMA is still too complicated and not cost effective for developing countries.

Concerning xylene, it is an aromatic hydrocarbon widely used in industry and medical technology as a solvent. Health and safety authorities in most countries, including Australia, recommend a threshold limit value (TLV) of 100 ppm in the working environment [47]. Xylene vapour is absorbed rapidly in the lungs, and xylene liquid and vapour are absorbed slowly through the skin [47]. Xylene in high concentrations acts as a narcotic, inducing neuropsychological and neurophysiological dysfunction. Respiratory tract symptoms are also frequent [47]. More chronic, occupational exposure has been associated with anemia, thrombocytopenia, leukopenia, chest pain with ECG abnormalities, dyspnea and cyanosis, in addition to CNS symptoms [47]. Recently, the amount of the major metabolite of xylene, methylhippuric acid (MHA), in urine has been recommended as a better indicator of exposure [47].

An important consideration for the toxic hydrocarbon pollutants is that these volatile hydrocarbons usually present as co-pollutants and therefore, the toxic effects are the complexes of each pollutant. The monitoring of the biomarker for the set of volatile hydrocarbons is proper. Langman indicated that concomitant exposure to xylene and other solvents, including toluene, affected hematological parameters, liver size, liver enzymes, auditory memory, visual abstraction, and vibration threshold in the toes [47]. In 1998, Hristeva-Mirtcheva studied a total of 171 workers with occupational exposure to benzene, toluene, xylene and ethylbenzene and found anemia in combination with thrombocytopenia or leukocytosis with decreased enzyme activity of the granulocyte alkaline phosphatase in these workers [48]. In this study, no definite relationship between changes in peripheral blood elements and length of service of the workers was found, but workers with over 20 years' exposure to aromatic hydrocarbons suffered from more severe forms of anemia [48].

Control of the industrial-related anemia must be based on the principle of occupational medicine. Conclusively, the preventive measurement as well as the monitoring of exposure via biomarker should be used. This combination should be set as the specific act [23, 40]. Of interest, the basic problems of many developing countries in the tropics are the lack of funds for and no systematic control of the use of the specific act. In addition, the extrapolation of basic occupational medicine to the real practice must be done. Grieco said that part of the scientific heritage of occupational medicine should be used to the fullest to plan and carry out prevention measures that have led to improved working conditions in many sectors of industry [49]. Grieco mentioned that the areas where scientific bio-medical knowledge could be used were: a) planning of prevention measures on a vast social scale; b) variables and indicators for planning and assessing services designed for diagnosis and prevention of occupational risks and diseases; and c) development of training programs [49].

References

[1]   Tarasova LA, Kuz'mina LP, Kasparov AA. The problem of genetic-biochemical basis of individual sensitivity in occupational medicine. *Med Tr Prom Ekol* 1998;(4):1-4.

[2]   Fleming AF. Agriculture-related anaemias. *Br J Biomed Sci* 1994;51:345-57.

[3]   Graber DR, Jones WJ, Johnson JA. Human and ecosystem health: the environment-agriculture connection in developing countries. *J Agromedicine* 1995;2:47-64.

[4]   Suyaphan A, Wiwanitkit V. The prevalence of anaemia among the hilltriber in Mae Jam district, Northern Thailand. *Haema* 2003; 6: 260 – 1.

[5]   Igbedioh SO. Undernutrition in Nigeria: dimension, causes and remedies for alleviation in a changing socio-economic environment. *Nutr Health* 1993;9:1-14.

[6]   Gilgen DD, Mascie-Taylor CG, Rosetta LL. Intestinal helminth infections, anaemia and labour productivity of female tea pluckers in Bangladesh. *Trop Med Int Health* 2001;6:449-57.

[7]   Carr-harris J. Eco-health in the rural environment. *Health Millions* 1993;1:2-6.

[8]   Chandiwana SK, Bradley M, Chombo F. Hookworm and roundworm infections in farm-worker communities in the large-scale agricultural sector in Zimbabwe. *J Trop Med Hyg* 1989;92:338-44.

[9] Wiwanitkit V, Waenlor W, Suyaphan A. Contamination of soil with parasites in a tropical hilltribe village in Northern Thailand. *Trop Doct* 2003;33:180-2.

[10] Kimerling ME, Houth H, Hilderbrand K, Goubert L. Identifying malaria control issues: a district hospital-based evaluation. *Southeast Asian J Trop Med Public Health* 1995;26:611-9.

[11] Akenzua GI, Ihongbe JC, Imasuen IW, Nwobi BC. Anaemia in children: a survey in (Obadan) a rural community in the rain forest zone of Nigeria. *J Trop Pediatr* 1985;31:20-4.

[12] Suyaphun A, Wiwanitkit V, Suwansaksri J, Nithiuthai S, Sritar S, Suksirisampant W, Fongsungnern A. Malaria among hilltribe communities in northern Thailand: a review of clinical manifestations. *Southeast Asian J Trop Med Public Health* 2002;33 Suppl 3:14-5.

[13] Soogarun S, Wiwanitkit V, Suwansaksri J. Report on blood cholinesterase among vegetable growers. *Southeast Asian J Trop Med Public Health* 2003;34:687-9.

[14] Soogarun S, Wiwanitkit V, Suyaphan A, Suwansaksri J, Pathompattama N. Decreased serum cholinesterase levels among a sample of a rural Thai population. *MedGenMed* 2003;5:30.

[15] Rugman FP, Cosstick R. Aplastic anaemia associated with organochlorine pesticide: case reports and review of evidence. *J Clin Pathol* 1990;43:98-101.

[16] Muir KR, Chilvers CE, Harriss C, Coulson L, Grainge M, Darbyshire P, Geary C, Hows J, Marsh J, Rutherford T, Taylor M, Gordon-Smith EC. The role of occupational and environmental exposures in the aetiology of acquired severe aplastic anaemia: a case control investigation. *Br J Haematol* 2003;123:906-14.

[17] Thummachinda S, Kaewpongsri S, Wiwanitkit V, Suwansaksri J. High urine ttMA levels among fishermen from a Thai rural village. *Southeast Asian J Trop Med Public Health* 2002;33:878-80.

[18] Harrison P. Healthy land--healthy people. *Earthwatch* 1990;(39):13-5.

[19] Lisiewicz J. Immunotoxic and hematotoxic effects of occupational exposures. *Folia Med Cracov* 1993;34:29-47.

[20] Grandjean P. Widening perspectives of lead toxicity. A review of health effects of lead exposure in adults. *Environ Res* 1978;17:303-21.

[21] Srianujata S. Lead--the toxic metal to stay with human. *J Toxicol Sci* 1998;23 Suppl 2:237-40.

[22] Suwansaksri J, Teerasart N, Wiwanitkit V, Chaiyaset T. High blood lead level among garage workers in Bangkok, public concern is necessary. *Biometals* 200215:367-70.

[23] Suwansaksri J, Wiwanitkit V. Monitoring of lead exposure among mechanics in Bangkok. *Southeast Asian J Trop Med Public Health* 2001;32:661-3.

[24] Lubran MM. Lead toxicity and heme biosynthesis. *Ann Clin Lab Sci* 1980;10:402-13.

[25] Rothstein A. Mercurials and red cell membranes. *Prog Clin Biol Res* 1981;51:105-31.

[26] Hall AH. Chronic arsenic poisoning. *Toxicol Lett* 2002;128:69-72.

[27] Benramdane L, Bressolle F, Vallon JJ. Arsenic speciation in humans and food products: a review. *J Chromatogr Sci* 1999;37:330-44.

[28] Bernard A, Roels H, Buchet JP, Cardenas A, Lauwerys R. Cadmium and health: the Belgian experience. *IARC Sci Publ* 1992;(118):15-33.

[29] Parkpian P, Leong ST, Laortanakul P, Thunthaisong N. Regional monitoring of lead and cadmium contamination in a tropical grazing land site, Thailand. *Environ Monit Assess* 2003;85:157-73.

[30] Hays EF, Margaretten N. Long-term oral cadmium produces bone marrow hypoplasia in mice. *Exp Hematol* 1985;13:229-34.

[31] Agency for Toxic Substances and Disease Registry (ATSDR). (1997) *Toxicological Profile for Benzene.* Atlanta, G.A.: U.S. Department of Health and Human Services, Public Health Service.

[32] Biro A, Pallinger E, Major J, Jakab MG, Klupp T, Falus A, Tompa A. Lymphocyte phenotype analysis and chromosome aberration frequency of workers occupationally exposed to styrene, benzene, polycyclic aromatic hydrocarbons or mixed solvents. *Immunol Lett* 2002;81:133-40.

[33] Wiwanitkit V, Suwansaksri J, Soogarun S. The urine trans, trans muconic acid biomarker and platelet count in a sample of subjects with benzene exposure. *Clin Appl Thromb Hemost* 2004;10:73-6.

[34] Bogadi-Sare A, Turk R, Karacic V, Zavalic M, Trutin-Ostovic K. Red blood cell glycerol lysis and hematologic effects in occupational benzene exposure. *Toxicol Ind Health* 1997;13:485-94.

[35] Joo WA, Kang MJ, Son WK, Lee HJ, Lee DY, Lee E, Kim CW. Monitoring protein expression by proteomics: human plasma exposed to benzene. *Proteomics* 2003;3:2402-11.

[36] Chen Y, Li G, Yin S. Individual susceptibility to hematotoxicity from benzene exposure and the genetic polymorphism of metabolic enzymes. *Wei Sheng Yan Jiu* 2002;31:130-2.

[37] Suwansaksri J, Wiwanitkit V. Urine trans,trans-muconic acid determination for monitoring of benzene exposure in mechanics. *Southeast Asian J Trop Med Public Health* 2000;31:587-9.

[38] Scherer G, Renner T, Meger M. Analysis and evaluation of trans,trans-muconic acid as a biomarker for benzene exposure. *J Chromatogr B Biomed Sci Appl* 1998; 717:179-99.

[39] Wiwanitkit V, Suwansaksri J, Nasuan P. Feasibility of urinary trans, trans-muconic acid determination using high performance liquid chromatography for biological monitoring of benzene exposure. *J Med Assoc Thai* 2001; 84 Suppl 1: S263-8.

[40] Wiwanitkit V, Suwansaksri J, Srita S, Fongsoongnern A. High levels of hippuric acid in the urine of Thai press workers. *Southeast Asian J Trop Med Public Health* 2002;33:624-7.

[41] Klavis G. Symptomatic hemolytic jaundice after exposure to trinitrotoluene. *Arch Toxikol* 1957;16:257-60.

[42] Agnisetta S. Acute hemoglobinuric hemolytic anemia caused by trinitrotoluene. *Riforma Med* 1955;69:873-8.

[43] Crawford MA. Aplastic anaemia due to trinitrotoluene intoxication. *Br Med J* 1954;4885:430-7.

[44] Wiwanitkit V, Suwansaksri J, Srita S, Fongsoongnern A. The effect of cigarette smoking on urinary hippuric acid concentration in Thai workers with occupational exposure to toluene. *J Med Assoc Thai* 2002;85 Suppl 1:S236-40.

[45] Amorim LC, Alvarez-Leite EM. Determination of o-cresol by gas chromatography and comparison with hippuric acid levels in urine samples of individuals exposed to toluene. *J Toxicol Environ Health* 1997;50:401-7.

[46] Inoue O, Kanno E, Kasai K, Ukai H, Okamoto S, Ikeda M. Benzylmercapturic acid is superior to hippuric acid and o-cresol as a urinary marker of occupational exposure to toluene. *Toxicol Lett* 2004;147:177-86.

[47] Langman JM. Xylene: its toxicity, measurement of exposure levels, absorption, metabolism and clearance. *Pathology* 1994;26:301-9.

[48] Hristeva-Mirtcheva V. Changes in the peripheral blood of workers with occupational exposure to aromatic hydrocarbons. *Int Arch Occup Environ Health* 1998;71 Suppl:S81-3.

[49] Grieco A. The contribution of science to health promotion in the workplace. *Med Lav* 1993;84:3-17.

Chapter 16

Anemia in the Pregnant in the Tropical Countries

Introduction to Anemia of Pregnancy

Anemia of pregnancy is an important problem in obstetrics. The operative definition of anemia of pregnancy is the condition that a pregnant has a hemoglobin level less than 10 g/dL [1 – 2]. Centers for Disease Control (CDC) gives the cutoff value for anemia of pregnancy in the first and the third trimester as the hemoglobin level less than 11 g/dL while in the second trimester as the hemoglobin less than 10.5 g/dL[3 - 4]. The prevalence of anemia of pregnancy varies in different settings due to many factors. However, the anemia of pregnancy is still a public health problem in most developing tropical countries. Brabin *et al.* noted that the average estimates for all-cause anemia attributable mortality, both direct and indirect, were 6.37, 7.26 and 3.0% for Africa, Asia and Latin America, respectively [5]. Case fatality rates, mainly for hospital studies, varied from <1% to >50% [5]. The relative risk of mortality associated with moderate anemia was 1.35 and for severe anemia was 3.51 [5]. A report issued by the World Health Organization's Maternal Health and Safe Motherhood Program revealed alarming rates of anemia among pregnant women in developing countries [6].

The pregnant subjects with anemia of pregnancy usually develop the signs and symptoms, similar to those of non-pregnant cases [1 – 2]. In mild cases, there may be no signs and symptoms [1 – 2]. In the severe cases, heart failure can be the serious manifestation which can lead to death [1 – 2]. It is noted that the 3-7% of pregnant women in the Third World who suffer from several anemia, under 7 g/dL, were at risk of mortality from heart failure [6]. Even women with moderate levels of anemia are in danger of severe health consequences as a result of the small amount of blood lost during a normal pregnancy [6]. A cycle of deteriorating health from pregnancy to pregnancy occurs when these women are unable to replace the blood lost during childbirth and their anemia becomes exacerbated by the demands of breastfeeding [6]. To avoid the severe blood loss during labor, normal labor is recommended for all cases with anemia of pregnancy [1 – 2].

Molecular and Genetic Basis of Anemia of Pregnancy

The anemia of pregnancy can be due to both acquired and genetic disorders. Concerning the genetic disorders, thalassemia, hemoglobinopathy and hemolytic anemia are the common causes. The molecular diagnosis of these genetic disorders can help physicians manage these cases effectively. Since all of the genetic anemic disorders in the pregnant subjects are old underlying diseases, increased risk for them is not as high as that for their fetus. Most of the investigations for these cases are aiming at antenatal diagnosis of fetal anemia [7]. Generally, fetal anemia may result from hemolytic disease, hemorrhage, suppression of erythropoiesis, infection especially for parvovirus B19, or trauma [7]. The present clinical laboratory plays an essential role in the evaluation of these disorders by way of the use of various hematologic, biochemical, serologic, cytometric, and molecular genetics methods [7 - 8].

Concerning the antenatal screening test, the hematocrit is recommended as a basic necessary test in any antenatal clinic. This screening test can screen the cases of anemia in pregnancy. In cases where the anemias are detected, further investigation for the etiologies are recommended. Iron supplementation as a therapeutic trial for diagnosis of iron deficiency anemia should be considered. In areas with a high prevalence of genetic disorders leading to anemia in pregnancy, thalassemia and hemoglobinopathies, the screening tests for these genetic disorders are also recommended. However, the basic rules in laboratory medicine, good history taking, good physical examination and good laboratory investigation must be followed. Breymann *et al.* noted that the first important steps for diagnosing anaemia in a pregnant patient include a thorough check of her medical history and a medical examination [9]. They mentioned that this procedure often laid the basis for a correct diagnosis [9].

Pathogenesis of Anemia in Pregnancy

Physiologically, the most predominant hematological change in the pregnant is the increasing of total blood volume to 45 % of normal [1 – 2]. During the course of pregnancy, the red cell mass increases about 450 mL and this requires iron about 500 mg [1 – 2]. It should be noted that the increased total blood volume is not proportional to the increased red blood cell mass leading to the hemodilution and consequently low hematocrit and hemoglobin [1 – 2]. Since hemodilution is physiologically normal during the second half of pregnancy, at a gestational age of 18 weeks and above, Wiersma *et al.* noted that only a haemoglobin-level of 6.5 mmol/l or less justifies the diagnosis of anemia, and only then should treatment be commenced [10]. In the normal pregnancy, 1 gram of iron is totally necessary: 50 mg for production of red blood cell mass in the mother, 300 mg for fetus and 200 mg for normal loss [1 – 2]. Therefore, in pregnancy, the serum iron and serum ferritin decrease in the second and third trimester while the total iron binding capacity increases [1 – 2]. Any conditions disturbing the described normal regulation process can lead to anemia of pregnancy [1 – 2]. Those abnormalities can be the old underlying disorders in the pregnant or the new ones. Both acquired and genetic disorders can be seen [1 – 2].

The anemia of pregnancy can lead to several complications of pregnancy. Underlying genetic disorders in the pregnant can bring the inherited disorder to the fetus in utero [1 – 2]. Thalassemia and hemoglobinopathy are good examples for those cases. Some reports mentioned that the anemia of pregnancy can lead to preterm labor, abortion, low birth weight and perinatal death. Allen said that iron deficiency anemia in pregnancy was a risk factor for preterm delivery and subsequent low birth weight, and possibly for inferior neonatal health [11]. Scholl and Reilly said that when maternal anemia is diagnosed before midpregnancy, it had been associated with an increased risk of preterm delivery while maternal anemia detected during the later stages of pregnancy, especially the third trimester, often reflects the expected and necessary expansion of maternal plasma volume [12]. They said that third-trimester anemia usually was not associated with increased risk of preterm delivery [12]. They noted that high hemoglobin concentration, elevated hematocrit and increased levels of serum ferritin late in pregnancy, however, all had been associated with increased preterm delivery and this increased risk might reflect in part the failure to expand maternal plasma volume adequately, thus diminishing appropriate placental perfusion [12]. Hamalainen *et al.* noted that maternal anemia detected in the first trimester is associated with low birth weight [13]. According to their study, the frequency of anemia was 2.6%, with 0.3% occurring in the first trimester [13]. After controlling for confounding factors, anemia detected in the first trimester was associated with low-birth-weight infants whereas the mid- and third-trimester anemia groups showed no significantly different outcomes when compared with the non-anemic women [13]. In addition, first trimester anemia was not significantly associated with small birth weight for gestational age or with premature delivery <37 weeks [13].

It is accepted that anemia is one of the most common risk factors in the area of obstetrics and perinatal medicine [1 – 2, 9]. Anemia progresses through 3 stages: compensation, with breathlessness on exertion only; decompensation, with breathlessness at rest and hemoglobin below about 7 g/L; cardiac failure, with Hb below about 4 g/L [1 – 2]. During pregnancy and in the puerperium, anemia is associated with an increased incidence of both maternal and fetal morbidity and mortality, the extent of which is dependent upon the severity of anaemia and the resulting complications [9]. Anemia of pregnancy brings several problems for the mother. The three common complications of anemia of pregnancy in the mother are infection, bleeding and heart failure [14 - 15]. Brabin *et al.* said that population-attributable risk estimates could be defended on the basis of the strong association between severe anemia and maternal mortality but not for mild or moderate anemia [5]. Durgamba and Qureshi studied the causes of maternal mortality in 431 Indian cases and noted that major causes were hemorrhage, preeclampsia, eclampsia, sepsis, and anemia, in that order [16]. In addition, Anand said that anemia was a major cause of maternal mortality in India [17]. In 1990, 19% of the maternal deaths were related to anemia [17]. Anand also noted that anemia of pregnancy was also a contributory factor to maternal deaths caused by hemorrhage, septicemia, and eclampsia [17]. However, for the fetus, apart from the inheritance disorders, anemia of pregnancy had little effect on since most of the hemoglobin in the fetus is hemoglobin F, which poses high affinity in oxygen binding [1 – 2].

Common Etiologies of Anemia of Pregnancy

Anemia in pregnancy is a major public health problem in developing countries. Recently, van den Broek *et al.* comprehensively assessed the full spectrum of nutritional and nonnutritional factors associated with pregnancy anemia [18]. In their study, iron, folate, vitamin B-12, and vitamin A were measured in serum in a cross-sectional study of 150 pregnant women in Blantyre, Malawi [18]. In addition, bone marrow aspirates were evaluated, peripheral blood films were examined for malaria parasites, stool and urine samples were examined for helminthic infection, and tests were done for genetic disorders and for HIV infection and C-reactive protein (CRP) concentrations and erythrocyte sedimentation rates were measured as markers of inflammation [18]. Of the 150 anemic women, 23% were iron deficient with no evidence of folate, vitamin B-12, or vitamin A deficiencies; 32% were deficient in iron and one or more of the other micronutrients; 26% were not iron deficient but had evidence of one of the other micronutrient deficiencies, most often vitamin A; and 19% were not deficient in any of the micronutrients studied [18]. CRP concentrations were notably high in 54% of the anemic women with no nutritional deficiencies and in 73.5% of the anemic women who were iron replete by bone marrow assessment [18]. Conclusively, van den Broek *et al.* noted the role of chronic inflammation as a possible contributing factor to anemia in pregnancy [18]. Dreyfuss *et al.* studied 336 pregnant women in Nepal and found that 72.6% were anemic, 19.9% had moderate to severe anemia (hemoglobin < 90 g/L) and 80.6% had iron deficiency [19]. They found that 88 % of cases of anemia were associated with iron deficiency and more than half of the women (54.2%) had a low serum retinol concentration (<1.05 micromol/L), 74.2% were infected with hookworms and 19.8% had *Plasmodium vivax* malaria parasitemia [19]. They also noted that hemoglobin, erythrocyte protoporphyrin (EP) and serum ferritin concentrations were significantly worse and the prevalence of anemia, elevated EP and low serum ferritin was increased with increasing intensity of hookworm infection [19]. According to this study, hookworm infection intensity was the strongest predictor of iron status, especially of depleted iron stores [19]. In addition, low serum retinol was most strongly associated with mild anemia, whereas *P. vivax* malaria and hookworm infection intensity were stronger predictors of moderate to severe anemia [19]. Based on these findings, Dreyfuss *et al.* mentioned the need for programs to consider reducing the prevalence of hookworm, malaria infection and vitamin A deficiency where indicated, in addition to providing iron supplements to effectively control anemia [19].

Breymann *et al.* noted that in order to correctly diagnose the type and degree of anemia, a prerequisite for selection of the proper therapy, one had to first of all correctly differentiate between the relative, especially for the physiological anemia of pregnancy due to the normal plasma volume increase during pregnancy, and real anaemias with various different pathophysiological causes [9]. In addition, when defining the Hb cutoff value for anaemia in pregnancy, the extent of the plasma volume changes with respect to the gestational age must be taken into consideration [9]. Breymann *et al.* said that it had been found that haemoglobin values < 11.0 g/dl in the first and third trimesters, and < 10.5 g/dl in the second trimester might point to an anaemic situation which should be further clarified [9].

1. Iron Deficiency Anemia

Anemia caused by lack of iron is the commonest nutritional deficiency in the world [16]. As already mentioned, the total iron needed during pregnancy is about 1000 mg [1 – 2]. The daily requirements for iron, as well as folate, are 6 times greater for a woman in the last trimester of pregnancy than for a non-pregnant woman [1 – 2, 16]. In healthy, well-nourished women with adequate iron stores, about half the total requirement of iron during pregnancy may come from maternal reserves [17]. If the diet is not supplemented with extra iron, a woman will become progressively depleted of iron during pregnancy, and anemia will result [17]. In the developing countries, where malnutrition is still an important health problem, iron deficiency due to insufficient intake can be expected. Similar to iron deficiency anemia in non-pregnant women, lack of iron directly affects the immune system; it diminishes the number of T-cells and the production of antibodies [17]. The World Health Organization (WHO) defined 3 stages of iron-deficiency: decreased storage of iron without any other detectable abnormalities; iron stores are exhausted, but anemia has not occurred yet; and overt iron deficiency when there is a decrease in the concentration of circulating hemoglobin [17].

The diagnosis of iron deficiency anemia in the pregnant is similar to that of non-pregnant cases. First, the diagnosis of hypochromic microcytic anemia can be performed. Then the specific investigations as EP and serum ferritin can be used as gold standards for diagnosis of iron deficiency anemia in the pregnant (EP > 70 micromol/mol heme or serum ferritin < 10 microg/L). In addition, the importance of the differential diagnosis of the hypochromic microcytic anemia due to thalassemia and hemoglobinopathy, should also be considered. In general practice, the therapeutic diagnosis by iron supplementation is also recommended for the setting with limited resource. Breymann *et al.* said that the current gold standard to detect iron deficiency remained the serum ferritin value [9]. To be reliable, they noted that this requires the ruling out of an infection, either chronic or acute, as a cause of the anemia [9]. They also recommendd a complete laboratory test for the exact haematological status as well as the assessment of specific chemical laboratory parameters; these should include a palette of additional, promising new parameters such as hypochromic red cells and transferrin receptors, which allow more accurate detection of iron deficiency and differential diagnosis of iron deficiency anemia [9].

After correct diagnosis, major emphasis should be put on safe and effective treatment of anemia which again depends on the severity of anemia, time for restoration and patients' characteristics [9]. The principle for treatment of iron deficiency anemia in the pregnant subjects is similar to the non-pregnant cases. Oral iron treatment is the most widely used therapeutic method [1 – 2]. In severe cases, blood transfusion is indicated [1 – 2]. Indeed, iron supplementation, calcium supplements, and a high-protein diet should be given to any women in the developing countries during pregnancy [17]. Although controlled trials of iron supplementation during pregnancy have consistently demonstrated positive effects on maternal iron status at delivery, they have not demonstrated reductions in factors that are associated with maternal anemia including increased risk of preterm delivery and infant low birth weight [12]. In addition, recent concerns have been voiced about harmful effects of iron supplementation during pregnancy [12]. Large doses of iron are most often prescribed and are associated with side effects and with increased oxidative damage [20]. However, Scholl and Reilly mentioned that no adverse effects of iron supplementation on pregnancy outcome had been demonstrated to date [12]. Beard said that interventions were often designed to prevent the decrease in hemoglobin concentration and the decline in iron stores associated with pregnancy [20]. They mentioned that enrichment and fortification of food items, and dietary changes resulting from education interventions, had met with some success in developed countries, but not often in the developing world [20]. They also said that a therapeutic approach to iron supplementation, rather than a public health-based approach, is used throughout much of the world but suffers from real, or perceived, problems of compliance [20]. Beard said that daily iron intervention provided more protection against a decline in the storage iron pool in pregnant women than did an intermittent schedule, but the latter is generally associated with fewer side effects, better compliance, and possibly a reduction in risk of oxidative damage [20]. In addition to oral iron treatment, parenteral iron treatment is also available. Indications for the use of parenteral iron are limited to conditions in which the oral supplementation of iron is not possible or fails [21]. When parenteral iron supplementation is required, careful attention to proper dosing and administration is necessary to optimize efficacy and safety [21]. Perewusnyk et al. said that the use of parenteral Fe-sucrose in cases of severe iron deficiency anemia during pregnancy was an efficient and safe treatment and considerably reduced the rate of blood transfusion to below 1 % of patients per year [22]. Today effective alternatives to oral iron only or blood transfusion such as parenteral iron sucrose complex and, in selected cases, also recombinant erythropoietin have been investigated and show promising results concerning effective treatment of anemia during pregnancy and postpartum [1 –2, 12, 17].

Apart from the malnutrition in underprivileged groups, the other common causes of iron deficiency anemia in the pregnant in the tropics are hemorrhoids and hookworm infestation. Hemorrhoids are often seen in pregnancy due to the fact that increased progesterone induces venodilation [1 – 2, 23 - 24]. In addition, the increased progesterone also induces constipation [1 – 2, 23 - 24]. Also, oral iron supplementation can be another contributing factor to constipation [1 –2, 23 – 24]. The anti-hemorrhoidal suppository drug is recommended especially in severe cases [23 – 24]. In non-severe cases, laxative and dietary modification are recommended [23 – 24]. The cessation of the oral iron supplement suspected of causing constipation is also necessary. In these cases, the parenteral iron supplementation may be used if necessary. Concerning hookworm infestation, Nurdia et al. investigated 442 pregnant women in Indonesia and found that most pregnant women (69.7%) were infected with at least one species of pathogenic intestinal helminths [25]. In this study, the most common helminth detected was Trichuris trichiura followed by hookworm and Ascaris lumbricoides and a significant negative association was found between hookworm infection and serum ferritin at the first trimester [25]. They concluded that hookworm infection could interfere with iron stores in pregnancy [25]. For treatment, no specific antihelminthic treatment is recommended in mild cases. However, in severe cases, the antihelminthic drug is recommended. Pyrantel palmoate 10 mg/kg is the recommended regimen [1 – 2]. However, Nurdia et al. said that antihelminthic therapy could be given to all infected women before conception as a public health strategy to improve iron status [25].

2. Hemoglobinopathy

Hemoglobinopathies are the most common class of single gene disorders worldwide [7]. In some tropical areas, hemoglobinopathies are common and becomes a public health problem for both pregnant and non-pregnant subjects. Examples of those hemoglobinopathies are hemoglobin E in Southeast Asia and hemoglobin S in Africa. Most problematic cases in pregnancy are due to the trait forms of these disorders. Although the mothers have no serious manifestation, the fetus had several disorders which could result in death in utero. The screening tests for these genetic disorders are therefore recommended in the highly endemic area. Concerning hemoglobin E disorder, although heterozygotes and homozygotes for HbE are microcytic, minimally anemic, and asymptomatic [26] the combination between beta-thalassemia trait and hemoglobin E trait can lead to thalassemia major, a problematic tropical anemia [27]. Therefore, screening of the spouse for the trait forms of these disorders are recommended in the endemic area. Of several screening tests, the basic biochemical test namely Dichlorophenolindophenol (DCIP) precipitation test is the most effective test [28]. Concerning hemoglobin S, the heterozygous Hb S has a mild clinical manifestation while homozygous Hb S has a severe manifestation. In addition, the combination between heterozygous Hb S with other hemoglobinopathies, can also lead to severe manifestation [29]. Pregnancy in a woman with sickle-cell anaemia may induce a sickle-cell crisis [30]. The maternal morbidity and mortality and perinatal mortality are high, in spite of a pronounced decrease due to improved care [30].

3. Thalassemia

Similar to thalassemia hemoglobinopathy is an important genetic disorder leading to anemia in pregnancy. Generally, the homozygotes of thalassemia are usually severe, transfusion dependant and pregnancy should be avoided. The problematic cases are those with heterozygote thalassemia. Similar to hemoglobinopathy, trait mother and trait father can bring the homozygous disorder to their child. Therefore, screening of the spouse for the trait forms of these disorders are recommended in the endemic area. The recommended screening test for the pregnant is osmotic fragility test (OF) [31]. Since, hemoglobinopathy and thalassemia usually co-occur in the endemic area, the combined screening test is recommended. In Southeast Asia, the combination between hemoglobin E and beta thalassemia is common, therefore, the recommended screening tests are combined DCIP with OF test [32]. This combined screening test is confirmed for its effectiveness [32]. In addition, Wiwanitkit *et al.* also reported that this combined test is a cost – effective one [33]. Concerning the outcome of pregnancy in the cases with thalassemia minor, Sheiner *et al.* found that the course of pregnancy of patients with thalassemia minor, including perinatal outcomes, was favorable [34]. However, because higher rates of intrauterine growth retardation (IUGR) were found, they recommend ultrasound surveillance of fetal weight for early detection of IUGR [34].

4. Vitamin B12 Deficiency

Vitamin B12 deficiency can lead to megaloblastic anemia in the pregnant subjects. Pregnant women who have been strict vegetarians for only a few years, and even those who consume low amounts of animal products, are more likely to become vitamin B12 deficient during pregnancy and lactation, to give birth to an infant who develops clinical or biochemical signs of B12 deficiency, and/or to have low levels of this vitamin in their breast milk [35]. Changes in B12 metabolism during pregnancy affect intestinal absorption, changes in plasma concentrations, and placental transport [35]. The recommended dietary allowance (RDA) during pregnancy is an increase from 2.0 mcg/day to 2.2 mcg/day to cover fetal storage [35]. The World Health Organization (WHO) advises an increase of 0.4 mcg/day to a total of 1.4 mcg/day [35]. Allen said that it was possible that vitamin B12 deficiency was more common in pregnant and lactating women and their young children in developing countries than had been recognized previously, due primarily to malabsorption [35].

Concerning treatment of vitamin B12 deficiency, the cyanocobalamine 1000 microgram intramuscular injection weekly for 6 weeks is recommended [1 – 2].

5. Folic Acid Deficiency

In pregnant women, the daily requirement of folic acid increases from 50 - 10 µg/day to 150 - 300 µg /day [1 – 2]. The increased estrogen and progesterone also disturb the absorption of folic acid [1 – 2]. Similar to vitamin B12 deficiency, folic acid deficiency can lead to megaloblastic anemia in the pregnancy. Folic acid deficiency in the pregnancy can be caused by several disorders. Malabsorption, some drugs (phenobarbital, phnytoin, pyimethamine and isoniazid), hemolytic anemia, malabsorption and twin pregnancy [36] are the examples.Hall *et al.* studied 123 cases of twin pregnancies and found that the incidence of low haemoglobin levels was found to be greater than in a single pregnancy; evidence of iron and folic acid deficiency was common in sternal marrow aspirates but not in peripheral blood films [36]. Concerning the treatment, folic acid supplement is recommended. The recommended dosage is 0.4 - 1 mg/day [1 –2, 37 - 38]. It is noted that the supplementation of folic acid at dosage 4 mg/day can help prevent recurrent neural tube defect [37 - 38].

6. Malarial Anemia

Malarial anemia is common in the tropical areas. Therefore, there is no doubt that malarial anemia can be seen in pregnant subjects in the tropics. Malaria in pregnancy is one of the most important preventable causes of low birthweight deliveries worldwide [39]. It is also a major cause of severe maternal anaemia contributing to maternal mortality [39]. In holoendemic malarious areas with a 5% severe anemia prevalence (hemoglobin <70 g/L), it was estimated that in primigravidae, there would be 9 severe-malaria anemia-related deaths and 41 nonmalarial anemia-related deaths, mostly nutritional, per 100,000 live births [5 – 6]. Shulman and Dorman said estimates show that 40% of the world's pregnant women were exposed to malaria infection during pregnancy [39]. Basically, the clinical features of P. falciparum malaria in pregnancy depend to a large extent on the immune status of the woman, which in turn is determined by her previous exposure to malaria [39]. In pregnant women with little or no pre-existing immunity, such as women from non-endemic areas or travellers to malarious areas, infection is associated with high risks of severe disease with maternal and perinatal mortality [39].

Recently, Garner and Gulmezoglu performed a systematic review to assess the effects of anti-malarial interventions in pregnant women living in malarial areas on the mother and the infant [40]. They found that drugs given regularly and routinely were associated with fewer episodes of fever in the mother, fewer women with severe anemia antenatally, and higher average birthweight in infants, and these effects appear to be greater in primigravidae [40]. They concluded that drugs locally effective for malaria when given routinely for malaria during pregnancy might reduce the incidence of low birth weight and anemia and this effect appeared to be limited to low parity women [40].

7. Acute Blood Loss

Acute blood loss in the pregnancy is generally due to obstetric complications including abortion, molar pregnancy, placenta previa, abruptio placenta, retained placenta, rupture uterine and uterine atony [1 –2]. These conditions can cause massive hemorrhage and result in an abrupt decrease of hemoglobin [1 – 2]. Klufio *et al.* said that immediate and late complications of primary postpartum hemorrhage include hypovolemic shock, cerebral anoxia, renal failure, anemia, puerperal sepsis, and Sheehan's syndrome [41]. In addition, the antepartum hemoglobin status and the rate of blood loss influence hemorrhage outcome [41]. Usually, emergency treatment for anemia is needed in these cases [1 – 2]. The common treatment is the red blood cell replacement [1 – 2]. The whole blood transfusion or packed red cell transfusion are usually indicated. After successful stopping of hemorrhage, the continuous replacement by oral iron supplementation is also recommended [1 – 2].

8. Hemolytic Anemia

Several disorders can lead to hemolytic anemia in the pregnancy. Those underlying disorders may be genetic disorders, such as glucose-6-phosphate dehydrogenase (G-6-PD) deficiency and pyruvate kinase deficiency, or acquired disorders such as autoimmune hemolytic anemia and paroxysmal noctural hemoglobinuria [1 – 2]. Although the G-6-PD deficiency is common in the tropics it is not a serious problem among the pregnant. Since the G-6-PD deficiency is an X-linked inherited disorder, the occurrence of hemolytic anemia due to G-6-PD deficiency in the pregnancy is not seen often [1 – 2]. In addition, hemolytic anemia as an obstetric complication should be mentioned. HELLP, the most serious form of eclampsia is associated with hemolytic anemia [42].

9. Anemia of Chronic Disease

Several underlying chronic diseases can lead to anemia in pregnancies [1 – 2]. Those chronic diseases, which can be seen in the tropics, are tuberculosis, systemic lupus erythrematosus (SLE) and rheumatoid arthritis (RA) [1 – 2]. These anemic diseases are usually presented as normochromic normocytic anemia and usually not severe [1 – 2]. Although the oral iron supplementation does not directly solve the underlying problems, it is still indicate in this case [1 – 2]. Folic acid supplementation accompanied with iron supplementation is also recommended [1 – 2].

10. Aplastic Anemia

Pregnancy-induced aplastic anemia is a rare entity and the association is not well explained [43]. Only a few cases have been documented all over the world. Recently Choudhry et al. studied the aplastic anemia in 11 pregnant subjects in India. According to their study, pallor and bleeding manifestations were the most common presenting complaints and 9 out of 11 (81%) pregnancies were successful of which 7 were full term and 2 were premature [43]. Two babies were small for their delivery dates. One spontaneous abortion and one intra uterine death (IUD) were observed [43]. Two out of 11 mothers died due to disease after delivery [43]. Two of the 8 surviving mothers had spontaneous partial response (22%); 4 mothers were asymptomatic after therapy with immunosuppressives given for 6 months; and 3 were lost to follow up without response [43]. Choudhry et al. concluded that pregnancy associated aplastic anemia was a rare association and spontaneous remission could occur in 25-30% of patients [43]. They noted that pregnancy could be terminated in the first trimester patients while the advanced pregnancy patients could be followed up with stringent supportive care [43]. They said that cyclosporin might be a safe drug antenatally in such patients [43]. Finally, the patients with established aplastic anemia should avoid pregnancy [43].

11. Anemia in the Pregnant with Human Immunodeficiency Virus Infection

Human immunodeficiency virus infection is the great infectious problem of the world at present. The high rate of HIV infection among the pregnant in the tropics, especially those living in the extremely underprivileged areas [44], is mentioned. HIV impacts on direct (obstetrical) causes of maternal mortality by an associated increase in pregnancy complications such as anaemia, post-partum haemorrhage and puerperal sepsis [45]. Similar to the non-pregnant the anemia in the HIV-infected pregnant subjects is an important health problem. Belperio and Rhew said that anemia had been shown to be a statistically significant predictor of progression to the acquired immunodeficiency syndrome and was independently associated with an increased risk of death in patients with HIV [46]. Resolution of HIV-related anemia has been shown to improve quality of life, physical functioning, energy, and fatigue in individuals with HIV [46]. Similar to non-pregnant HIV-infected cases, treatment of anemia with epoetin-alpha has resulted in significantly fewer patients requiring transfusion as well as decreases in the mean number of units of blood transfused [46]. More recently, the use of highly active antiretroviral therapy has also been associated with a significant increase in hemoglobin concentrations and a decrease in the prevalence of anemia [46].

Summary of Anemia in the Pregnant in the Tropical Countries

It can be said that the anemia of pregnancy is a common obstetrics complication in the tropics. Anemia is often multifactorial, with the different causes interacting in a vicious cycle of depressed immunity, infection and malnutrition [47]. Three-quarters of pregnant women in southern Asia and over half of those in Africa have hemoglobin levels under 11 g/dL, compared with 17% of their counterparts in Europe and North America [6]. Concerning the other tropical areas, 39% of pregnant women in Latin America and 71% of those in Oceania, excluding Australia and New Zealand, are anemic [6]. Without treatment, over half of the women with haematocrit less than 0.13 and heart failure die [47].

Major causes of anemia in pregnancy in tropical Africa are malaria, iron deficiency, folate deficiency and haemoglobinopathies: and also now the acquired immune deficiency syndrome [47]. Maternal anemia, malaria and deficiencies of iron and folate cause intrauterine growth retardation, premature delivery and, when severe, perinatal mortality [47]. Fleming said that treatment with blood transfusions was even more hazardous since the advent of AIDS, and should be limited to saving the life of the mother [47]. Of several anemic disorders in pregnancy in Africa, malarial anemia is an important problematic disorder. According to a recent study of Guyatt and Snow in 2001, 18 studies from areas with stable malaria transmission in sub-Saharan Africa suggested that the median prevalence of severe anemia in all-parity pregnant women was approximately 8.2% [48]. Assuming that 26% of these cases are due to malaria, Guyatt and Snow suggested that as many as 400,000 pregnant women might have developed severe anemia as a result of infection with malaria in sub-Saharan Africa [48]. Concerning malarial anemia in pregnancy, Fleming said that treatment of malaria was complex as chloroquine-resistant strains are now common [47]. Fleming said that prevention of anemia of pregnancy in Africa remained relatively easy with proguanil and supplements of iron and folic acid and was highly cost-effective in the improvement of maternal and infant health; it was more important than ever as it avoided the unnecessary exposure of women and infants to HIV transmitted through blood transfusion [47].

Concerning Southeast Asia, that region has causes of anemia of pregnancy similar to those of Africa; iron deficiency, folate deficiency, malnutrition and HIV infection can be seen. To combat the iron deficiency anemia in pregnancy, universal iron supplementation has been the major strategy for pregnant women, using village health volunteers to encourage continuation of the antenatal care schedule and encouraging a preventive approach by health service providers [49]. Winichagoon said that program obstacles had included lack of access to iron tablets by some populations and lack of understanding of the importance of anemia [49]. In addition, women's compliance was complicated by fear of having a large fetus, forgetfulness and side effects [49]. However, the most problematic anemia of pregnancy at present is due to the highly endemicity of thalassemia and hemoglobin E disorders. Although these disorders do not directly affect the pregnant they can cause problematic anemic infants, which lead to a great public health problem. There are several attempts to control these inheritable diseases. Antenatal screening test is recommended as an effective strategy for control of inherited hemoglobin disorders [33, 50]. Recently, Wanapirak *et al.* proposed the strategies to control severe thalassemia in pregnancy in Thailand including (1) carrier identification by retrospective (history review) and prospective screening program; (2) the couples at risk were counseled and offered cordocentesis; (3) analysis of fetal blood with high performance liquid chromatography (HPLC) or electrophoresis; and (4) counseling for termination of pregnancy in case of an affected fetus [50]. They proved that these strategies were effective and should be used [50].

Concerning South Asia, iron deficiency, folate deficiency and malnutrition are still the common leading causes of anemia in pregnancy. There are several attempts to fight the anemia of pregnancy in this area. Fighting malnutrition becomes a common strategy for this purpose. Kumar said that plans should focus on three vital strategies: promotion of regular consumption of foods rich in iron, provisions of iron and folate supplements in the form of tablets to the high risk groups, and identification and treatment of severely anemic cases [51]. Pregnant women are recommended to have one big tablet per day for 100 days after the first trimester of pregnancy; a similar dose applies to lactating women and IUD acceptors [51]. In addition to control of malnutrition-related anemia of pregnancy, the control for other leading causes are also necessary.

References

[1]   Cunningham FG, MacDonald PC, Gant NF, Levono KJ, Gastrap LC. Williams *Obstetrics*. 19th ed. Connecticut: Appleton and Lange, 1993; 220 - 5, 1171 -99.

[2]   Laros RK. *Blood Disorders in Pregnancy*. Philadelphia: Lea and Fabriger, 1986; 1 – 84

[3]   CDC criteria for anemia in children and childbearing-aged women. *MMWR Morb Mortal Wkly Rep* 1989;38:400-4.

[4]   CDC releases new reference criteria for anemia screening. *Am Fam Physician* 1989;40:303, 306, 308.

[5]   Brabin BJ, Hakimi M, Pelletier D. An analysis of anemia and pregnancy-related maternal mortality. *J Nutr* 2001;131(2S-2):604S-614S.

[6]   Anaemia during pregnancy - a major public health problem. *Safe Mother* 1993;(11):1-2.

[7]   Rubin LP, Hansen K. Testing for hematologic disorders and complications. *Clin Lab Med* 2003;23:317-43.

[8]   Old JM, Ludlam CA. Antenatal diagnosis. *Baillieres Clin Haematol* 1991;4:391-428.

[9]   Breymann C; Anaemia Working Group. Current aspects of diagnosis and therapy of iron deficiency anemia in pregnancy. *Schweiz Rundsch Med Prax* 2001;90:1283-91.

[10]   Wiersma TJ, Daemers DO, Oldenziel JH, Flikweert S, Assendelft WJ; Nederlands Huisartsen Genootschap. Summary of the practice guideline 'Pregnancy and

puerperium' from the Dutch College of General Practitioners. *Ned Tijdschr Geneeskd* 2004;148:65-72.

[11] Allen LH. Anemia and iron deficiency: effects on pregnancy outcome. *Am J Clin Nutr* 2000;71(5 Suppl):1280S-4S.

[12] Scholl TO, Reilly T. Anemia, iron and pregnancy outcome. *J Nutr* 2000;130(2S Suppl):443S-447S.

[13] Hamalainen H, Hakkarainen K, Heinonen S. Anaemia in the first but not in the second or third trimester is a risk factor for low birth weight. *Clin Nutr* 2003;22:271-5.

[14] McFee JG. Anemia: a high-risk complication of pregnancy. *Clin Obstet Gynecol* 1973;16:153-71.

[15] Scott DE. Anemia in pregnancy. *Obstet Gynecol Annu* 1972;1:219-44.

[16] Durgamba KK, Qureshi S. Maternal mortality at government maternity hospital. Hyderabad, Andhra Pradesh (a review of 431 cases). *J Obstet Gynaecol India* 1970;20:450-1.

[17] Anand A. Anaemia -- a major cause of maternal death. *Indian Med Trib* 1995;3:5, 8.

[18] van den Broek NR, Letsky EA. Etiology of anemia in pregnancy in south Malawi. *Am J Clin Nutr* 2000;72(1 Suppl):247S-256S.

[19] Dreyfuss ML, Stoltzfus RJ, Shrestha JB, Pradhan EK, LeClerq SC, Khatry SK, Shrestha SR, Katz J, Albonico M, West KP Jr. Hookworms, malaria and vitamin A deficiency contribute to anemia and iron deficiency among pregnant women in the plains of Nepal. *J Nutr* 2000;130:2527-36.

[20] Beard JL. Effectiveness and strategies of iron supplementation during pregnancy. *Am J Clin Nutr* 2000; 71(5 Suppl):1288S-94S.

[21] Kumpf VJ. Parenteral iron supplementation. *Nutr Clin Pract* 1996;11:139-46.

[22] Perewusnyk G, Huch R, Huch A, Breymann C. Parenteral iron therapy in obstetrics: 8 years experience with iron-sucrose complex. *Br J Nutr* 2002 ;88:3-10.

[23] Abramowitz L, Sobhani I. Anal complications of pregnancy and delivery. *Gastroenterol Clin Biol* 2003;27(3 Pt 1):277-83.

[24] Wald A. Constipation, diarrhea, and symptomatic hemorrhoids during pregnancy. *Gastroenterol Clin North Am* 2003;32:309-22.

[25] Nurdia et al said that anthelminthic therapy could be given to infected women before conception as public health strategy to improve iron status. *Southeast Asian J Trop Med Public Health* 2001;32:14-22.

[26] Dode C, Berth A, Bourdillon F, Mahe C, Labie D, Rochette J. Haemoglobin disorders among Southeast-Asian refugees in France. *Acta Haematol* 1987;78:135-6.

[27] Rees DC, Styles L, Vichinsky EP, Clegg JB, Weatherall DJ. The hemoglobin E syndromes. *Ann N Y Acad Sci* 1998;850:334-43.

[28] Kulapongs P, Tawarat S, Sanguansermsri T. Dichlorophenolindophenol (DCIP) precipitation test : a simple screening test for hemoglobin E and alpha thalassemia (Thalassemia Conference In Memorial of Dr. Sa-nga Pootrakul At the Mahidol University Faculty of Medicine Siriraj Hospital February 10-11, 1977). *J Med Assoc Thai.* 1978; 61: 62-63.

[29] Lonergan GJ, Cline DB, Abbondanzo SL. Sickle cell anemia. *Radiographics* 2001;21:971-94.

[30] Radder CM, Statius van Eps LW, Kagie MJ. Sickle cell anemia during pregnancy. *Ned Tijdschr Geneeskd* 1998;142:2530-2.

[31] Wiwanitkit V. Osmotic fragility test for screening for thalassaemia in Thai pregnant subjects: a re-evaluation. *Haema* 2004; 7:205-207.

[32] Wiwanitkit V. Combined osmotic fragility and dichlorophenol-indolphenol test for hemoglobin disorder screening in Thai pregnant subjects: an appraisal. *Lab Hematol* 2004;10:119-20.

[33] Wiwanitkit V, Suwansaksri J, Paritpokee N. Combined one-tube osmotic fragility (OF) test and dichlorophenol-indolphenol (DCIP) test screening for hemoglobin disorders, an experience in 213 Thai pregnant women. *Clin Lab* 2002;48:525-8.

[34] Sheiner E, Levy A, Yerushalmi R, Katz M. Beta-thalassemia minor during pregnancy. *Obstet Gynecol.* 2004 Jun;103:1273-7.

[35] Allen LH. Vitamin B12 metabolism and status during pregnancy, lactation and infancy. *Adv Exp Med Biol* 1994;352:173-86.

[36] Hall MH, Campbell DM, Davidson RJ. Anaemia in twin pregnancy. *Acta Genet Med Gemellol* (Roma) 1979;28:279-82.

[37] Refsum H. Folate, vitamin B12 and homocysteine in relation to birth defects and pregnancy outcome. *Br J Nutr* 2001;85 Suppl 2:S109-13.

[38] Geisel J. Folic acid and neural tube defects in pregnancy: a review. *J Perinat Neonatal Nurs* 2003;17:268-79.

[39] Shulman CE, Dorman EK. Importance and prevention of malaria in pregnancy. *Trans R Soc Trop Med Hyg* 2003;97:30-5.

[40] Garner P, Gulmezoglu AM. Prevention versus treatment for malaria in pregnant women. *Cochrane Database Syst Rev* 2000;(2):CD000169.

[41] Klufio CA, Amoa AB, Kariwiga G. Primary postpartum haemorrhage: causes, aetiological risk factors, prevention and management. *P N G Med J* 1995;38:133-49.

[42] Severe Alvarez Navascues R, Marin R. maternal complications associated with pre-eclampsia: an almost forgotten pathology? *Nefrologia* 2001;21:565-73.

[43] Choudhry VP, Gupta S, Gupta M, Kashyap R, Saxena R. Pregnancy associated aplastic anemia--a series of 10 cases with review of literature. *Hematology* 2002;7:233-8.

[44] Wiwanitkit V, Suyaphan A. A note on the anti-HIV seroprevalence of the mothers in the labor room at a rural Thai hospital. *Arch Gynecol Obstet.* 2003 Aug 22.

[45] McIntyre J. Mothers infected with HIV. *Br Med Bull* 2003;67:127-35.

[46] Belperio PS, Rhew DC. Prevalence and outcomes of anemia in individuals with human immunodeficiency virus: a systematic review of the literature. *Am J Med* 2004;116 Suppl 7A:27S-43S.

[47] Fleming AF. Tropical obstetrics and gynaecology. 1. Anaemia in pregnancy in tropical Africa. *Trans R Soc Trop Med Hyg* 1989;83:441-8.

[48] Guyatt HL, Snow RW. The epidemiology and burden of Plasmodium falciparum-related anemia among pregnant women in sub-Saharan Africa. *Am J Trop Med Hyg* 2001;64(1-2 Suppl):36-44.

[49] Winichagoon P. Prevention and control of anemia: Thailand experiences. *J Nutr* 2002;132(4 Suppl):862S-6S.

[50] Wanapirak C, Tongsong T, Sirivatanapa P, Sa-nguansermsri T, Sekararithi R, Tuggapichitti A. Prenatal strategies for reducing severe thalassemia in pregnancy. *Int J Gynaecol Obstet* 1998;60:239-44.

[51] Kumar A. National nutritional anaemia control programme in India. *Indian J Public Health* 1999;43:3-5, 16.

Chapter 17

Anemia in Infancy and Childhood in the Tropical Countries

Introduction to Pediatric Anemia

1. Anemia in Neonate

Anemia is an important problem in neonatology. In the term neonate, anemia is diagnosed if the hemoglobin from capillary blood determination is less than 14.5 g/dL. Physiologically, up to one-third of the blood in the neonate at birth is at the placenta. It is proposed that delayed umbilical cord clamp and cutting can increase blood distribution to the neonate. Generally, hemoglobin level in the cord blood is about 16.8 g/dL and the hemoglobin of the neonate in the first 3 hours can increase up to 22.8 g/dL then it is physiologically diluted, with rapid expansion of the blood volume, to the level equal to that of the umbilical cord [1 – 3]. It should be noted that hemoglobin, hematocrit and mean corpuscular volume tend to be higher in newborns and they further increase in the first 2 days of life [1 – 2]. These blood indices also depend on the gestational age, day of life, maternal factors, mode of delivery and site of blood collection [2]. Physiologic anemia is a common and normal finding in newborn infants [1 - 2]. However, the extreme decrease of the hemoglobin level in the newborn implies the possible pathology [1 – 3]. Generally, pathological anemia in the newborn is usually caused by either hemorrhage or hemolysis and rarely due to decreased production [2]. In the newborn, hemorrhage can be ante or intra or post natal and it could be external or internal and it could be acute or chronic [2]. Management of acute severe hemorrhage includes packed cell transfusion [2]. Hemolysis is usually due to isoimmune hemolysis, glucose-6-phosphate dehydrogenase (G6PD) deficiency or rarely due to the hemoglobinopathy like alpha-thalassemia or due to spherocytosis [2]. Usually patients will have indirect hyperbilirubinemia which needs phototherapy or exchange transfusion [2, 4]. Rarely congenital pure red cell aplasia can present at birth with physical anomalies and anemia. Treatment of neonatal anemia depends on the arteriology [2]. The anemia in the first day of a newborn is usually related to the hemorrhage due to obstetric complication or immune hemolytic anemia, while the anemia after the first day of the newborn usually relates to the non-hemolytic anemia or hemorrhage. Reticulocytosis and presence of nucleated red cells are normally seen in the first week of life [2]. Persistent elevation of reticulocyte count indicates the pathological process, especially for hemolytic anemia [2, 4]. Concerning treatment of neonatal anemia, the basic principle of anemia management should be used. The red blood cell replacement by blood transfusion is indicated in severe cases. Humbert and Wacker noted that erythropoietin therapy, often at doses much higher than those used in the adult, should be seriously considered in most cases of non-hypoplastic neonatal anemias, to minimize maximally the use of transfusions [3]. Concerning the newborns with the anemia due to hemolysis, the awareness and prevention of the complication of hyperbilirubinemia is necessary [4].

Table 17.1. Common causes of placenta neonatal anemia [1 – 3]

Groups	Examples
1. Hemorrhage	o twin-to-twin transfusions, feto-maternal transfusions, vasa previa
2. Hemolysis	o ABO incompatibility (frequent [3]), Rh incompatibility (nearly disappeared following the use of anti-D immunoglobulin in postpartum Rh-negative mothers [3]), hereditary spherocytosis and G-6-PD deficiency
3. Erythropoiesis defect (hypoplastic anemia)	o Parvovirus B19 (predominates [3]), Diamond-Blackfan anemia, alpha-thalassemia and sideroblastic anemias (rare [3])

In preterm infants, anemia of prematurity is usually the result of the normal physiologic process compounded by the morbidity of prematurity [1]. The multifactorial anemia of prematurity develops principally as a result of plasma volume expansion in this group of patients [3]. Premature infants also reach their nadir hemoglobin level sooner and at a lower level than term infants [1]. In addition, the same pathological disorders described for the term newborns can be the problems for the preterm newborns as well. Due to the lower tolerance than the term newborn, the special management of anemia of prematurity is necessary. Mahapatra and Choudhry noted that premature infants were among the most frequently transfused groups of patients, usually receiving red cells [5]. The immaturity of the immune system, its lesser ability to cope with a metabolic load and the presence of maternal antibodies, all complicate the picture [5]. Conservation of blood to minimize losses and the need for replacement transfusion is an important strategy that has already been successful in reducing the need for transfusion on neonatal units [5]. Ohls said that decreasing phlebotomy losses and instituting standardized transfusion guidelines have both been shown significantly to decrease the transfusion requirements of preterm infants [6]. Mahapatra and Choudhry said that the advent of erythropoietin provided another strategy for reducing the need for transfusion [5]. Ohls said that the administration of erythropoietin likely decreased transfusion requirement [6]. Ohlas also mentioned that it was likely that the combination of instituting rigorous and standardized transfusion guidelines, decreasing phlebotomy losses, and the appropriate use of erythropoietin would have the greatest impact in decreasing transfusion requirements in all preterm and term neonates, regardless of the cause of their anemia [6]. However, Mahapatra and Choudhry said that it was unfortunate that the sickest patients who required the most transfusion responded poorly to erythropoietin [6]. In those cases, Mahapatra and Choudhry noted that the main concern was the long-term consequences of transfusion and the aim of decision making should be to minimize transfusion risks and give transfusions only when they were indicated [5].

2. Anemia in Infant

In infants, anemia is an important hematological problem. Apart from the hemolytic disorders, there are several underlying causes of infantile anemia. Those disorders include infection and malnutrition – induced anemia. Concerning infection, since the infant has low immunity, they can easily get infected by several pathogens. Therefore, the anemia due to the infectious diseases can be expected in the infant. As indicated in previous chapters, several bacterial and viral infections in the infants can lead to anemia [7]. Some examples of the common infection-induced anemia in the infant are cytomegalovirus related anemia, pneumococcal related anemia and meningococcal related anemia [7]. Concerning the malnutrition-related anemia in the infant, the two common underlying factors are the mothers have no food for their children or the mothers have poor basic knowledge of infantile feeding. Since the infants cannot feed themselves, therefore, the correction of the malnutrition-related anemia should focus on their mother. Nutritional surveillance, both as the follow up at the well baby clinic and community survey, should be applied [8 - 9]. Nutritional supplementation for the risk infants is indicated [8]. Concerning the treatment of infantile anemia, the same principle as described in the neonatal anemia should be used.

3. Anemia in Children

Similar to the adulthood anemia, there are several etiologies of childhood anemia [10]. However, some etiologies are more frequent in childhood [10]. Those etiologies include some common infection in childhood and some severe inherited diseases, of which the affected children died before becoming adults. In addition, some anemic disorders due to the insufficiency of some specific nutrients and the side effect of recommended immunization in childhood, can be seen. Concerning the infection-induced anemia, some infections are common in childhood, especially CMV infection [7]. Concerning the inherited disorders, the common anemic disorders, which are usually overt in childhood, include thalassemia major and several hemoglobinopathies. These disorders are usually severe and the affected children usually die young. The iron overload is the most common cause of death among transfusion-dependent subjects affected by thalassemia major and other congenital anemias [11]. Energy, protein, vitamin A, iron and zinc are samples of basic requirements in daily childhood nutrition [12]. These specific nutrients are necessary for erythropoiesis. Tarini *et al.* suggested that dietary scores were relevant but that the diversity of food eaten might be a better determinant of growth status if energy intake is close to meeting dietary requirements and multiple dietary inadequacies were frequent among children from developing countries so scores of overall dietary quality might be more appropriate indicators than the intakes of specific nutrients [12]. Finally, some vaccinations for children, especially the DPT vaccine [13], have been mentioned for their side effects as induction of anemia.

The principles of treatment for childhood anemia are similar to anemia in other age groups. New drugs, recently available for treatment of different forms of anemia, have somehow changed the therapeutic scenario in pediatric hematology [14]. Erythropoietin, the specific growth factor of red cell precursors, is now an established option for anemia of chronic renal failure, bone marrow transplantation and chemotherapy [6, 14]. Hemoglobin analogues are currently under investigation, in order to obtain a synthetic oxygen-carrier that can substitute blood transfusions [14]. Finally drugs that are able to increase the production of hemoglobin F have been used in thalassemias and hemoglobinopathies [14]. For patients with sickle cell disease, hydroxyurea is proven to be effective in terms of both clinical and hematological improvement [14 - 15].

4. Anemia in Adolescent

Anemic disorders in adolescents is similar to those of adults. However, some specific problems in the adolescent can be seen. Some inherited hematological disorders run to the end stage on the adolescent life of the patients. In addition some anemic problems are related to the biopsychosocial changes in the teenages. The teenage pregnancy has an increased chance of anemia, pregnancy-induced hypertension, low birth weight, prematurity, intra-uterine growth retardation and neonatal mortality [16]. Some teenagers are addicted to some drugs or substances that can lead to anemia. The problem of drug abuse is also the present social problem in many developing countries. The role of practitioner is to provide continuity of care, and to advocate in the policy arena for development and funding of comprehensive and efficacious programs to help prevent or treat substance abuse in those adolescents [17].

Important Tropical Neonatal Anemia

1. Anemia Due to Obstetric Complication

Hemorrhage can result from many obstetric complications.

Intrapartum hemorrhage can be a serious problem and can bring anemia to both mother and newborn. During intrapartum hemorrhage, the pregnant uterus becomes a vital source of blood volume during hypovolemic events because it is not considered a vital organ [18]. The pregnancy itself may become burdensome, and birth may occur as an intrinsic maternal compensatory mechanism and the resultant fetal hypoxemia may also stress the fetus into initiating labor [18]. The affected newborns are not only anemic but also suffer from asphyxia, and these can lead to neonatal death. Of interest is the high neonatal mortality rate due to the neonatal asphyxia mentioned in the developing countries [19]. Good labor practices to prevent the intrapartum hemorrhage is necessary. In addition to intrapartum hemorrhage, the antenatal blood loss can be the underlying cause of neonatal anemia as well. Fetus blood losses due to twin-twin transfusion and feto-maternal transfusion are documented. These anemias are serious and may be life-threatening or disabling due to hypovolaemia and tissue hypoxaemia in the fetus or newborn [20]. These neonatal hemorrhagic disorders can be the important leading causes of neonatal death. Although the obstetric complication can be seen elsewhere, the poorer management can be seen in the developing countries. Borghi *et al.* performed a study in Ghana and Benin and noted that the economic burden of hospital-based delivery care in Ghana and Benin was likely to deter or delay women's use of health services. They noted that if a woman developed severe obstetric complications while in labor, the relatively high costs of hospital care could have a potentially catastrophic impact on the household budget [21]. Of interest, Brabin *et al.* said that with good antenatal and obstetric care most anemia-related deaths were preventable, and policies to reduce anemia prevalence should not be divorced from efforts to provide adequate antenatal and delivery facilities for women in developing countries [21].

2. Anemia Due to Hemolytic Disease of the Newborn

Hemolytic disease of the newborn (HDN) is an important condition in neonatology. These anemias are serious and may be life-threatening or disabling due to the risk of a possible hyperbilirubinaemia after birth [4]. Those hemolytic disorders can be divided into two main groups, immune hemolytic and non - immune hemolytic disorders. As previously mentioned, immune hemolytic disorder occurs earlier than non – immune hemolytic disorder. Concerning the immune hemolytic disorder in the newborn, the blood group incompatibilities are the common problems. ABO incompatibility is the most frequent incompatibility (Table 17.1). Brown said that ABO incompatibility was common in Kenya and becomes a consideration for the health care in the country [22]. Augustine and Bhatia studied the records of all the infants admitted during the first 7 days of life in the Pediatrics Ward of JIPMER hospital, India for the neonatal mortality and found that ABO incompatability accounted for 1.18 % of neonatal mortality [23]. Dudin *et al.* studied the blood group in Palestinian newborns and found that 30 % of A or B infants born to O Rh(D)-positive mothers had a positive direct antiglobulin test with the presence of allo-immune A or B antibody in infant serum [24]. They concluded that ABO incompatibility was a major reason for phototherapy during the 1st week of life [24]. Due to the fact that ABO compatibility is common and can be the cause of neonatal anemia and subsequently hyperbilirubinemia, the mother's and newborn's blood group examinations are recommended as routine practice in all neonatal units [4].

Table 17.1. Possibility of ABO incompatibility

Mother's blood group	Father's blood group			
	A	B	AB	O
A	No	Yes	Yes	No
B	Yes	No	Yes	No
AB	No	No	No	No
O	Yes	Yes	Yes	No

Another less common blood group incompatability is Rh incompatibility. Although less common, Rh incompatibility is usually more severe than ABO incompatibility. According to the study of Augustine and Bhatia, Rh incompatability accounted for 2.37 % of neonatal mortality [23]. Genetically, the Rh antigens are encoded by the RHD and RHCE genes [25]. In RhD negative individuals, the RHD gene is absent or grossly deleted [25]. Routinely, Rh typing is performed by haemagglutination [25]. However, Cotorruelo *et al.* noted that there were some clinical situations in which serological techniques are not suitable for determining the red blood cell phenotype accurately [25]. They noted that DNA-based analyses might be better than serological typing to infer the appropriate phenotype in those cases. They also noted that agglutination methods were also of limited use for determining the red blood cell phenotype of a fetus at risk of haemolytic disease of the newborn [25]. In addition, molecular RHD typing using amniocytes or DNA obtained from maternal plasma might obviate the need of amniocentesis during pregnancy when the fetus was RhD negative, thus providing an important tool in managing possible sensitization by fetal erythrocytes [25]. The serious hemolytic episodes in the Rh incompatibility occur in the Rh-negative mothers with Rh-positive fathers and have their first sensitization in their first gestations (Figure 17.1). The recommendation for prevention of Rh alloimmunization is Anti-D Ig 300 microg IM or IV should be given within 72 hours of delivery to a postpartum nonsensitized Rh-negative woman delivering an Rh-positive infant [26]. Additional anti-D Ig may be required for fetomaternal hemorrhage (FMH) greater than 15 mL of fetal red blood cells (about 30 mL of fetal blood) [26]. Luckily due to the great concern and nuptial screening, Rh incompatibility has nearly disappeared following the use of anti-D immunoglobulin in postpartum Rh-negative mothers [3].

Concerning non-immune hemolytic anemia, hereditary spherocytosis and G-6-PD deficiency are the two common examples. Hereditary spherocytosis is the most common member of inherited disorders of the red cell membrane skeleton: the other are hereditary elliptocytosis, and hereditary pyropoikilocytosis [27]. Hereditary spherocytosis is a Mendelian dominant, genetically determined disorder of the erythrocyte membrane [28]. There is commonly a family history and a typical clinical and laboratory blood picture so that the diagnosis is usually easily made without additional laboratory tests [29]. The classical blood picture in peripheral blood examination is the presence of numerous isocytosis spherocytic red blood cell, different from autoimmune hemolytic anemia, which contain anisocytosis spherocytes. Atypical cases may require measurement of membrane proteins and molecular genetics to clarify the nature of the membrane disorder [29]. Bolton-Maggs noted that it was particularly important to rule out stomatocytosis because splenectomy was contraindicated because of the thrombotic risk [29]. Concerning treatment, mild hereditary spherocytosis can be managed without folate supplements and does not require splenectomy while moderately and severely affected individuals are likely to benefit from splenectomy, which should be performed after the age of 6 and with appropriate counselling about the risk of infection [29]. Bolton-Maggs also noted that careful dialogue between physician, child and the family was essential in all cases [29]. However, the hereditary spherocytosis is relatively common in Caucasian populations and most individuals have mild or only moderate disease [29].

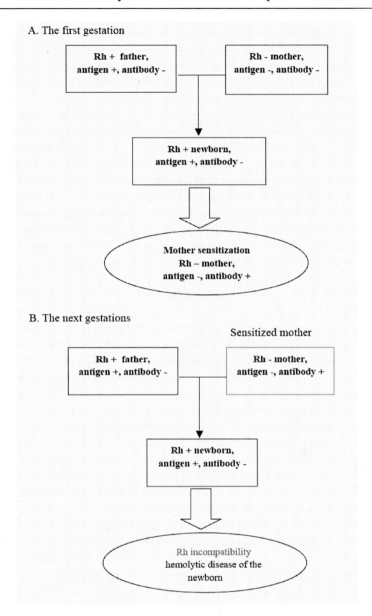

Figure 17.1 The diagram showing the pathogenesis of Rh incompatibility

Concerning G-6-PD deficiency in the newborn, it is a common cause of hemolytic anemia as mentioned in the previous chapter. G-6-PD deficiency is common in the tropical population and is one of a main causes of hemolytic anemia [30 - 31]. Screening for G-6-PD deficiency is of concern. Chuu *et al.* recently indicated that severe neonatal jaundice can be effectively prevented by neonatal screening for G-6-PD deficiency [32]. Many deficient variants of G-6-PD have been described [33]. DNA sequence analysis has shown that the vast majority of these are caused by single amino acid substitutions [33]. The screening test for G-6-PD deficiency in cord blood is recommended in the endemic area [4]. It should also be noted that there is a large difference in activity between newborns and adults for G-6-PD activity [34]. In newborn infants, Jansen *et al.* noted that there was an almost linear and steep decline of hexokinase (HK), pyruvate kinase (PK), and G-6-PD activity with a decreasing number of reticulocytes [35]. These data are therefore illustrative for a biphasic activity decay pattern of HK, PK, and G-6-PD during neonatal red cell aging [35]. The details of hemolytic anemia in the tropics can be found in the previous chapter.

Apart from the G-6-PD deficiency, the PK deficiency is the other widely mentioned enzymatic disorder that can induce anemia. The gene encoding for PK (PK-LR) has been localized to the long arm of chromosome I; the cDNA of R-type is 2060 bp long and codes for 574 amino acids [36]. More than 130 different mutations, mostly missense, have so far been described in association with PK deficiency [36]. PK deficiency is the most frequent enzyme abnormality of the Embden-Meyerhof pathway causing hereditary non-spherocytic hemolytic anemia [36]. The degree of hemolysis varies widely, ranging from very mild or fully compensated forms, to life-threatening neonatal anaemia and jaundice necessitating exchange transfusions [36].

Zanella and Bianchi said that splenectomy should be reserved for young patients who require regular blood transfusions [36]. The PK deficiency is also common in the tropics. The possible correlation between PK deficiency and malaria in the tropics is widely mentioned as well. Recently, Min-Oo *et al.* performed an animal experimental study and found a significant correlation between PK deficiency and malaria [37].

3. Hypoplastic Anemia

Hypoplastic anemias in the newborn are also important anemic disorders in the tropics. Several anemic disorders including parvovirus B19 infection and alpha-thalassemia are common in the tropics. Human parvovirus B19 (B19) infection causes human bone marrow failure, by affecting erythroid-lineage cells [38]. However, the anemia induced by B19 infection is of minor clinical significance in healthy subjects, however, it becomes critical in those afflicted with hemolytic diseases [38]. The details of anemia in parvovirus B19 infection can be found in the previous chapter. Concerning alpha-thalassemia, the homozygous form usually results in hydrop fetalis. This disorder can bring very high mortality to the affected cases. Concerning the epidemiology of alpha-thalassemia, alpha(+)-thalassemia is prevalent throughout tropical and subtropical regions of the world, whereas alpha(0)-thalassemia occurs at higher frequency in Southeast Asia [39]. Antenatal screening program for this disorder is recommended in the endemic area [40]. The details of anemia in alpha-thalassemia can be found in the previous chapter. In addition to these common hypoplastic anemias, there are also other uncommon hypoplastic anemias in neonates.

Diamond-Blackfan Anemia (DBA) a rare congenital hypoplastic anemia often diagnosed early in infancy, is an example [41]. In DBA, a moderate to severe aregenerative anemia is found in association with erythroblastopenia in an otherwise normocellular bone marrow [41]. Recent molecular studies have identified mutations in the gene encoding the ribosomal protein RPS19 on chromosome 19 in 25% of patients with DBA and linkage analysis has also identified another locus on chromosome 8p in association with DBA in another subset of patients [41]. A majority of patients with DBA respond to steroid therapy [41].

4. Anemia Due to Congenital Infection

Many congenital infections can bring anemia to the newborn. Examples for those congenital infections are parvovirus B19, syphilis and malaria. The congenital parvovirus B19 is mentioned for the correlation to the severe congenital aplastic anemia [42]. Intravenous administration of immunoglobulins is recommended in the patients with aplastic anemia due to congenital parvovirus B19 infection [42]. The PCR monitoring of the presence of parvovirus B19 DNA in blood and bone marrow cells during and after the treatment of congenital aplastic anemia caused by parvovirus B19 chronic infection becomes the necessity for rational therapy [42]. Concerning congenital syphilis, anemia is a common finding. Hollier *et al.* studied 24 cases of fetal syphilis and found anemia in 26% [43]. More details on the syphilis-related anemia can be seen in the previous chapter. Considering congenital malaria, fever, respiratory distress, pallor and anemia, hepatomegaly, and jaundice are common signs and symptoms [44]. Of interest, the malaria is prevalent in many developing tropical countries. Therefore, the high prevalence of congenital anemia as well as its anemic complication can be expected. Steketee *et al.* estimated that each year 75,000 to 200,000 infant deaths were associated with malaria infection in pregnancy [45]. They noted that failure to apply known effective antimalarial interventions through antenatal programs continued to contribute substantially to infant deaths globally [45]. Of interest, the described congenital infections are common infections in the tropics, therefore, good antenatal care and screening can be the best preventive method.

Important Tropical Infantile Anemia

1. Infection-Related Anemia

As already mentioned, several infections can induce anemia in the infant. Briefly, CMV infection in infants can lead to hemolytic anemia [46]. Treatment with intravenous CMV immune globulin is indicated in the infected infant [46]. Parvovirus B19 infection can lead infantile anemia as already mentioned. Pneumococcal infection in infants can also induce hemolytic anemia. Cochran *et al.* said that pneumococcus-induced hemolytic uremic syndrome (HUS) carried an increased risk of mortality and renal morbidity compared with *E. coli*-induced HUS [47]. Pathogenically, the pneumococcal organism produces an enzyme, which can expose an antigen (T-antigen) present on erythrocytes, platelets, and glomeruli; and antibodies to the T-antigen, normally found in human serum, bind the exposed T-antigen, and the resultant antigen-antibody reaction (T-activation) can lead to HUS and anemia [47].

Meningococcal infections in infant can also produce HUS [48 - 49]. More details of infection-related anemias are described in the previous chapters.

2. Malnutrition-Related Anemia

The infants cannot feed themselves, therefore, they pose a risk for malnutrition if they are not well fed. Infantile anemia due to malnutrition is common in the tropical countries. Presently, the FAO, UNICEF and the WHO joined forces to deal with the problem of children suffering from protein-calorie malnutrition in those developing countries [50]. Several nutrient deficiencies can be seen in the far rural communities. Fighting malnutrition including anemia should be global strategies at present [9]. As already mentioned, the training for good infantile feeding is necessary to face up with infantile anemia in the tropics. Adoption of the recommended breast-feeding and complementary feeding behaviors and access to the appropriate quality and quantity of foods are essential components of optimal nutrition for infants [51]. More details on the nutritional-related anemia are provided in the previous chapter.

Important Tropical Childhood Anemia

1. Anemia Due to Malnutrition in Childhood

Malnutrition is still the big problem of the developing countries at present.

Anemia is the most common disorder in hospital patients in tropical countries, and it is demonstrated in up to 70% of inpatients [52]. Similar to adulthood, iron deficiency is the most common cause of nutritional anemia. Kasili said that as many as 40% of the children younger than 15 years of age, 63% of these being younger than 3 years, were anemic [52]. Kasili also said that although the anemia was multifactorial in etiology, the interplay between malnutrition as well as infection was still the most important element in causing the morbidity and mortality attributed to childhood anemia in Africa [52]. In addition to nutritional supplementation, correction for other common causes of anemia in childhood, especially those due to the parasitic infestations, are necessary in coping with anemia in childhood in the tropics.

For more details, the readers can investigate the previous chapter.

2. Anemia Due to Advance Stage of Inherited Anemic Disorders

The important inherited anemic disorders in the tropics, which present overt abnormalities in late childhood, include thalassemic and sickle cell disorders.

The treatment for these disorders in the tropics, where resources are limited, is still the blood transfusion. The totally unwanted complication as secondary hemochromatosis, which is the common cause of death, can be expected [53]. In order to improve the quality of life and life span of the affected children, the supportive chelation therapy is recommended [53]. More details on these anemic disorders can be taken from the previous chapter.

3. Anemia Due to Immunization

Some vaccinations can lead to anemia. The common problematic vaccine is DPT [13]. The other vaccines reported for the causing of anemia include hepatitis B vaccine (hemolytic anemia) [54] and measles vaccine (paroxysmal noctural hemoglobinuria) [55]. However, those vaccine-induced anemias are rare and do not disturb the recommendation for usage of the vaccines.

Table 17.2. Some abusive drugs and substances that can cause anemia

Drugs or substances	Major hematotoxicity	Type of anemia
1. Volatile solvent or glue	The major toxicity is usually due to the disturbance of bone marrow by the important hydrocarbon, benzene [57].	Aplastic anemia (in chronic usage)
2. Alcohol	Chronic and heavy alcohol consumption can lead to anemia due to liver impairment and vitamin malabsorption [58].	Non megaloblastic macrocytic anemia
3. Amphetamine	Exposure to Ecstasy (MDMA, 3,4 methylenedioxymethamphetamine) can induce bone marrow suppression [59].	Aplastic anemia
4. Marihuana	If marihuana is administrated intravenously, the anemia accompanied with thrombocytopenia and leukocytosis can be found [60].	Normocytic anemia (in intra-venous usage only)
5. Cocaine	The proposed pathogenetic mechanisms include: (1) cocaine-induced vasoconstriction and endothelial damage and (2) procoagulant effects of cocaine can lead to the clinical syndrome of microangiopathic hemolytic anemia, thrombocytopenia and acute renal failure [61].	HUS

Important Tropical Adolescent Anemia

1. Anemia in Drugs and Substance Abuse

Several drug and substance abuses are mentioned in the teenager with familial problems. Drug addiction becomes the great problem in many tropical countries [56]. The anemia in drug abusers can be the direct effect of many abusive drugs or substances [57 – 61] (Table 17.2). In addition to the hematotoxic effect, several toxicities on other organ systems of abusive substances are documented. Finally, the following social problems and criminal events are the unwanted outcomes. How to cope with the usage of abusive substances in the tropics should be included in the present global public health strategies.

References

[1]   Salsbury DC. Anemia of prematurity. *Neonatal Netw* 2001;20:13-20.

[2]   Lokeshwar MR, Dalal R, Manglani M, Shah N. Anemia in newborn. *Indian J Pediatr* 1998;65:651-61.

[3]   Humbert J, Wacker P. Common anemias in neonatology. *Schweiz Rundsch Med Prax* 1999;88:164-71.

[4]   Wiwanitkit V. Laboratory investigation in neonatal jaundice. *Med J Ubon H*osp 2001; 22: 231-239.

[5]   Mahapatra M, Choudhry VP. Blood transfusion in newborn. *Indian J Pediatr* 2003;70:909-14.

[6]   Ohls RK. The use of erythropoietin in neonates. *Clin Perinatol* 2000;27:681-96.

[7]   McCarthy PL, Bachman DT, Shapiro ED, Baron MA. Fever without apparent source on clinical examination, lower respiratory infections in children, bacterial infections, and acute gastroenteritis and diarrhea of infancy and early childhood. *Curr Opin Pediatr* 1995;7:107-25.

[8]   Morali A, Vidailhet M. Current topics in pediatric nutrition. *Arch Pediatr* 2002;9:726-32.

[9]   Wiwanitkit V. Nutritional Surveillance in rural countries. Presented at MILANOPEDIATRIA 2004. Milan, Italy.

[10] Hirt A. Diagnosis of anemia in childhood. *Schweiz Rundsch Med Prax* 2002;91:1845-9.

[11] Musumeci S, Romeo MA, Di Gregorio F, Schiliro G, Russo G. Chelating therapy in beta-thalassemia. *Pediatr Med Chir* 1982;4:55-9.

[12] Tarini A, Bakari S, Delisle H. The overall nutritional quality of the diet is reflected in the growth of Nigerian children. *Sante* 1999 ;9:23-31.

[13] Downes KA, Domen RE, McCarron KF, Bringelsen KA. Acute autoimmune hemolytic anemia following DTP vaccination: report of a fatal case and review of the literature. *Clin Pediatr* (Phila) 2001;40:355.

[14] La Spina M, Russo G. New drugs for childhood anemia. *Minerva Pediatr* 2003;55:483-93, 493-8.

[15] Amrolia PJ, Almeida A, Halsey C, Roberts IA, Davies SC. Therapeutic challenges in childhood sickle cell disease. Part 1: current and future treatment options. *Br J Haematol* 2003;120:725-36.

[16] Cunnington AJ. What's so bad about teenage pregnancy? *J Fam Plann Reprod Health Care* 2001;27:36-41.

[17] Schiffman RF. Drug and substance use in adolescents. *MCN Am J Matern Child Nurs* 2004 ;29:21-7.

[18] Curran CA. Intrapartum emergencies. *J Obstet Gynecol Neonatal Nurs* 2003;32:802-13.

[19]   Brabin B, Prinsen-Geerligs P, Verhoeff F, Kazembe P. Anaemia prevention for reduction of mortality in mothers and children. *Trans R Soc Trop Med Hyg* 2003;97:36-8.

[20]   Hernandorena X. Anemia in the newborn infant. *Rev Prat* 1989;39:2128-32.

[21]   Borghi J, Hanson K, Acquah CA, Ekanmian G, Filippi V, Ronsmans C, Brugha R, Browne E, Alihonou E. Costs of near-miss obstetric complications for women and their families in Benin and Ghana. *Health Policy Plan* 2003;18:383-90.

[22]   Brown MS. Health care in Africa. *Nurse Pract* 1984;9:38-43.

[23]   Augustine T, Bhatia BD. Early neonatal morbidity and mortality pattern in hospitalised children. *Indian J Matern Child Health* 1994;5:17-9.

[24]   Dudin AA, Rambaud-Cousson A, Badawi S, Da'na NA, Thalji A, Hannoun A. ABO and Rh(D) blood group distribution and their implication for feto-maternal incompatibility among the Palestinian population. *Ann Trop Paediatr* 1993;13:249-52.

[25]   Cotorruelo CM, Biondi CS, Garcia Borras S, Racca AL. Clinical aspects of Rh genotyping. *Clin Lab* 2002;48:271-81.

[26]   Fung Kee Fung K, Eason E, Crane J, Armson A, De La Ronde S, Farine D, Keenan-Lindsay L, Leduc L, Reid GJ, Aerde JV, Wilson RD, Davies G, Desilets VA, Summers A, Wyatt P, Young DC; Maternal-Fetal Medicine Committee, Genetics Committee. Prevention of Rh alloimmunization. *J Obstet Gynaecol Can* 2003;25:765-73.

[27]   Lux SE, Wolfe LC. Inherited disorders of the red cell membrane skeleton. *Pediatr Clin North Am* 1980;27:463-86.

[28]   Weed RI. Herediatary spherocytosis. A review.: *Arch Intern Med* 1975;135:1316-23.

[29]   Bolton-Maggs PH. The diagnosis and management of hereditary spherocytosis. *Baillieres Best Pract Res Clin Haematol* 2000;13:327-42.

[30]   Kaplan M, Hammerman C. Glucose-6-phosphate dehydrogenase deficiency: a potential source of severe neonatal hyperbilirubinaemia and kernicterus. *Semin Neonatol* 2002;7:121-8.

[31]   Evdokimova AI, Ryneiskaia VA, Plakhuta TG. Hemostatic changes in hereditary hemolytic anemias in children. *Pediatriia.* 1979;8:17-21.

[32]   Chuu WM, Lin DT, Lin KH, Chen BW, Chen RL, Lin KS. Can severe neonatal jaundice be prevented by neonatal screening for glucose-6-phosphate dehydrogenase deficiency?--a review of evidence. *Zhonghua Min Guo Xiao Er Ke Yi Xue Hui Za Zhi.* 1996;37:333-41.

[33]   Mehta A, Mason PJ, Vulliamy TJ. Glucose-6-phosphate dehydrogenase deficiency. *Baillieres Best Pract Res Clin Haematol* 2000;13:21-38.

[34]   Mohrenweiser HW, Fielek S, Wurzinger KH. Characteristics of enzymes of erythrocytes from newborn infants and adults: activity, thermostability, and electrophoretic profile as a function of cell age. *Am J Hematol* 1981;11:125-36.

[35]   Jansen G, Koenderman L, Rijksen G, Cats BP, Staal GE. Characteristics of hexokinase, pyruvate kinase, and glucose-6-phosphate dehydrogenase during adult and neonatal reticulocyte maturation. *Am J Hematol* 1985;20:203-15.

[36]   Zanella A, Bianchi P. Red cell pyruvate kinase deficiency: from genetics to.clinical manifestations. *Baillieres Best Pract Res Clin H*aematol 2000;13:57-81.

[37] Min-Oo G, Fortin A, Tam MF, Nantel A, Stevenson MM, Gros P. Pyruvate kinase deficiency in mice protects against malaria. *Nat Genet* 2003;35:357-62.

[38] 38. Chisaka H, Morita E, Yaegashi N, Sugamura K. Parvovirus B19 and the pathogenesis of anaemia. *Rev Med Virol* 2003;13:347-59.

[39] Bhardwaj U, Zhang YH, Blackburn W, McCabe LL, McCabe ER. Rapid confirmation of Southeast Asian and Filipino alpha-thalassemia genotypes from newborn screening specimens. *Am J Hematol* 2002;71:56-8.

[40] Old JM. Screening and genetic diagnosis of haemoglobin disorders. *Blood Rev* 2003;17:43-53.

[41] Da Costa L, Willig TN, Fixler J, Mohandas N, Tchernia G. Diamond-Blackfan anemia. *Curr Opin Pediatr* 2001;13:10-5.

[42] Veprekova L, Jelinek J, Zeman J. Congenital aplastic anemia caused by parvovirus B19 infection. *Cas Lek Cesk* 2001;140:178-80.

[43] Hollier LM, Harstad TW, Sanchez PJ, Twickler DM, Wendel GD Jr. Fetal syphilis: clinical and laboratory characteristics. *Obstet Gynecol* 2001;97:947-53.

[44] Ibhanesebhor SE. Clinical characteristics of neonatal malaria. *J Trop Pediatr* 1995;41:330-3.

[45] Steketee RW, Nahlen BL, Parise ME, Menendez C. The burden of malaria in pregnancy in malaria-endemic areas. *Am J Trop Med Hyg* 2001;64(1-2 Suppl):28-35.

[46] Murray JC, Bernini JC, Bijou HL, Rossmann SN, Mahoney DH Jr, Morad AB. Infantile cytomegalovirus-associated autoimmune hemolytic anemia. *J Pediatr Hematol Oncol* 2001;23:318-20.

[47] Cochran JB, Panzarino VM, Maes LY, Tecklenburg FW. Pneumococcus-induced T-antigen activation in hemolytic uremic syndrome and anemia. *Pediatr Nephrol* 2004;19:317-21.

[48] Khodasevich LS, Dobrodeev KG. Hemolytic-uremic syndrome in meningococcal infection. *Pediatriia* 1991;(1):86-8.

[49] Reynes Muntaner J, Gomez Rivas B, Vidal Palacios C, Marti Mauri D, Allue Martinex X, Mas Delgado JM, Labay Matias MV. Hemolytic uremic syndrome associated with meningococcal sepsis. *An Esp Pediatr* 1983;19:204-6.

[50] Nutrition: a review of the WHO programme. II. *WHO Chron* 1972;26:195-206.

[51] Lutter CK, Rivera JA. Nutritional status of infants and young children and characteristics of their diets. *J Nutr* 2003;133:2941S-9S.

[52] Kasili EG. Malnutrition and infections as causes of childhood anemia in tropical Africa. *Am J Pediatr Hematol Oncol* 1990;12:375-7.

[53] Marx JJ. Pathophysiology and treatment of iron overload in thalassemia patients in tropical countries. *Adv Exp Med Biol* 2003;531:57-68.

[54] Lliminana C, Soler JA, Melo M, Roig I. Hemolytic anemia and thrombocytopenic purpura after the administration of the recombinant hepatitis B vaccine. *Med Clin* (Barc) 1999;113:39.

[55] Bunch C, Schwartz FC, Bird GW. Paroxysmal cold haemoglobinuria following measles immunization. *Arch Dis Child* 1972;47:299-300.

[56] Health DB. Culture and substance abuse. *Psychiatr Clin North Am* 2001;24:479-96, vii-viii.

[57] Flanagan RJ, Ives RJ. Volatile substance abuse. *Bull Narc* 1994;46:49-78.

[58] Davenport J. Macrocytic anemia. *Am Fam Physician* 1996;53:155-62.

[59] Marsh JC, Abboudi ZH, Gibson FM, Scopes J, Daly S, O'Shaunnessy DF, Baughan AS, Gordon-Smith EC. Aplastic anaemia following exposure to 3,4-methylenedioxymethamphetamine ('Ecstasy'). *Br J Haematol* 1994;88:281-5.

[60] Payne RJ, Brand SN. The toxicity of intravenously used marihuana. *JAMA* 1975;233:351-4.

[61] Tumlin JA, Sands JM, Someren A. Hemolytic-uremic syndrome following "crack" cocaine inhalation. *Am J Med Sci* 1990;299:366-71.

Chapter 18

Anemia in the Elderly in the Tropical Countries

Introduction to Geriatric Anemia

Aging is an important process in all living-things. Degeneration can be seen in the aging process, which occurs after birth. The elderly become the important group of population, who is attacked with several health problems. Some problems are due to the normal aging process, the other are due to the pathological process. As the aging population and the incidence of age-related health conditions increase, the cost of healthcare is also expected to rise [1]. Anemia commonly occurs in the elderly, and is associated with a number of health conditions such as falls, weakness, and immobility [1]. Ershler said that anemia was one of the characteristics of the frailty phenotype and was often observed in elderly patients [2]. During aging, modulation of hematopoiesis becomes disordered, impairing the ability of older people to respond appropriately to the physiological demand for blood cell replacement triggered by stimuli such as blood loss or cytoreductive chemotherapy [3]. Rothstein said that these might contribute to the increase in the prevalence of anemia that was observed during aging [3]. They also said that various age-related events, such as genomic mutations secondary to oxidative stress and impaired regulation of cytokine production, might contribute to or cause the emergence of abnormal clones of hematopoietic cells, therefore, normal hematopoiesis was disrupted [3]. These disorders are so tightly associated with aging that they are considered to be geriatric disorders; they can lead to anemia, neutropenia, and thrombocytopenia and to the development of acute nonlymphoblastic leukemia [3].

Concerning geriatric anemia, it is a common concern in geriatric health, but its exact incidence and prevalence are unclear [4]. Beghe et al. noted that several studies had addressed the rate of geriatric anemia with discrepant results [4]. They noted that estimates of anemia prevalence reported in the articles ranged from 2.9% to 61% in elderly men and from 3.3% to 41% in elderly women and most existing reports indicated that elderly men had higher rates of anemia than did elderly women, but the threshold values were, in general, higher for men than for women [4]. They also noted that incidence of anemia rose with age; some studies reported a particularly notable increase in prevalence of anemia in the oldest subjects, those > or =85 years of age [4]. As previously mentioned, several pathologies can be seen in the elderly and those disorders can lead to anemia. Similar underlying pathologies of anemia such as iron deficiency, blood loss and parasitic infestations, can be seen. However, some specific disorders are common in the elderly including chronic diseases (both infectious and non-infectious) and cancers. The prevalence of vitamin B12 deficiency due to reduced absorption of food-bound vitamin B12 also increases with aging [5].

Balducci said that anemia could also be a result of the presence of comorbid conditions that could mask the symptoms of anemia [5]. Therefore, appropriate diagnosis and management strategies of anemia in the elderly need to be identified, particularly because anemia may indicate the presence of other serious diseases [5].

Although anemia in people of advancing age can often be attributed to underlying etiologies such as iron deficiency or chronic disease, some cases do not have any identifiable cause [2]. Therefore, it has been suggested that the aging process, degeneration-related, itself might be an intrinsic factor in the development of anemia, possibly through the age-related dysregulation of certain proinflammatory cytokines such as interleukin-6 (IL-6) [2]. Ershler said that although the mechanism underlying the association between increased IL-6 and anemia had not been fully elucidated, it had been suggested that, like with other cytokines, it involved direct inhibition of erythropoietin production or interaction with the erythropoietin receptor [2]. Rothstein said that dysregulation of mechanisms controlling hematopoiesis was an important characteristic of the hematopoietic system in the elderly, but the response of progenitor cells to humoral stimulators was preserved and accounted for the effectiveness of recombinant hematopoietic growth factors used as emerging treatment modalities for hematopoietic disorders in the elderly [3]. In addition, a primary deficiency of erythropoietin may be at fault in at least some of the geriatric anemic cases since the response of erythropoietin to anemia may decrease in individuals over age 70 [5]. In addition to a thorough history and physical examination, laboratory investigations are needed for diagnosis and classification of anemia in the elderly. Several laboratory investigations such as red cell indices and morphology, reticulocyte count, hematinic assays and occasionally bone marrow examination, will detect the underlying pathology in most cases.

A rise in the aging population has been predicted, and, as a result, it is expected that the incidence of age-related health conditions will also increase [5]. Although common in the elderly, anemia is often mild and asymptomatic and rarely requires hospitalization [5]. However, anemia is associated with symptoms ranging from weakness and fatigue to increased falls and depression, and in severe cases can lead to congestive heart failure [1 – 4]. It can also lead to more-serious complications such as neurological impairments [1]. Consequently, anemia can have a significant effect on healthcare requirements and healthcare expenditure [1]. Balducci said that untreated anemia could be detrimental, because it was associated with increased mortality, poor health, fatigue, and functional dependence and could lead to several complications [5]. The general principle for treatment of anemia can be applied for the geriatric population. The treatment of anemia should aim to correct the underlying cause of the disorder and to improve the quality of the blood. Regular blood transfusion may be required for some elderly patients with chronic anemia. However, the attendant risks of this procedure, such as iron overload human immunodeficiency virus and viral hepatitis transmission, should be considered.

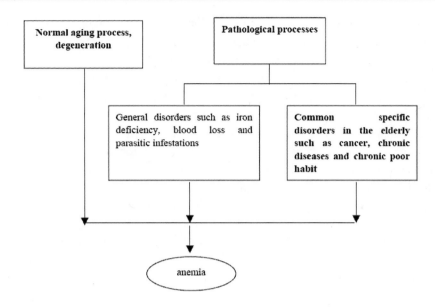

Figure 18.1. Diagram showing the underlying cause of anemia in the elderly

Important Geriatric Anemia

1. Cancer-Related Anemia

Anemia is common in patients with cancer. Cancer-related anemia often develops from the infiltration of marrow by malignant cells, impaired hemoglobin production related to chemotherapy or radiation therapy, iron deficiency, or low endogenous erythropoietin levels [6]. However, Balducci said that anemia should not necessarily be ascribed to cancer or aging and the causes of anemia should be pursued and reversed [7]. The signs and symptoms of anemia can be seen in any cases with cancer-related anemia. In addition, the patients with cancer-related anemia may also experience cognitive dysfunction including decreased mental alertness, poor concentration, and memory problems [6]. Cunningham said that these symptoms often are exacerbated in the elderly patient with cancer and related to underlying low hemoglobin concentrations [6]. Balducci said that anemia was an issue of concern in the management of older patients with cancer [7]. In this age group, the incidence and prevalence of both cancer and anemia increase with age [7]. Steensma said that low hemoglobin levels were associated with diminished quality of life and possibly decreased overall survival [8]. Aapro *et al.* said that age as a covariate in multiple linear regression analysis failed to reach significance for most measures of function and quality of life (QOL), including measures of energy, activities, mental health, general cancer-related QOL, and overall QOL in a study of anemic elderly cancerous patients [9]. They also said that other factors, including cancer progression, hemoglobin change, and baseline hemoglobin levels, were much more important in determining change in functional and quality-of-life scores [9].

Concerning treatment of cancer-related anemia, restoring Hb levels via the administration of iron supplements, blood transfusions, or, more recently, erythropoiesis-stimulating therapy (epoetin alfa) results in significant improvement [6]. The use of epoetin alfa as a treatment option for patients with chemotherapy-associated anemia and an hemoglobin concentration less than 10 g/dL has been recommended by the American Society of Clinical Oncology and the American Society of Hematology [6]. Erythropoiesis-stimulating therapies are a promising treatment option for cancer-related anemia that may improve cognitive function and quality of life for patients with cancer [6]. Balducci said that hemoglobin levels should be maintained at a minimum of 12 g/dL in cancer patients undergoing chemotherapy who are responsive to erythropoietin [7]. However, Steensma noted that there were some new concerns in cancer patients for the risk of thromboembolism in cancer patients with higher hemoglobin levels who were receiving epoetin, and possible immunosuppressive effects of blood product transfusions that might have relevance to neoplasia progression [8]. Since anemia is a correctable pathologic finding in elderly people, prompt treatment of cancer-related anemia in the elderly is recommended [9]. Successful treatment of anemia has undeniable benefits for patients, often yielding dramatic symptomatic improvement [9].

2. Iron Deficiency Anemia

Aging is often associated with dysregulation of immune response even among healthy elderly; some of these changes may be secondary to deficiencies of macronutrients (energy and protein) and micronutrients (notably, vitamins B6, B12, and folic acid as well as iron and zinc) [10]. Nutrient needs of the elderly are unique and complex [11]. Older individuals often have multiple nutrient deficiencies because of physiological, social and economic factors. Similar to other age groups, iron deficiency anemia is common in the elderly [12]. Iron deficiency can lead not only to anemia but to decreased work capacity, abnormal neurotransmitter function, and altered immunologic and inflammatory defenses [13]. Recently Lukito *et al.* performed a study to examine the relationship between lymphocyte subsets and nutritional status, and total mortality in an institutionalized elderly population, 115 permanent elderly residents were drawn from a large geriatric institution in Melbourne, Australia [14]. They reported positive correlations of serum ferritin with the number of CD8 (T-suppressor cell) and of serum iron with CD56 (natural killer, NK cells) in men and proposed that the number of CD4 T-cells might be useful in the prediction of total mortality in an institutionalized elderly population [14]. Risk for iron deficiency is a function of iron loss, iron intake, iron absorption, and physiologic demands [13].

Concerning iron loss, iron deficiency in the elderly almost always results from blood loss. Luman and Ng found a much higher incidence of gastrointestinal disorders in the group of male and postmenopausal women than in the group with premenopausal women [15]. Indeed, gastrointestinal blood loss in the geriatric population is an important health problem. The iron deficiency can be a manifestation in an elder with gastrointestinal tract cancer. According to the study of Luman and Ng, they recommended bidirectional endoscopy for postmenopausal women with iron deficiency anemia [14]. Concerning iron intake, the low iron intake is still an important nutritional problem in the elderly, especially those in the developing countries. Park *et al.* found that the low-income urban elderly Korean people had a low energy intake, less than 5300 kJ/day, with an inadequate intake of iron, thiamin, riboflavin and niacin in addition to calcium and vitamin A [16]. Indeed, malnutrition in ill elderly subjects is common in hospitals, nursing homes, and home care [17]. Depending on the type and composition of the groups of patients under consideration, the prevalence of malnutrition is cited at up to 60%. With advancing age, the amounts of food consumed daily diminish and become significantly smaller than the amounts consumed by the younger population [17]. Basically, the elderly mostly eat food of low nutrient density [17]. Seiler said that malnutrition prolonged hospital stays, imposed enormous costs on health services, and caused considerable mortality [17]. To overcome the problem of iron deficiency anemia due to inadequate intake in the elderly, the iron supplementation is suggested [18]. Concerning the abnormality in iron absorption in the geriatric population, one of the most remarkable changes in the gastrointestinal tract with aging is the frequent development of atrophic gastritis and the inability to secrete gastric acid [19]. Saltzman and Russell said that this process affected approximately a third of older adults in the United States and only recently was recognized to be due to infection by *Helicobacter pylori* in the majority of cases [19]. The lack of gastric acid in atrophic gastritis may lead to small intestinal bacterial overgrowth and influences the absorption of a variety of micronutrients, including iron, folate, calcium, vitamin K, and vitamin B12 [19]. Although not well documented, the effect of age on iron absorption and iron excretion appears to be small, and body stores of iron increase with age [20]. Concerning physiologic demand in the elderly, the increased iron requirement can be expected due to the impairment of iron absorption by the gastrointestinal tract. However, Johnson *et al.* noted that the studies of noninstitutionalized elderly individuals reported mean iron intakes that meet current Recommended Dietary Allowances for iron [20]. They also noted that dietary practices that might decrease iron bioavailability, and hence iron stores in the body, include low intakes of ascorbic acid or high intakes of calcium, and decreased consumption of highly available iron from meat, fish, and poultry [20].

Of interest, the iron deficiency anemia in the elderly is more common in the tropics. This finding might be due to many factors, especially those environmental factors. Although iron deficiency anemia is not a major health problem in developed countries, iron deficiency is still a problem for the elderly, however, about 10% of Caucasians carry the mutation for hereditary hemochromatosis and are at risk for iron overload [21]. Concerning the diagnosis of iron deficiency anemia, the similar process as indicated in the previous chapter for the general population should be followed. However, there are some specific notifications that should be mentioned. Firsl, specific concern in cases with positive occult blood test for the occult gastrointestinal malignancy is necessary [22]. Second, serum ferritin is the most useful test to differentiate iron deficiency anemia from anemia of chronic disease. Ferritin depletion is the hallmark for diagnosis of iron deficiency [23]. A serum ferritin level that is diagnostic is the level less than 18 micrograms/L and suggestive is the level between 18 and 45 micrograms/L [23]. However, the tests used to diagnose iron deficiency have certain limitations regarding their ability to detect iron deficiency before the overt anemia occurs [24]. The tests which diagnose iron deficiency most accurately are low serum ferritin and reduced iron staining of a bone marrow aspirate [24]. Finally, Besa said that surveys have shown that there is no increase in iron deficiency with age, and the majority of elderly patients with mild anemia show no demonstrable cause and are unresponsive to therapy [25].

Besa noted that the statement that anemia was often a presenting sign of a serious underlying illness and that patients with anemia had to undergo a complete work-up should be reconsidered in the elderly, and the criteria for anemia should be redefined to prevent unnecessary studies for individuals who fell in the lower limits of normalcy because of age [25]. Besa proposed that asymptomatic elderly patients with mild anemia might not be anemic if the general practitioner adjusted the expected levels for the elderly and, in doing so, the general practitioner could save 95 per cent of these patients from undergoing unnecessary testing [25].

Johnson *et al.* said that it was difficult to estimate the prevalence of iron deficiency in elderly persons, because impaired iron status can be the result of iron deficiency or chronic disease [20]. They said that further study was necessary to determine whether red blood cell ferritin and serum transferrin receptors might be useful biochemical markers to differentiate the anemia of chronic disease from iron deficiency anemia [20]. Schultz and Freedman also noted that there was evidence to suggest that iron deficiency may predispose individuals to certain infections [24]. Other information points to the promotion of certain bacterial and parasitic infections after rapid correction of iron deficiency, thus, elderly patients having iron replacement therapy should be followed closely [24]. Smieja *et al.* found that of 66 (36%) of 183 admitted eligible elderly patients in their study had anemia, in 47 cases (71%) the anemia was documented by house staff or attending physicians [26]. Of the 66 anemic patients 49 had a non-macrocytic anemia of unknown cause: 26 had their serum ferritin level measured, 5 underwent bone-marrow aspiration, and 21 were referred for gastrointestinal endoscopy [26]. In this study, six of eight patients with probable iron deficiency underwent endoscopy, two were found to have cancer of the stomach or cecum [26]. They said that anemia was common among elderly patients in hospitals, however, iron deficiency was usually underrecognized and underinvestigated [26].

Concerning the clinical manifestations of iron deficiency anemia in the elderly, similar findings to the non - geriatric population can be seen. Because iron is present in many metabolic processes besides the production of hemoglobin, iron deficiency results in a variety of defects which are manifested at biochemical, tissue, and functional levels [24]. Iron deficiency results in tissue defects, including those affecting the gastrointestinal tract, and defects of mitochondria and lymphocytes. A deficiency of iron, independent of the anemia, results in reduced exercise capacity that can be measured in both physiological and economic terms [24]. A deficiency of iron has also been shown to result in certain behavioural and learning abnormalities [24]. In addition, iron deficiency has been shown to result in impaired control of body temperature, resulting in an increase in catecholamine levels and the impairment in heat-generating ability was shown to result from reduced conversion of T4 to T3 in the peripheral tissues [24]. Schultz noted that elderly patients complaining of increased fatigue should therefore be screened for iron deficiency [24]. However, Garry et al. recently proposed that the health status, race, socioeconomic status, diet, and region are more important than age as explanations for the high prevalence of anemia seen in many previous studies [27]. Concerning the treatment of iron deficiency anemia in the elderly, principles similar to those for the general population, as indicated in the previous chapter, can be applied.

3. Anemia Due to Blood Loss

As previously mentioned, chronic occult gastrointestinal blood loss is an important cause of iron deficiency anemia in the elderly with a gastrointestinal malignancy. The details of iron deficiency anemia due to blood loss in the elderly has already been mentioned in the former topic. However, acute blood loss in the elderly can also be the underlying cause of anemia. In the elderly, anaemia with an absolute reticulocytosis is due either to acute blood loss or hemolysis [28].

4. Anemia Due to Parasitic Infestations

Parasitic infestations can be the etiology of geriatric anemia. In the tropics, common parasitic infestations including malaria, babesia and hookworm infections can be the cause of anemia in the elderly. Stich *et al.* suggested a higher risk for a severe course of malaria including malarial anemia in the elderly [29]. They also proposed providing extensive advice on the correct use of exposure- and chemoprophylaxis of malaria for travellers above the age of 60 [29]. Alward *et al.* noted that babesia infection was often subclinical but might be fulminant, especially in the elderly [30]. They noted that babesiosis in an elderly subject is usually manifested by high fevers, confusion, hemolytic anemia, and thrombocytopenia [30]. Elias *et al.* reported a strong inverse association among the elderly subjects between intensity of hookworm infection (unciniasis) and hemoglobin levels but only at intensities greater than 2,000 eggs/gram feces [31]. More details on parasitic-related anemic disorders can be found in the previous chapter.

5. Megaloblastic Anemia

Megaloblastic anemia in the elderly is usually due to vitamin B12 deficiency. As previously mentioned, vitamin B12 (cobalamine) is the micronutrient which is usually deficient in the geriatric population [10]. This is because of the increased prevalence of cobalamin malabsorption in this age group, which is mainly caused by autoimmune atrophic body gastritis [32]. Elderly individuals with cobalamin deficiency may present with neuropsychiatric or metabolic deficiencies, without frank macrocytic anemia [32]. An investigation of symptoms and signs should include the diagnosis of deficiency as well as any underlying cause [32]. Nilsson-Ehle noted that vitamin B12 deficiency states could still exist even when serum vitamin B12 levels are higher than the traditional lower reference limit [32]. Smith noted that not all cases of vitamin B12 deficiency could be identified by low vitamin B 12 serum levels and proposed that the serum methylmalonic acid (MMA) level might be more useful for diagnosis of vitamin B12 deficiency in the elderly [33]. Nilsson-Ehle said that cobalamin-responsive elevations of MMA and homocysteine were helpful laboratory tools for the diagnosis, however, the health-related reference ranges for homocysteine and MMA appear to vary with age and gender [32].

Nilsson-Ehle said that the patients who are at risk from cobalamin deficiency included those with a gastrointestinal predisposition (such as atrophic body gastritis or previous partial gastrectomy), autoimmune disorders (type 1 or insulin-dependent diabetes mellitus and thyroid disorders), those receiving long term therapy with gastric acid inhibitors or biguanides, and those undergoing nitrous oxide anesthesia [32]. Predominantly, the high prevalence of poor vitamin B12 status is caused by the increasing prevalence of atrophic gastritis type B, which occurs with a frequency of approximately 20-50% in elderly subjects [34]. Nilsson-Ehle said that atrophic body gastritis could be indirectly diagnosed by measuring serum levels of gastrin and pepsinogens, and the atrophic body gastritis could cause dietary cobalamin malabsorption despite a normal traditional Schilling's test [32]. Concerning treatment, Vitamin B12 deficiency is effectively treated with oral vitamin B12 supplementation [33]. To date, inadequate Vitamin B12 intake has not proven to be a major risk factor [33]. However, it can be a problem in some elderly populations with specific eating patterns, such as vegetarianism due to religious belief [34]. Elderly patients respond to cobalamin treatment as fully as younger patients, with complete haematological recovery and complete or good partial resolution of neurological deficits [33]. Chronic dementia responds poorly but should, nevertheless, be treated if there is a metabolic deficiency (as indicated by elevated homocysteine or MMA levels) [33]. Nilsson-Ehle said that cobalamin supplementation was affordable and nontoxic, and it might prevent irreversible neurological damage if started early [32].

Apart from vitamin B12 deficiency, folate deficiency can be the cause of megaloblastic anemia in the elderly. Wolters *et al.* said that 3-60% of the elderly were classified as vitamin B12 deficient and about 29% as folate deficient [35]. In contrast to vitamin B12, folic acid intake among elderly subjects is generally well below the recommended dietary reference values [35]. Similar to vitamin B12 deficiency, depression, dementia, and mental impairment are often associated with folate deficiency [35]. Concerning treatment, folate deficiency is treated with 1 mg of folic acid daily [33].

6. Anemia Due to Myelodysplastic Syndrome

As previously mentioned, the abnormal erythropoiesis can be seen in the elderly, and it can lead to the myelodysplatic syndrome as well as anemia [3]. Generally, the myelodysplastic syndromes are characterized by hemopoietic insufficiency associated with cytopenias leading to serious morbidity plus the additional risk of leukemic transformation [36]. Generation of abnormal sideroblast formation appears to be due to the malfunction of the mitochondrial respiratory chain, attributable to mutations of mitochondrial DNA, to which aged individuals are most vulnerable [36].

7. Anemia Due To Chronic Poor Habitual Practice

Since the elderly have lived longer and, practiced more habits than younger people, they can get many adverse effects from poor habitual practice. Those poor habitual practices include poor sanitation habits, which are a risk for chronic infection, ingestion or use of things toxicant to their health, and few concerns about their health. A good example of poor habitual practice is chronic alcoholic consumption. Indeed, chronic alcoholic consumption can lead to subsequent liver disease, which can be the cause of anemia. In addition, alcohol consumption itself can directly cause anemia. Recently, Latvala *et al.* noted that alcohol abuse resulted in diverse patterns of hematological effects and affects several cell lines [37]. They noted that the incidence of anemia was 51% in the alcohol abusers, as compared with 69% in the nonalcoholics [37].

8. Anemia Due to Chronic Diseases

Anemia of chronic disease is an important group of anemic disorders in the elderly. The important key of anemia of chronic disease is the long duration, therefore, the elderly who have lived the longest have a higher risk of having anemia of chronic disease than the younger. Aging is usually associated with an increase in chronic disease as well as infections and associated morbidity and this is often thought to be secondary to immunosenescence [10]. In general, aging is associated with a decline in activity and an increase in chronic inflammatory as well as cardiovascular disorders [20]. These alter not only red blood cell production but also plasma volume, leading to an increased frequency of a lower hemoglobin concentration and hematocrit level [20]. It is noted that all patients with chronic conditions be adequately treated and counseled for their condition. Indeed, several chronic diseases can lead to anemia including renal, hepatic and cardiac disorders. Chronic diseases can not only directly lead to anemia but also indirectly cause complications, fatigue, anorexia and wasting which can all lead to anemia.

Chronic renal disease is common in the elderly and can lead to anemia. Indeed, several degenerative disorders in the elderly especially diabetes mellitus [38] and hypertension [39] can lead to chronic renal disease and subsequently anemia. Anemia can worsen renal function and cause a more rapid progression to end stage renal disease and dialysis than is found in patients without anemia [38 – 40]. Anemia is the main problem in the patients with end stage renal disease (ESRD). In patients with ESRD, high levels of pro-inflammatory cytokines and increased oxidative stress are common features and may contribute to the development of malnutrition, anemia, resistance to recombinant human erythropoietin (epoetin) and atherosclerosis [40]. The onset of inflammation is multi-factorial and is a predictor of poor outcome in ESRD [40]. Pathophysiologically, inflammation and the acute-phase response interact with the haematopoietic system at several levels, resulting in reduced erythropoiesis, accelerated destruction of erythrocytes and blunting of the reactive increase in erythropoietin in response to reduced hemoglobin levels [40]. Stenvinkel said that epoetin resistance had been linked with inflammation In patients with ESRD, which was often associated with a state of functional iron deficiency and the patients with ESRD were thought to have a reduced capacity in their control of oxidative stress and there was evidence that suggests that a relationship might exist between inflammation, oxidative stress and the treatment of anemia with epoetin [40]. Parfrey said that the burden of disease in ESRD is high and the cost of ESRD therapy is also high [41]. Parfrey noted that the age and co-morbidity of patients was increasing, and many patients were started on therapy with little hope of rehabilitation, and with a high likelihood of death within a short period of time [41]. Of interest, anemia due to chronic renal disease is common among the elderly. Artz et al. noted that occult renal dysfunction is the main mechanisms of unexplained anemia among the elderly in the nursing home [42]. Concerning the therapeutic method, recombinant human erythropoietin has revolutionized the treatment of anemia associated with chronic renal failure, while its role in other anemias is currently under investigation [28]. In addition, the National Kidney Foundation recently published guidelines stating that regular use of intravenous iron therapy will prevent iron deficiency and promote better erythropoiesis than oral iron therapy in patients with end stage renal disease (ESRD) who are undergoing hemodialysis [43]. This regimen was proved to be highly effective with low adverse effects [43].

Concerning chronic liver disease, cirrhosis is well documented for the correlation to anemia. Spur cell anemia is the common type of anemic disorder in the patients with severe cirrhosis. In those patients, erythrocytes of peripheral blood showed typical spiculated cells on light microscopic and scanning electron microscopic studies [44]. Free-cholesterol/phospholipid ratio of the erythrocyte membrane was elevated, and the level of chenodeoxycholic acid increased in serum [44]. An important complication as chronic disseminated intravascular coagulopathy (DIC) in these patients are mentioned [44]. In addition, hemolysis is also documented in the cases with chronic liver diseases. Liver disease, particularly alcoholic cirrhosis, is associated with a number of interesting chemical changes which result in structural and metabolic abnormalities of the erythrocyte membrane leading to microscopically observable cell shape changes and hemolytic anemia varying from very mild to potentially lethal [45]. An increase in unesterified serum cholesterol owing to lecithin cholesterol acyl transferase (LCAT) deficiency in cirrhosis leads to expansion of the lipid bilayer and macrocytosis without megaloblastic changes in precursors and the substitutions of phosphatidyl choline (PC) moieties in the erythrocyte lipid bilayer lead to echinocytes (disaturated PC) or to stomatocytes (diunsaturated PC) [45]. The most severe hemolysis in liver disease is associated with acanthocytes (spur cells) and a marked imbalance in cholesterol-phospholipid ratio. These patients usually have hypersplenism, as well as rigid erythrocyte membrane transformations which are irreversible [45].

Concerning chronic heart diseases, chronic heart failure is proved to relate to anemia [46 - 48]. Anemia can increase the severity of CHF and is associated with a rise in mortality, hospitalization and malnutrition [46]. Uncontrolled CHF can cause rapid deterioration of renal function and anemia [46]. Aggressive therapy against CHF with all the conventional medications at the accepted doses often fails to improve the CHF if anemia is also present but is not treated [46]. The triad of anemia, chronic kidney insufficiency (CKI) and CHF is known as the cardio-renal anemia syndrome [46 - 48]. The three conditions form a vicious circle, in which each condition is capable of causing or being caused by another [46 - 48]. CKI can also cause anemia, as well as worsen the severity of CHF, and is associated with increased mortality and hospitalization in patients with CHF [46 - 48]. Silverberg et al. said that the nephrologists should assess the cardiac status of all patients with CKI carefully, and this includes an echocardiogram along with possibly measuring the levels of B-type natriuretic peptide [46].

Geriatric Anemia in the Tropics

Similar to other age groups, the geriatric populations in the tropics have a high prevalence of anemia. In 1993, Prayurahong *et al.* studied the anemia among the Thai elderly and found that anemia could be detected in 15 % [49]. They suggested that folate deficiency might play a role in the occurrence of anemia in elderly people, and therefore, dietary counseling and supplementation of folic acid are recommended [49]. A similar study was preformed in India by Parasulamula *et al.* [50]. According to this study, the high prevalence of anemia associated with the low social status of the elderly could be demonstrated [50]. Allain *et al.* also performed a similar study in Zimbabwe and found that 23% were anemic, 3% with microcytic and 20% with macrocytic indices [51]. They found that folate levels were significantly lower in urban subjects and B12 levels were significantly lower in rural subjects [51]. According to these studies, the high prevalence of anemia among the elderly in the tropical developing countries can be confirmed.

Table 18.1. Anemia and common tropical cancers in the elderly

Cancers	Brief specific details about anemia
Cholangiocarcinoma	o Cholangiocarcinoma is a cancerous disease with a very high prevalence in Southeast Asia [53]. Pinyosophan and Wiwanitkit studied the co-morbidity of anemia and cholangiocarcinoma, and they found that the prevalence of anemia among the cholangiocarcinoma patients was as high as 18.2 % [54]. Rea *et al.* also noted that the factors associated with tumor recurrence included: male sex, tumor grade 3 or 4, a low hemoglobin level both at diagnosis and preoperatively, and a low preoperative prothrombin time and low alkaline phosphatase level at diagnosis and preoperatively [55].
Hepatoma	o Hepatoma is common in the tropics due to the high prevalence of viral hepatitis infection. Hepatoma usually follows cirrhosis, therefore, a similar finding to cirrhosis-related anemia can be seen [44 – 45]. o
Cervical carcinoma	o Cervical carcinoma is common in the tropical developing countries where the population lacks knowledge and has low concern for screening tests. Cervical carcinoma usually relates to menstruation disorders and this can lead to anemic presentation. Obermair *et al.* noted that a low nadir hemoglobin level was highly predictive of shortened progression-free survival in the patients undergoing chemoradiation for cervical carcinoma [56].

Concerning several types of geriatric anemic disorders, some are common in the tropics. These include the parasitic – related anemias, anemias due to chronic poor habitual practice and some specific cancer-related anemias. Concerning parasitic-related anemias, there is no doubt that the high prevalence of this type of geriatric anemia is high in the tropics since parasitic infestations are common in tropical developing countries. Concerning the anemias due to chronic poor habitual practice, low education and low socioeconomic status are the two main underlying factors. Health promotion and supportive services for the elderly in the underprivileged rural communities in tropical countries is still necessary [52]. Concerning cancer-related anemia, the high prevalence of anemia is also reported in the common cancerous diseases of the elderly in the tropics. The details of anemia in those common tropical cancers in the geriatric populations are presented in Table 18.1.

References

[1] Robinson B. Cost of anemia in the elderly. *J Am Geriatr Soc* 2003;51(3 Suppl):S14-7.

[2] Ershler WB. Biological interactions of aging and anemia: a focus on cytokines. *J Am Geriatr Soc* 2003;51(3 Suppl):S18-21.

[3] Rothstein G. Disordered hematopoiesis and myelodysplasia in the elderly. *J Am Geriatr Soc* 2003;51(3 Suppl):S22-6.

[4] Beghe C, Wilson A, Ershler WB. Prevalence and outcomes of anemia in geriatrics: a systematic review of the literature. *Am J Med* 2004;116 Suppl 7A:3S-10S.

[5] Balducci L. Epidemiology of anemia in the elderly: information on diagnostic evaluation. *J Am Geriatr Soc* 2003 ;51(3 Suppl):S2-9.

[6] Cunningham RS. Anemia in the oncology patient: cognitive function and cancer. *Cancer Nurs* 2003;26(6 Suppl):38S-42S.

[7] Balducci L. Anemia, cancer, and aging. *Cancer Control* 2003;10:478-86.

[8] Steensma DP. Management of anemia in patients with cancer. *Curr Oncol Rep* 2004;6:297-304.

[9] Aapro MS, Cella D, Zagari M. Age, anemia, and fatigue. *Semin Oncol* 2002;29(3 Suppl 8):55-9.

[10] Ahluwalia N. Aging, nutrition and immune function. *J Nutr Health Aging* 2004;8:2-6.

[11] Van Grevenhof J, Funderburg K. Prevention of nutritional deficiencies in the elderly. 1: *J Okla State Med Assoc* 2003;96:150-3.

[12] Mukhopadhyay D, Mohanaruban K. Iron deficiency anaemia in older people: investigation, management and treatment. *Age Ageing* 2002;31:87-91.

[13] Ross EM. Evaluation and treatment of iron deficiency in adults. *Nutr Clin Care* 2002;5:220-4.

[14] Lukito W, Wattanapenpaiboon N, Savige GS, Hutchinson P, Wahlqvist ML Nutritional indicators, peripheral blood lymphocyte subsets and survival in an institutionalised elderly population. *Asia Pac J Clin Nutr* 2004;13:107-12.

[15] Luman W, Ng KL. Audit of investigations in patients with iron deficiency anaemia. *Singapore Med J* 2003;44:504-10.

[16] Park YH, de Groot LC, van Staveren WA. Dietary intake and anthropometry of Korean elderly people: a literature review. *Asia Pac J Clin Nutr* 2003;12:234-42.

[17] Seiler WO. Clinical pictures of malnutrition in ill elderly subjects. *Nutrition* 2001;17:496-8.

[18] Pfeiffer AF, Einig Ch. Disease prevention by vitamins and trace elements. *Dtsch Med Wochenschr* 2002;127:2251-2.

[19] Saltzman JR, Russell RM. The aging gut. Nutritional issues. *Gastroenterol Clin North Am* 1998;27:309-24.

[20] Johnson MA, Fischer JG, Bowman BA, Gunter EW. Iron nutriture in elderly individuals. *FASEB J* 1994;8:609-21.

[21] Marx JJ. Iron deficiency in developed countries: prevalence, influence of lifestyle factors and hazards of prevention. *Eur J Clin Nutr* 1997;51:491-4.

[22] Chamberlain SA, Soybel DI. Occult and obscure sources of gastrointestinal bleeding. *Curr Probl Surg* 2000;37:861-916.

[23] Wiwanitkit V. Electrochemiluminescence immunoassay for ferritin analysis. *Buddhachinaraj Med J* 2000; 17: 151 – 7.

[24] Schultz BM, Freedman ML. Iron deficiency in the elderly. Baillieres Clin Haematol 1987;1:291-313

[25] Besa EC. Approach to mild anemia in the elderly. *Clin Geriatr Med* 1988;4:43-55.

[26] Smieja MJ, Cook DJ, Hunt DL, Ali MA, Guyatt GH. Recognizing and investigating iron-deficiency anemia in hospitalized elderly people. *CMAJ* 1996;155:691-6.

[27] Garry PJ, Goodwin JS, Hunt WC. Iron status and anemia in the elderly: new findings and a review of previous studies. *J Am Geriatr Soc* 1983;31: 389-99.

[28] Murphy PT, Hutchinson RM. Identification and treatment of anaemia in older patients. *Drugs Aging* 1994;4:113-27.

[29] Stich A, Zwicker M, Steffen T, Kohler B, Fleischer K. Old age as risk factor for complications of malaria in non-immune travellers. *Dtsch Med Wochenschr* 2003;128:309-14.

[30] Alward W, Javaid M, Garner J. Babesiosis in a Connecticut resident. *Conn Med* 1990;54:425-7.

[31] Elias D, Wolff K, Klassen P, Bulux J, Solomons NW. Intestinal helminths and their influence on the indicators of iron status in the elderly. *J Nutr Health Aging* 1997;1:167-73.

[32] Nilsson-Ehle H. Age-related changes in cobalamin (vitamin B12) handling. Implications for therapy. *Drugs Aging* 1998;12:277-92.

[33] Smith DL. Anemia in the elderly. *Am Fam Physician* 2000;62:1565-72.

[34] Obeid R, Geisel J, Schorr H, Hubner U, Herrmann W. The impact of vegetarianism on some haematological parameters. *Eur J Haematol* 2002;69:275-9.

[35] Wolters M, Strohle A, Hahn A. Age-associated changes in the metabolism of vitamin B(12) and folic acid: prevalence, aetiopathogenesis and pathophysiological consequences. *Z Gerontol Geriatr* 2004;37:109-35.

[36] Greenberg PL, Young NS, Gattermann N. Myelodysplastic syndromes. *Hematology* (Am Soc Hematol Educ Program) 2002;:136-61.

[37] Latvala J, Parkkila S, Niemela O. Excess alcohol consumption is common in patients with cytopenia: studies in blood and bone marrow cells. *Alcohol Clin Exp Res* 2004;28:619-24.

[38] Jenkins K, Van Waeleghem JP. Awareness of anaemia in diabetes patients. *EDTNA ERCA J* 2003;29:160-2.

[39] Heptinstall RH. Hypertension and vascular diseases of the kidney. *Monogr Pathol* 1979;20:281-94.

[40] Stenvinkel P. Anaemia and inflammation: what are the implications for the nephrologist? *Nephrol Dial Transplant* 2003;18 Suppl 8:viii17-22.

[41] Parfrey PS. Clinical epidemiology in chronic uremia. *Clin Invest Med* 1994;17:466-73.

[42] Artz AS, Fergusson D, Drinka PJ, Gerald M, Bidenbender R, Lechich A, Silverstone F, McCamish MA, Dai J, Keller E, Ershler WB. Mechanisms of Unexplained Anemia in the Nursing Home. *J Am Geriatr Soc* 2004;52:423-427.

[43] Hood SA, O'Brien M, Higgins R. The safety of intravenous iron dextran (Dexferrum) during hemodialysis in patients with end stage renal disease. *Nephrol Nurs J* 2000;27:41-2.

[44] Fukuda T, Baba Y, Tanaka M, Ishibashi H, Hirata Y, Okamura T, Kudo J, Niho Y, Yamanaka M. Severe alcoholic cirrhosis associated with spur cell anemia and DIC. *Fukuoka Igaku Zasshi* 1991 ;82:398-402.

[45] Morse EE. Mechanisms of hemolysis in liver disease. *Ann Clin Lab Sci* 1990;20:169-74.

[46] Silverberg D, Wexler D, Blum M, Wollman Y, Iaina A. The cardio-renal anaemia syndrome: does it exist? *Nephrol Dial Transplant* 2003;18 Suppl 8:viii7-12.

[47] Silverberg D, Wexler D, Blum M, Schwartz D, Iaina A. The association between congestive heart failure and chronic renal disease. *Curr Opin Nephrol Hypertens* 2004;13:163-70.

[48] Silverberg DS, Wexler D, Blum M, Wollman Y, Schwartz D, Sheps D, Keren G, Iaina A. The interaction between heart failure, renal failure and anemia - the cardio-renal anemia syndrome. *Blood Purif.* 2004;22:277-84.

[49] Prayurahong B, Tungtrongchitr R, Chanjanakijskul S, Lertchavanakul A, Supawan V, Pongpaew P, Vudhivai N, Hempfling AA, Schelp FP, Migasena P. Vitamin B12, folic acid and haematological status in elderly Thais. *J Med Assoc Thai* 1993;76:71-8.

[50] Parasuramalu BG, Vastrad SA, Shivaram C. Prevalence of anaemia in the aged population in selected slums of Hubli City. *Indian J Public Health* 1990;34:117-8.

[51] Allain TJ, Gomo Z, Wilson AO, Ndemera B, Adamchak DJ, Matenga JA. Anaemia, macrocytosis, vitamin B12 and folate levels in elderly Zimbabweans. *Cent Afr J Med* 1997 ;43:325-8.

[52] Sima Zue A, Chani M, Ngaka Nsafu D, Carpentier JP. Does tropical environment influence morbidity and mortality? *Med Trop* (Mars) 2002;62:256-9.

[53] Wiwanitkit V. Clinical findings among 62 Thais with cholangiocarcinoma. *Trop Med Int Health* 2003 ;8:228-30.

[54] Pinyosophon A, Wiwanitkit V. Co - morbidity between anaemia and cholangiocarcinoma; a retrospective summary. *Haema* 2003; 6: 415 – 6.

[55] Rea DJ, Munoz-Juarez M, Farnell MB, Donohue JH, Que FG, Crownhart B, Larson D, Nagorney DM. Major hepatic resection for hilar cholangiocarcinoma: analysis of 46 patients. *Arch Surg* 2004;139:514-23.

[56] Obermair A, Cheuk R, Horwood K, Neudorfer M, Janda M, Giannis G, Nicklin JL, Perrin LC, Crandon AJ. Anemia before and during concurrent chemoradiotherapy in patients with cervical carcinoma: Effect on progression-free survival. *Int J Gynecol Cancer*2003;13:633-9.

Chapter 19

Emerging and Reemerging Anemic Diseases in the Tropics

Introduction to Emerging and Reemerging Diseases

Presently, there are several emerging and reemerging diseases. Those diseases are usually the infectious diseases. Emerging infectious diseases pose a significant but underappreciated threat to public health [1]. Pollard said that in a world where international travellers, immigrants, and refugees could carry dangerous organisms almost anywhere, no region should be considered free from risk [1]. Pollard noted that outbreaks of disease might be caused by newly recognized pathogens and drug-resistant organisms and these outbreaks demonstrated the need for improved worldwide surveillance and for improved compliance with guidelines for the use of antimicrobial agents [1 - 2]. The emerging diseases can be either new emerging or reemerging infections. Moren *et al.* noted that there were the evolutionary properties of pathogenic microorganisms and the dynamic relationships between microorganisms, their hosts and the environment [3]. Basically, several underlying factors can lead to the emerging of the infectious diseases as shown in Table 19.1

Table 19.1. Some underlying causes of emerging infectious diseases

New emerging disease	Reemerging disease
1. Mutation of known non -pathogenic organism to the new pathogenic one	1. Travelling and transmission of previously controlled disease from the uncontrolled area to the disease-free area
2. New identified pathogen or vector travelling and transmission of pathogens or vectors from endemic to non-endemic area	2. Impairment of host immunity
3. Impairment of host immunity	

Concerning those emerging infectious diseases some are zoonosis or vector-borne and the others are human-to-human transmission diseases. New emerging or re-emerging zoonoses is a relatively complex topic [2]. The concept covers not only new or recently identified zoonotic agents but also agents that are already known but appear in regions and/or species in which they have not been previously observed and agents that disappear then reappear in a country in the form of an epidemic outbreak [2]. Many wild or domestic species and almost all infectious agents may be involved [2]. In general intervention either by vaccination or by elimination of suspect or contaminated individuals is easier in domestic animals than in wild animals especially since the latter may belong to an endangered species [2]. Meslin noted that because of the wide range of pathogenic agents, animal vectors and target populations, there were a wide variety of epidemiological patterns, and adapted surveillance and control strategies should be used with various degrees of success [2]. The emerging vector-borne disease shares a similar problem to the emerging zoonosis disease. The control of vectors is sometimes difficult. However, human-to-human transmission emerging disease is a more serious emerging infectious problem because of possible direct transmission of diseases from a patient to members of a healthy population. For example, human immunodeficiency virus infection, a well-known new emerging infectious disease in the 1980's has been widespread throughout the world since it was first discovered [4]. Morens et al. said that infectious diseases have for centuries ranked with wars and famine as major challenges to human progress and survival, and they remained among the leading causes of death and disability worldwide [3]. Moren et al. also mentioned that against a constant background of established infections, epidemics of new and old infectious diseases periodically emerged, greatly magnifying the global burden of infections [3].

However, not only the infectious diseases but also several non-infectious diseases become new emerging problems for the world. Accidents [5 - 6], drug abuse [7 - 8], psychiatric problems [8], intoxication [9 - 10], metabolic and degenerative diseases [11 - 13] are those problems. Of interest, the problems are rising in the tropical countries which are industrialized. These problems should also be of concern and need specific management at present.

Important Emerging and Reemerging Diseases and Tropical Anemia

Several new emerging and reemerging diseases can lead to anemia. Those infectious emerging diseases are the focus at present. In addition, anemic diseases can be an emerging problem as well. Many tropical anemias can be the new emerging diseases in non-tropical areas. Due to the good transportation system at present, anemic disease due to infection can be transmitted from the endemic to the non-endemic area. In addition, some inherited anemic disorders can also be transferred to the new areas due to worldwide migration. The concept of travelling medicine can be a good explanation for these phenomena [14]. Here, the details of new emerging and reemerging diseases and their correlation to anemia are presented with special focus on the tropical region.

A. Anemia and Infectious Emerging Diseases

1. Anemia in Emerging Virus Disease

Severe Acute Respiratory Syndrome and Anemia

Severe acute respiratory syndrome (SARS) is a new human infectious disease caused by coronavirus. The first world outbreak occured in 2002, starting in China and then moving through many countries including Hong Kong, Canada and Singapore [15 – 16]. The incubation period for this disease is commonly 3-5 days [15 – 16]. The disease usually begins with simple respiratory symptoms described as fever and cough for 2-3 days and atypical pneumonia develops on day 4-5 [15 – 16]. Similar to other viral infections, this disease has many effects on the hematology system. Yang et al. proposed that the possible mechanisms of SARS for this hematologic finding may include directly infecting blood cells and bone marrow stromal cells via CD13 or CD66a; and inducing auto-antibodies and immune complexes to damage these cells [17]. Lymphopenia among the SARS patients has been reported [18]. Wong et al. noted that the depletion of T lymphocyte subsets might be associated with disease activity [18]. Decreased platelet count, prolonged partial thromboplastin time and disseminated intravascular coagulation (DIC) can be seen as well [18]. Concerning anemia, Avendano et al. said that severe hemolytic anemia might be a feature of SARS or might be a complication of therapy, possibly with ribavirin [19].

Here, the author performs a further analysis to document the magnitude of the hemolytic anemia in the clinical course of SARS by way of a metanalysis study. The author performed a literature review on the previous descriptive study concerning the prevalence of anemia among SARS patients from various countries using PubMed (www.pubmed.com) as a search engine. The reports with complete data on the prevalence of anemia among SARS patients were selected. The prevalence rate reported from all detected reports were recorded and used as primary data for further analysis. Concerning metanalysis, the overall prevalence rate was calculated by pooled summary of the reported prevalence rate from each included report. Two available reports concerning the prevalence of anemia in SARS among different populations [20 - 21] were selected for further analysis in this study. The quoted prevalence rate pattern is shown in Table 19.2. Overall 399 SARS patients were retrospectively analyzed and 191 cases presented anemia. According to this study, the overall prevalence rate of anemia in SARS is 47.7 %. According to this analysis, we found that the anemia is a common hematological manifestation in the patients with SARS. However, Li et al. recently studied 18 cases of pediatric SARS in Beijing and did not find significant lower hemoglobin and platelet levels [22].

Table 19.2. Reports on the prevalence of anemia in SARS patients

Author	Subjects		Prevalence of anemia (%)
	Country	Number	
Sung *et al*, 2004 [20]	Hong Kong	132	37.1
Choi *et al*, 2003 [21]	Hong Kong	267	53.0

Concerning hemolytic anemia as the adverse effect of SARS therapy, Booth et al. recently reported their experience in a total of 126 patients treated with ribavirin, and found hemolysis in 76% and a decrease in hemoglobin of 2 g/dL in 49 % of the patients [23]. Knowles *et al.* also reported a similar finding in their SARS patients treated with ribavirin that 61 % of the patients had evidence of hemolytic anemia [24].

West Nile Virus Infection and Anemia

West Nile virus infection has quickly become a feared cause of neurologic disability and death, particularly when it presents with encephalitis [25]. It is a mosquito-related disease. Recent epidemics in endemic regions of Eurasia and Africa, as well as its recent spread to North America, have highlighted the need for all physicians to be aware of its clinical presentation and course [25]. Bledsoe noted that since its identification in New York City in 1999, the West Nile virus has spread to 45 states and caused human infections in at least 44 states [26]. West Nile virus is difficult to correctly diagnose without a high level of clinical suspicion and can cause severe debilitation or death in those with the most severe symptoms [26]. Brandt *et al.* said that because of the increased susceptibility of West Nile virus infection during outdoor activities, as well as during travel to the Middle East and Southeastern Europe, military physicians should be informed about case recognition, management, and prevention to maintain the health of soldiers and their families [25].

Huhn *et al.* noted that West Nile virus infection has no characteristic findings on routine laboratory tests, although anemia, leukocytosis, or lymphopenia might be present [27]. They noted that testing for IgM antibody to West Nile virus in serum or cerebrospinal fluid was the most common diagnostic method [27]. Concerning treatment, there is nothing specific but supportive services are available [27]. Although Ribavirin is mentioned for the possible usefulness in treatment of the infection, it is not confirmed and the hemolytic anemia due to the use of this drug is an unforgettably important adverse effect [28].

Avian Flu and Anemia

Although viruses of relatively few HA and NA subtype combinations have been isolated from mammalian species, all 15 HA subtypes and all 9 NA subtypes, in most combinations, have been isolated from birds [29]. In the 20th century the sudden emergence of antigenically different strains transmissible in humans, termed antigenic shift, has occurred on four occasions, 1918 (H1N1), 1957 (H2N2), 1968 (H3N2) and 1977 (H1N1), each time resulting in a pandemic [29]. Avian flu or bird flu has become an important public health problem in many countries, especially those in Asia, at present. It attacked millions of farmed chickens all over the world and there are some reports of human infections. Webster noted that the recent H5N1 bird flu incident in Hong Kong served to remind general practitioners that influenza is an emerging disease [30]. Capua and Alexander said that it might well be that infection of humans with avian influenza viruses occurs much more frequently than originally assumed, but due to their limited effect go unrecognized [29]. They said that for the human population as a whole the main danger of direct infection with avian influenza viruses appears to be if people infected with an 'avian' virus are infected simultaneously with a 'human' influenza virus [29]. However, the anemia relating the avian flu is not well documented and may not be an important problem.

Nipah Virus and Anemia

In 1998, an outbreak of acute encephalitis with high mortality rates among pig handlers in Malaysia, a tropical country in Southeast Asia, led to the discovery of a novel paramyxovirus named Nipah virus [31 – 32]. The outbreak caused widespread panic and fear because of its high mortality and the inability to control the disease initially [32]. There were considerable social disruptions and tremendous economic loss to an important pig-rearing industry [32]. Lam said that this highly virulent virus, believed to be introduced into pig farms by fruit bats, spread easily among pigs, and it was transmitted to humans who came into close contact with infected animals [32]. Lam also noted that from pigs, the virus was also transmitted to other animals such as dogs, cats, and horses [32]. Recently Wong *et al.* studied clinical and autopsy findings derived from a series of 32 fatal human cases of Nipah virus infection and found that the main histopathological findings included a systemic vasculitis with extensive thrombosis and parenchymal necrosis, particularly in the central nervous system [31]. According to their study, endothelial cell damage, necrosis, and syncytial giant cell formation were seen in affected vessels, and characteristic viral inclusions were seen by light and electron microscopy [31]. Abundant viral antigens were also seen in various parenchymal cells, particularly in neurons [31]. They concluded that infection of endothelial cells and neurons as well as vasculitis and thrombosis seemed to be critical to the pathogenesis of this new human disease [31]. However, the anemia is not well documented in this new emerging disease.

Ebola Virus and Anemia

Ebola hemorrhagic fever (EHF) is an acute viral syndrome that presents with fever and an ensuing bleeding diathesis that is marked by high mortality in human and nonhuman primates [33 - 34]. Due to its lethal nature, fatality rates are between 50% and 100%, this filovirus is classified as a biological class 4 pathogen [33 - 34]. Incubation ranges from 2 to 21 days [33 - 34]. Patients who are able to mount an immune response to the virus will begin to recover in 7 to 10 days and start a period of prolonged convalescence [33 - 34]. The disease directly affects the immune system and vascular bed, with correspondingly high mortality rates [35]. The patients with severe disease produce dangerously high levels of inflammatory cytokines, which destroy normal tissue and microcirculation, leading to profound capillary leakage, renal failure, and disseminated intravascular coagulation [35]. Concerning the pathogenesis, Fisher-Hoch *et al.* performed an animal experiment in a monkey model and found that marked neutrophilia, depletion of lymphocytes, and early failure of platelet aggregation preceded a consumption coagulopathy with a microangiopathic haemolytic anaemia, thrombocytopenia, and failure of prostacyclin production by vascular endothelium could be seen in Ebola infected monkeys [36]. Supportive management of infected patients is the primary method of treatment, with particular attention to maintenance of hydration, circulatory volume, blood pressure, and the provision of supplemental oxygen [33].

Hepatitis TT Virus and Anemia

Hepatitis TT virus infection is a new emerging infectious disease. TT virus (TTV) was first described in 1997 by representational difference analysis of sera from a non-A to non-G post-transfusion hepatitis Japanese patient and hence intensively investigated as a possible addition to the list of hepatitis-inducing viruses [37]. Some reports also mentioned the high prevalence of TTV infection among the thalassemic patients, who were transfusion dependant [38 – 39]. The TTV genome is a covalently closed single-stranded DNA of approximately 3.8 kb with a number of characteristics typical of animal circoviruses, especially the chicken anemia virus [37]. TTV is genetically highly heterogeneous, which has led investigators to group isolates into numerous genotypes and subtypes and has limited the sensitivity of many PCR assays used for virus detection [37]. The most remarkable feature of TTV is the extraordinarily high prevalence of chronic viremia in apparently healthy people, up to nearly 100% in some countries [37]. Although aplastic anemia has been reported to occur after viral hepatitis of unknown etiology, Udomsakdi-Auewarakul argued against the role of this novel hepatitis-associated virus in the pathogenesis of aplastic anemia in Thailand [40].

2. Anemia in Emerging Rickettsial Disease

Erhlichiosis and Anemia

Ehrlichiosis is a term that has been used to describe infection with any of a number of related intracellular, vector-borne pathogens [41 - 43]. This infection is a rickettsial disease of animals and humans caused by various species of Ehrlichia [41 – 43]. A recent reclassification has resulted in the transfer of several species previously known as Ehrlichia to the genus Anaplasma or Neorickettsia [41 – 43]. Ehrlichia and Anaplasma are transmitted largely through the bite of infected ticks, while vectors for Neorickettsia include trematodes and the intermediate hosts (including fish, snails, and insects) involved in the trematode life cycle [41 – 43]. Dogs and cats are susceptible to infection with several of these pathogens, and veterinarians should be aware of the similarities and differences between *E canis* and related infections [41 – 43]. For animals in endemic areas, prevention of exposure to vectors can lessen the risk of disease for pets and might lessen the potential for animals to become carriers of disease to their human companions [41 – 43]. Diagnosis requires careful consideration of all circumstances and symptoms (history of tick bite and the presence of a flu-like syndrome with variable degrees of anemia, thrombocytopenia, and leukopenia, and elevated liver enzymes) [44]. Schutze and Jacobs studied the clinical presentation of 8 patients with human ehrlichiosis [45]. According to this study, the patients demonstrated thrombocytopenia (92%), elevated liver function tests (91%), lymphopenia (75%), hyponatremia (67%), leukopenia (58%), and anemia (42%) on the initial laboratory examination [45]. Weinstein also noted that the most common initial clinical findings of ehrlichiosis included fever, malaise, myalgia, headaches and rigors, while the most common laboratory findings were thrombocytopenia, leukopenia, anemia and elevated liver enzyme levels [46]. Doxycycline is the recommended drug of choice for ehrlichiosis.

3. Anemia in Emerging Bacterial Diseases

Mycobacterium Avium Complex (MAC) and Anemia

Tuberculosis (TB) and Mycobacterium avium complex (MAC) are the most important of the mycobacterioses in HIV-infected patients [47 - 48]. It is estimated that in 1999, HIV-related TB reached 1,000,000 cases and caused 30% of the 2,500,000 AIDS-related deaths [47]. Hanna said that MAC organisms caused disseminated disease in the patients with AIDS [48]. Severely immunocompromised patients with CD4-counts < 50/microliter are at greatest risk for the disease [49]. Pathophysiologically, the organisms penetrate the gastrointestinal mucosa by unknown mechanisms and are phagocytosed by macrophages in the lamina propria [48]. These cells cannot kill the organisms, and MAC spreads through the submucosal tissue [48]. Lymphatic drainage transports mycobacteria to abdominal lymph nodes, from which the organisms enter the bloodstream [48]. Hematogenous spread can occur to many sites, but spleen, bone marrow, and liver are the most common [48]. The leading symptom of MAC infection is fever eventually accompanied by weight lost, night sweats, enlarged lymph nodes, hepatosplenomegaly, abdominal pain and anemia [49]. Blood cultures are very sensitive and the most appropriate examination [49]. Concerning anemia in the AIDS patients with MAC infection, Flegg et al. studied the clinical features of AIDS patients with MAC infections compared with case-matched controls (AIDS cases without disseminated MAC)[50]. They found that weight loss, anemia, leucopenia, and elevated liver transaminases and alkaline phosphatase were significantly more common among cases than controls [50].

Phongsamart et al. studied 10 HIV-infected patients with MAC and found that common clinical findings included prolonged fever, weight loss, lymphadenopathy, hepatosplenomegaly, diarrhea, anemia and leukopenia [51]. Gordin et al. also mentioned that characteristics of MAC disease that occurred before bacteremia were weight loss, fever, and anemia and elevated lactate dehydrogenase [52].

Rhodococcosis and Anemia

Rhodococcosis, caused by *Rhodococcus equi*, is a new emerging disease [53]. More than 100 cases of this infection have been reported since the first description of human disease caused by this organism [54]. The vast majority of patients infected with *R. equi* are immunocompromised, and two-thirds have human immunodeficiency virus infection [54]. The clinical manifestations of rhodococcosis are diverse, although 80% of patients have some pulmonary involvement [53 – 54]. Concerning anemia, Knottenbelt studied the rhodococcosis in the foals and found that anemia was not a major finding in any case [55]. The organism is easily cultured from specimens of infected tissue or body fluid, but it may be misdiagnosed as a contaminant [53 – 54]. Treatment is often prolonged, and relapses at distant sites are common [54].

4. Anemia in Emerging Parasitic Diseases

Malaria and Anemia

Due to the changing pattern of malaria epidemiology, the malarial anemia can be the new emerging tropical anemic disorder in many non - tropical countries. Malaria in the Americas is a reemerging health issue [56]. In 1969, the World Health Organization shifted policy from malaria eradication to malaria control [56]. With this shift, vector control (house spraying with dichlorodiphenyltrichloroethane [DDT]) was deemphasized [56]. Since that time, house spray rates have decreased and malaria rates have increased [56]. The new emergence of the drug-resistant malaria is another good example of the changing pattern of infectious disease at present. Since the first reports of chloroquine-resistant falciparum malaria in southeast Asia and South America almost half a century ago, drug-resistant malaria has posed a major problem in malaria control [57]. By the late 1980s, resistance to sulfadoxine-pyrimethamine and to mefloquine was also prevalent on the Thai-Cambodian and Thai-Myanmar (Thai-Burmese) borders, rendering them established multidrug-resistant (MDR) areas [57]. Chloroquine resistance spread across Africa during the 1980s, and severe resistance is especially found in east Africa [57].

5. Anemia and Prion Diseases

Creutzfeldt-Jakob Disease and Anemia

The protein-only theory of transmission of the prion diseases remains controversial and other mechanisms such as the virus, virino, and viroid hypotheses are still under consideration [58]. All these fit in the concept of 'slow' infections that had been proposed in 1954 by Bjorn Sigurdsson, an Icelandic pathologist [58]. Regardless of the exact mode of infection, the presence of prions in the brain has served to unite Creutzfeldt-Jakob disease (CJD) as well as scrapie and a number of other animal diseases, into a single pathological entity, the transmissible spongiform encephalopathies [58]. Will said that the actual cause of sporadic Creutzfeldt-Jakob disease (CJD) was unknown, hereditary cases were associated with mutations of the prion protein gene and acquired forms were caused by the transmission of infection from human to human or, as a zoonosis, from cattle to human [59]. Although acquired forms of human prion disease are rare, the transmission of a fatal and untreatable neurological disorder has had major implications for public health and public policy [59]. Spongioform encephalopathy is the hallmark pathology in the patients with CJD [60]. Concerning the anemia in CJD, there is no exact evidence that CJD can lead to anemia. Brusis reported on a 47-year-old male patient who developed persistent postoperational bleeding after tonsillectomy, which made tamponading of the pharynx necessary [61]. In this case, even though the patient left the hospital after one week with a haemoglobin value of 10.6 g% and without any complaints, he developed personality changes and later severe neurological symptoms which led to the diagnosis of hypoxic brain damage as suggested by a variety of neurologists and psychiatrists [61]. Brusis concluded that the accidental coincidence of the tonsillectomy and the beginning of the Jakob-Creutzfeldt disease had led to the incorrect diagnosis of an operation-caused brain damage [61].

Of interest, many emerging infectious diseases are common in the tropics and these diseases can sometimes lead to anemia. To cope with the tropical anemia in the present era, the awareness of these emerging infectious diseases is necessary. In addition, the bioterrorism, the new problem in the present day, becomes another issue of concern [62 – 63]. One of the common agents mentioned for bioterrorism is the *Bacillus anthrasis*, the corresponding organism for anthrax [62 – 63]. Of interest, anthrax is an organism, which can lead to anemia and can be the emerging cause of anemia due to the biological weapon [64].

B. Anemia and Non-Infectious Emerging Problems

Anemia and Accident

Traffic accident increases are prevalent in developing countries with rapid urbanization. Anemia due to an accident is mainly due to the acute hemorrhagic episode according to bleeding. In addition, the trauma itself can be the cause of hemolysis [65].

Anemia and Intoxication

Several toxic substances can lead to anemia. Due to the industrialization in many developing countries, the intoxication can be more frequently seen than in the past. The anemia can be the result of the intoxication, as the occupational health aspect. The details of anemia due to intoxication are already presented in the previous issue.

Anemia and Metabolic and Degenerative Diseases

The metabolic and degenerative diseases become the new emerging problems in the tropics. Some of those important diseases include diabetes mellitus (DM), dyslipidemia and hyperuricemia. Of these diseases, there are several evidences for the correlation between the anemia and DM. Concerning DM, Jenkins *et al.* said that the link between DM and anemia has been firmly established in the renal world [66]. The renal anemia as the complication of anemia, diabetic nephropathy is the current interesting topic [66]. Stevens *et al.* said that anemia had a significant impact on the quality of life of patients with DM [67]. They noted that although patients were aware of anemia, their awareness of being tested for anemia was low and a significant number of those in whom anemia was detected received no treatment [67]. They proposed that it was likely that anemia in the patients with DM was unrecognised, undetected and untreated [67]. Sidibe said that DM constituted a major financial burden in developing countries in Africa with relatively limited resources and that hyperleukocytosis and anemia were correlated with ineffective antibiotic therapy [68].

More details concerning anemia and DM can be seen in the previous chapter.

New Emerging Inherited Tropical Anemic Diseases

As previously mentioned, the changing of some inherited tropical anemic disorders can be seen. Weatherall said that over the next decade it would be essential to make the thalassemia problem more visible to governments and international health agencies that were involved in health care in the emerging countries [69]. In recent years, population shifts and rapid transportation have facilitated the spread of certain infectious and some inherited diseases from endemic to non-endemic areas [70]. Recently, Fujimoto *et al,* studied 423 subjects who immigrated from Southeast Asia, Africa, Central and South America, and other developing countries in tropical or subtropical areas to Japan and found that thalassemia-like hematological disorders were seen in 7.6 percent of the students, and intestinal parasites were revealed in 12.7 percent of them [70]. Fujimoto *et al.* concluded that international preventive strategies, education of people regarding new emerging diseases, and sufficient medical staffs for this purpose were urgently recommended [70].

References

[1] Pollard C. The emerging infectious diseases. *Physician Ass*ist 1995;19:73, 77-8, 80-1.

[2] Meslin FX. Emerging and re-emerging zoonoses. Local and worldwide threats. *Med Trop* (Mars) 1997;57(3 Suppl):7-9.

[3] Morens DM, Folkers GK, Fauci AS. The challenge of emerging and re-emerging infectious diseases. *Nature* 2004;430:242-9.

[4] Goldrick BA. 21st-century emerging and reemerging infections. *Am J Nurs* 2004;104:67-70.

[5] Accidents--an emerging health problem in India. *Indian J Public Health* 1967;11:177-9.

[6] Hyder AA, Ghaffar A, Masood TI. Motor vehicle crashes in Pakistan: the emerging epidemic. *Inj Prev* 2000;6:199-202.

[7] Weiss SR, Kung HC, Pearson JL. Emerging issues in gender and ethnic differences in substance abuse and treatment. *Curr Womens Health Rep* 2003;3:245-53.

[8] Smith J, Hucker S. Schizophrenia and substance abuse. *Br J Psychiatry* 1994;165:13-21.

[9] Bielecki J. Emerging food pathogens and bacterial toxins. *Acta Microbiol Pol* 2003;52 Suppl:17-22.

[10] Smital T, Luckenbach T, Sauerborn R, Hamdoun AM, Vega RL, Epel D. Emerging contaminants-pesticides, PPCPs, microbial degradation products and natural substances as inhibitors of multixenobiotic defense in aquatic organisms. *Mutat Res* 2004;552:101-17.

[11] Steinbaum SR. The metabolic syndrome: an emerging health epidemic in women. *Prog Cardiovasc Dis* 2004;46:321-36.

[12] Abbate R, Sofi F, Brogi D, Marcucci R. Emerging risk factors for ischemic stroke. *Neurol Sci* 2003;24 Suppl 1:S11-2.

[13] Smith SR, Ravussin E. Emerging paradigms for understanding fatness and diabetes risk. *Curr Diab Rep* 2002;2:223-30.

[14] Wiwanitkit V. Amazing Thailand Year 1998-1999 Tourist's health concepts. *Chula Med J* 1998; 42: 975 – 84.

[15] Hoheisel G, Wu A, Lee N, Wong KT, Ahuja A, Joynt GM, Chung SC, Sung JJ, Hui DS. Severe acute respiratory syndrome (SARS). *Pneumologie* 2003; 57:315-21.

[16] Wong KF, To TS, Chan JK. Severe acute respiratory syndrome (SARS). *Br J Haematol* 2003; 122: 171.

[17] Yang M, Hon KL, Li K, Fok TF, Li CK. The effect of SARS coronavirus on blood system: its clinical findings and the pathophysiologic hypothesis. *Zhongguo Shi Yan Xue Ye Xue Za Zhi* 2003; 11:217-21.

[18] Wong RS, Wu A, To KF, Lee N, Lam CW, Wong CK, Chan PK, Ng MH, Yu LM, Hui DS, Tam JS, Cheng G, Sung JJ. Haematological manifestations in patients with severe acute respiratory syndrome: retrospective analysis. *BMJ* ,326:1358-62, 2003.

[19] Avendano M, Derkach P, Swan S. Clinical course and management of SARS in health care workers in Toronto: a case series. *CMAJ* 2003;168:1649-60.

[20] Sung JJ, Wu A, Joynt GM, Yuen KY, Lee N, Chan PK, Cockram CS, Ahuja AT, Yu LM, Wong VW, Hui DS. Severe acute respiratory syndrome: report of treatment and outcome after a major outbreak. *Thorax* 2004;59:414-20.

[21] Choi KW, Chau TN, Tsang O, Tso E, Chiu MC, Tong WL, Lee PO, Ng TK, Ng WF, Lee KC, Lam W, Yu WC, Lai JY, Lai ST; Princess Margaret Hospital SARS Study Group. Outcomes and prognostic factors in 267 patients with severe acute respiratory syndrome in Hong Kong. *Ann Intern Med* 2003;139:715-23.

[22] Li ZZ, Shen KL, Wei XM, Wang HL, Lu J, Tian H, Sun GQ, Zeng JJ, Hu YH, Zhao SY, Yin J, Feng XL, Jiang ZF, Yang YH. Clinical analysis of pediatric SARS cases in Beijing. *Zhonghua Er Ke Za Zhi* 2003;41:574-7.

[23] Booth CM, Matukas LM, Tomlinson GA, Rachlis AR, Rose DB, Dwosh HA, Walmsley SL, Mazzulli T, Avendano M, Derkach P, Ephtimios IE, Kitai I, Mederski BD, Shadowitz SB, Gold WL, Hawryluck LA, Rea E, Chenkin JS, Cescon DW, Poutanen SM, Detsky AS. Clinical features and short-term outcomes of 144 patients with SARS in the greater Toronto area. *JAMA* 2003;289:2801-9.

[24] Knowles SR, Phillips EJ, Dresser L, Matukas L. Common adverse events associated with the use of ribavirin for severe acute respiratory syndrome in Canada. *Clin Infect Dis* 2003;37:1139-42.

[25] Brandt AL, Martyak N, Westhoff J, Kang C. West Nile virus. *Mil Med* 2004;169:261-4.

[26] Bled*soe GH. The West Nile virus: a lesson in emerging infections.* Wilderness Environ Med 2004;15:113-8.

[27] Huhn GD, Sejvar JJ, Montgomery SP, Dworkin MS. West Nile virus in the United States: an update on an emerging infectious disease. *Am Fam Physician* 2003;68:653-60.

[28] Snell NJ. Ribavirin--current status of a broad spectrum antiviral agent. *Expert Opin Pharmacother* 2001;2:1317-24.

[29] Capua I, Alexander DJ. Avian influenza and human health. *Acta Trop* 2002;83:1-6.

[30] Webster RG. The importance of animal influenza for human disease. *Vaccine* 2002;20 Suppl 2:S16-20.

[31] Wong KT, Shieh WJ, Kumar S, Norain K, Abdullah W, Guarner J, Goldsmith CS, Chua KB, Lam SK, Tan CT, Goh KJ, Chong HT, Jusoh R, Rollin PE, Ksiazek TG, Zaki SR; Nipah Virus Pathology Working Group. Nipah virus infection: pathology and pathogenesis of an emerging paramyxoviral zoonosis. *Am J Pathol* 2002;161:2153-67.

[32] Lam SK. Nipah virus--a potential agent of bioterrorism? *Antiviral Res* 2003;57:113-9.

[33] Casillas AM, Nyamathi AM, Sosa A, Wilder CL, Sands H. A current review of Ebola virus: pathogenesis, clinical presentation, and diagnostic assessment. *Biol Res Nurs* 2003;4:268-75.

[34] Titenko AM. Filovirus haemorrhagic fevers: Ebola fever. *Zh Mikrobiol Epidemiol Immunobiol* 2002;(5):116-22.

[35] Nyamathi AM, Fahey JL, Sands H, Casillas AM. Ebola virus: immune mechanisms of protection and vaccine development. *Biol Res Nurs* 2003;4:276-81.

[36] Fisher-Hoch SP, Platt GS, Lloyd G, Simpson DI, Neild GH, Barrett AJ. Haematological and biochemical monitoring of Ebola infection in rhesus monkeys: implications for patient management. *Lancet* 1983;2:1055-8.

[37] Bendinelli M, Pistello M, Maggi F, Fornai C, Freer G, Vatteroni ML. Molecular properties, biology, and clinical implications of TT virus, a recently identified widespread infectious agent of humans. *Clin Microbiol Rev* 2001;14:98-113.

[38] Sampietro M, Tavazzi D, Martinez di Montemuros F, Cerino M, Zatelli S, Lunghi G, Orlandi A, Fargion S, Fiorelli G, Cappellini MD. TT virus infection in adult beta-thalassemia major patients. *Haematologica* 2001;86:39-43.

[39] Kondili LA, Pisani G, Beneduce F, Morace G, Gentili G, Ballati G, Rapicetta M. Prevalence of TT virus in healthy children and thalassemic pediatric and young adult patients. *J Pediatr Gastroenterol Nutr* 2001;33:629-32.

[40] Udomsakdi-Auewarakul C, Auewarakul P, Permpikul P, Issaragrisil S. TT virus infection in Thailand: prevalence in blood donors and patients with aplastic anemia. *Int J Hematol* 2000;72:325-8.

[41] Cohn LA. Ehrlichiosis and related infections. *Vet Clin North Am Small Anim Pract* 2003;33:863-84.

[42] Pusterla N, Braun U, Leutenegger CM, Reusch C, Lutz H. Ehrlichiosis in Switzerland--significance for veterinary medicine. *Schweiz Arch Tierheilkd* 2000;142:367-73.

[43] Ungwatcharaprakarn V, Yamsuwan T, Wiwanitkit V, Soogarun S. Ehrlichiosis, literature review in human infection. *Songklanagarind Medical Journal* 2003; 21:301-305

[44] Blanco JR, Oteo JA. Human granulocytic ehrlichiosis in Europe. *Clin Microbiol Infect* 2002;8:763-72.

[45] Schutze GE, Jacobs RF. Human monocytic ehrlichiosis in children. *Pediatrics* 1997;100:E10

[46] Weinstein RS. Human ehrlichiosis. *Am Fam Physician* 1996;54:1971-6.

[47] Pozniak A. Mycobacterial diseases and HIV. *J HIV Th*er 2002;7:13-6.

[48] Hanna L. Mycobacterium avium complex disease. *BETA* 1995;:17-24.

[49] Fatkenheuer G, Salzberger B, Diehl V. Disseminated infection with Mycobacterium avium complex (MAC) in *HIV infection. Med Klin* (Munich) 1998;93:360-4.

[50] Flegg PJ, Laing RB, Lee C, Harris G, Watt B, Leen CL, Brettle RP. Disseminated disease due to Mycobacterium avium complex in AIDS. *QJM* 1995;88:617-26.

[51] Phongsamart W, Chokephaibulkit K, Chaiprasert A, Vanprapa N, Chearskul S, Lolekha R. Mycobacterium avium complex in HIV-infected Thai children. *J Med Assoc Thai* 2002;85 Suppl 2:S682-9.

[52] Gordin FM, Cohn DL, Sullam PM, Schoenfelder JR, Wynne BA, Horsburgh CR Jr. Early manifestations of disseminated Mycobacterium avium complex disease: a prospective evaluation. *J Infect Dis* 1997;176:126-32.

[53] Weinstock DM, Brown AE. Rhodococcus equi: an emerging pathogen. *Clin Infect Dis* 2002;34:1379-85.

[54] Boonchalermvichian C, Wiwanitkit V. Rhodococcus equi : the easily overlooked opportunistic organism in the AIDS era. *Chula Med J* 2000; 44: 137-150.

[55] Knottenbelt DC. Rhodococcus equi infection in foals: a report of an outbreak on a thoroughbred stud in Zimbabwe. *Vet Rec* 1993;132:79-85.

[56] Butler WP, Roberts DR. Malaria in the Americas: a model of reemergence. *Mil Med* 2000;165:897-902.

[57] Wongsrichanalai C, Pickard AL, Wernsdorfer WH, Meshnick SR. Epidemiology of drug-resistant malaria. *Lancet Infect Dis* 2002;2:209-18.

[58] Poser CM. Notes on the history of the prion diseases. Part II. *Clin Neurol Neurosurg* 2002;104:77-86.

[59] Will RG. Acquired prion disease: iatrogenic CJD, variant CJD, kuru. *Br Med Bull* 2003;66:255-65.

[60] Chesebro B. Introduction to the transmissible spongiform encephalopathies or prion diseases. *Br Med Bull* 2003;66:1-20.

[61] Brusis T. Brain damage after tonsillectomy? *Laryngorhinootologie* 1994;73:231-3.

[62] Peralta LA. Bioterrorism: an overview. *Semin Perioper Nurs* 2001;10:167-74.

[63] World MJ. Bioterrorism: the need to be prepared. *Clin Med* 2004;4:161-4.

[64] Freedman A, Afonja O, Chang MW, Mostashari F, Blaser M, Perez-Perez G, Lazarus H, Schacht R, Guttenberg J, Traister M, Borkowsky W. Cutaneous anthrax associated with microangiopathic hemolytic anemia and coagulopathy in a 7-month-old infant. *JAMA* 2002;287:869-74.

[65] Buzio M, Pigella S, Memore L, Olivero G. Hemolysis and multiple trauma. A clinical case report. *Minerva Chir* 1997;52:485-7.

[66] Jenkins K, Van Waeleghem JP. Awareness of anaemia in diabetes patients. *EDTNA ERCA J* 2003;29:160-2.

[67] Stevens PE, O'Donoghue DJ, Lameire NR. Anaemia in patients with diabetes: unrecognised, undetected and untreated? *Curr Med Res Opin* 2003;19:395-401.

[68] Sidibe EH. Main complications of diabetes mellitus in Africa. *Ann Med Interne* (Paris) 2000;151:624-8.

[69] Weatherall DJ. Thalassemia in the next millennium. Keynote address. Ann N Y Acad Sci 1998;850:1-9

[70] Fujimoto K, Momosaka Y, Uchida K, Ide H, Narisada H, Fujishiro K, Oda S, Okubo T. Implication of health checkups of students from developing countries in Japan. *Nippon Koshu Eisei Zasshi* 1999;46:476-86.

Chapter 20

Quality System of Hematology Laboratory in the Tropical Countries

Introduction to Laboratory Quality System

In laboratory medicine, the two main general aims are good service and good quality. In the previous day, good quality focused on good quality control and assessment in the analytical process. However, reliability cannot be achieved in a clinical laboratory through the control of accuracy in the analytical phase of the testing process alone [1]. Due to the good governance concepts, accountability of the whole laboratory process is the main focus of current concern in laboratory medicine [1]. Freedman said that clinical governance has, for the first time, placed the quality of healthcare as a direct responsibility of the Chief Executive and therefore the board of all hospitals, community providers and primary care or general practitioners [2].

Freedman also said that good governance should include clinical effectiveness and optimization of clinical care, clinical risk management, learning from complaints, professional development, good quality clinical data systems and involvement of patients and caregivers [2]. Hernandez said that the demand for proving the value of newer and more expensive medical technologies, including newer medical tests, would increase substantially [3]. Payers, including Medicare, commercial insurers, and employers, would demand accountability and elimination of the abuse and misuse of ineffective testing strategies [3]. Pathologists and laboratorians played a key role in guiding the most cost-effective use of testing strategies, including the judicious use of algorithms [3].

Basically, there should be a certification on the whole laboratory, but not on a single analytical process [1]. Precision and accuracy of analyses are not only determined by the analytical procedure but also by pre-analytical factors as well as post-analytical factors. In addition, at present, in case of a medical laboratory "good medical laboratory services" is preferred worldwide. Presently, external reviews and the accreditation of medical laboratories involve more than the mere assessment of conformance with standards for organizational process [4]. Dybkaer said that demonstrable quality of laboratory services entailed two parts [5]. First, one needs a quality policy statement, identification of user needs, choice of measurement procedures, reference measurement system to provide traceability, control materials, and proficiency testing with materials having reference-measurement-assigned values [5]. Second, it may be useful to obtain a recognition of competence in addition to the director's certificate, such as Good Laboratory Practice, ISO certification of a self-defined quality system, nongovernmental professional accreditation, or, most demanding, governmental accreditation [5]. The new approaches to quality improvement suggest that, rather than using inspection to correct unusual errors, there should be more emphasis on prevention or risk forecasting. Total quality management (TQM) of laboratory services is a concept widely used at present. Since, TQM concentrates not only on analytic performance and organizational issues, including specimen collection, reporting, and interpretation of results, but focuses also on the benefits to society related to the use of specific laboratory tests in prevention, early detection, and therapy monitoring, as well as on outcome measures, the good service and quality of the laboratory can be expected [4]. Many quality systems based on TQM have been adapted for usage in the medical laboratory.

General Aspects of Quality System for the Hematology Laboratory

1. General Principles for Hematology Laboratory Quality Management

Similar to other medical laboratories, the coagulation laboratory needs the TQM. A prerequisite to TQM are international and national standardization programs for the establishment of optimized and standardized methods, as well as for the development and evaluation of suitable reference materials [6]. In addition, Tatsumi *et al.* noted that high variation could be seen among reagents for hematological tests [7]. They noted that some quality improvement would be required [7]. Presently, it is accepted that all medical laboratories should put an emphasis on TQM and competence requirements for at least one quality system, which should agree with the policies of government agencies and national professional organizations. Those processes aim for the final global accreditation of medical laboratories. Last but not least, the good benefit for the patients can be derived [1]. A quality management protocol for hematology, as for other sections of the laboratory, should encompass both internal quality control and external quality assurance programs [8]. The extent to which a hematology laboratory should be involved depends upon various factors, including availability of facilities, financial resources, range of tests, workload, the number of staff and their levels of training, and the overall organization of the laboratory [8].

Gulati and Hyun said that the intralaboratory quality management program should include at least the minimal measures of monitoring and control at each step from collection of blood specimens, through the actual processing and analysis, to reporting of the results in order to ensure quality patient care [8]. Gulati and Hyun also noted that the quality management protocol should be written concisely and in simple language; the procedure manual should offer all of the pertinent information along with references; all concerned personnel should be well trained and competent; and adequate facilities and time should be available for the purpose of quality management [8]. They also noted that continuous education was an integral part of an effective quality management program [8].

Basically, two components, technical process and service process should be focuses. Concerning the technical process, the quality management should cover all phases in the laboratory cycle: pre-analytical process, analytical process and post-analytical process (Table 20.1).

In addition to the technical process, the quality management should also cover the service process. The first consideration is about the administration level of the laboratory. The proper resource management should cover all 4'M: man, material, money and management. The other aspects of service processes that usually get non-conformation to the standard are usually related to the statistical collection of the laboratory. The laboratory usually lacks for supportive evidences for corrective and preventive actions. Concerning the corrective actions, the surveillance system is necessary. Monitoring for some important key performance index including satisfaction, complaint, incident report, non-conforming specimen, non-conforming laboratory result, instrument error, labor workload and turnaround time is recommended.

Table 20.1. Brief details of quality management in the technical process of hematology laboratory

Phase	Brief details
1. Pre-analytical process	The pre-analytical phase error in hematology study shows higher incidence than the other following phases [1, 9]. The analytical process and the global laboratory quality are heavily influenced by the preanalytical phase, including biological material collection, identification, storage and transport of the specimen, preparation for analyses of the specimen through centrifugation, freezing and thawing, aliquoting and sampling [10]. Physiologic variables, such as lifestyle, age, and sex, and conditions such as pregnancy and menstruation, are some of the pre-analytic phase factors [11]. Good quality management for this phase is necessary. Wiwanitkit noted that the improper quality of specimen was the main problem in the quality system of the hematological study [1, 9]. Therefore, the control of specimen is recommended. Indeed, the laboratory should itself perform the specimen collection. The specimen collection for hematological study must be gently performed and well controlled. The risk management, especially for the universal precautions and patients first aid, must be prepared [12]. All personnel who practice as phlebotomists must be certified [12]. In case that the specimens are not collected and controlled by the laboratory, the specific protocol should be distributed. Indeed, although the specimens are collected by the laboratory, that protocol must be developed. The protocol should identify the details of the test, the collection technique, patient preparation technique, transportation, technique, precaution, turnaround time, reference, price and other necessary contact details. When the specimen reaches the laboratory, before analysis, another important process is specimen preparation. In this phase, the laboratory must look for the possible non-conforming specimens, especially for clot and hemolysis [9]. If the non-conforming specimen can be detected, rejections accompanied with suggestions for corrective method should be provided to the client [1].

Table 20.1. (Continued)

Phase	Brief details
2. Analytical process	o Gulati and Hyun said that the three very important aspects of quality control for laboratory analysis in hematology were calibration of automated instruments, monitoring of accuracy and precision of instruments and procedures, and verifying the reliability of test results [8]. As a rule, all analytical methods must be documented and traceable. All material including reagent and equipment should be well controlled. All personnel must be certified for their jobs: ones who relate to the result validation should be registered and authorized. Concerning the analytical methods, the common pitfalls usually relate to lack of method evaluation before and after start of service. The lack of reference values for the laboratory is another common pitfall. Indeed, the reference values of hematological study are very variable laboratory by laboratory [6 – 7]. Concerning the reagent, the evaluation before and after usage of each lot of reagent is necessary. The results of evaluation must be recorded and kept as evidence for traceability. The labeling of in use reagent is necessary; including opening data, expired date and lot number. A combination of commercial controls and retained or fresh patient blood specimens is recommended for monitoring of accuracy and precision on a long- and short-term basis [8]. Concerning the equipment, all equipment must have their own specific history, indicating manufacturer, supplier, history of fixing, maintenance, setting and movement. All equipment must be certified and calibrated: it should be noted that calibration must be performed. In addition, all analytical processes must be under the internal quality control and external quality assessment program, which international proficiency test is preferred. Participation in an external quality assessment program offers the most practical means of monitoring overall work performance in comparison with instrument, method, and/or reagent-based peer group data [8]. A laboratory may choose to participate in one or more national and/or regional quality control programs, depending upon the range of tests it performs and the requirements of accreditation and regulatory agencies [8]. However, in case that the resource is limited, inter-laboratory assessment is acceptable [8]. In addition, all documents relating to the quality control and assessment program must be collected and kept as evidence for traceability.
3. Post-analytical process	o After complete analysis, the laboratory must be systematically validated by the authorized medical personnel. The personnel who validate must sign for their responsibility. Repeated recheck for every step is recommended. In case that the laboratory information system (LIS) is used, the validation and maintenance for the LIS as well as recheck for the agreement of the results in intra-laboratory and extra-laboratory screens are necessary [13]. In case that the laboratory itself distributes the laboratory result, the process to prevent the lost of the results must be set. Also, there must be the process to keep the patient confidence.

Table 20.2. Resource management for the laboratory

Item	Brief details
1. Man	o The common pitfalls are due to lack of job description (JD) and job specification (JS) document, lack of organization chart and lack of future education plan for the laboratory personnel. Therefore, it is necessary to complete the mentioned aspects.
2. Material	o The common pitfalls are due to lack of good stocking system for laboratory material and lack of evaluation of suppliers. The specific protocols for purchasing, evaluation and monitoring of all laboratory materials are necessary.
3. Money	o The common pitfalls are due to lack of unit cost evaluation, lack of revenue analysis, lack of purchasing plan and lack of a future plan for proper workload of service. Wiwanitkit proposed that the "money" becomes an important factor in organizing of any laboratory setting at present, therefore, each laboratory should perform its own laboratory unit cost analysis [14]. Cost containment and budgeting becomes a necessity in laboratory management in this era [15].
4. Management	o The common pitfalls are lack of management review, lack of policies planning and review and lack of continuous TQM plan.

2. Some Aspects in Technical Process for Hemoglobin Determination

As mentioned in the previous chapter, the hemoglobin determination is the core hematology laboratory in the diagnosis of anemia. Similar to other hematological tests, the quality management in the pre-analytic phase for hemoglobin determination is necessary. First, the general principles for blood collection are necessary. Prolonged tourniquet may result in hemoconcentration. However, Campbell *et al.* said that there is no clinically significant difference in hemoglobin due to the hemoconcentration [16]. Some non-experienced practitioners might collect the blood sample from the site with intravenous fluid infusion and the hemodilution can be expected. Second, some interference factors including lipedmia and hyperbilirubinemia, for hemoglobin determination should be noted. Indeed, those interference factors usually make the detected hemoglobin level lower than the actual level. Concerning lipemia, it can not only affect the standard hemoglobin level but also the determination of specific forms of hemoglobin. Garrib *et al.* noted for the artifactually low glycated hemoglobin in the patient with type II diabetes mellitus and severe hypertriglyceridemia [17]. Concerning hyperbilirubinemia, Wong and Schenkel said that owing to the overlapping absorption bands of hemoglobin and bilirubin, spectrophotometric determination of plasma free hemoglobin has been plagued by the interference of bilirubin when the latter is present in significant concentration [18]. Finally, the laboratory should reject the non - conformance specimen, especially those with a clot since the detected hemoglobin level will be decreased.

Concerning analytical process, if the specimen is not well controlled for the interference and non - conformation, the incorrect laboratory result can be expected. The poor quality management for materials and instruments can also result in a false result. In addition, the usage of automated hematology analyzer can provide errors in hemoglobin determination in some cases such as high white blood cell count, incomplete red blood cell lysis in the analytical process and high fraction of carboxyhemoglobin. Of interest, these problems can be solved by the standard manual determination. Considering high white blood cell count, Du *et al.* noted that abnormally higher WBC might lead to increase of error in the detection of hemoglobin concentration; the ultimate result in close proximity to true hemoglobin concentration of whole blood samples with abnormally higher WBC could be acquired through the linear regression equation [19]. Considering incomplete red blood cell lysis, the incorrect low hemoglobin level can be seen. Concerning high carboxyhemoglobin level, it can turn to cyanmethemoglobin and consequently incorrect hemoglobin level can be expected. Concerning the reference value, although there are a variety of normal ranges in different settings, the standard criteria for diagnosis should be used.

Concerning post-analytical process, the result validation is important. The repeated recheck before reporting the result is necessary. In addition, it should be confirmed that the correct laboratory result reaches correct subject. The general practitioner should also focus on the possibility of incorrect laboratory result due to the incorrect reporting.

Quality System for the Hematology Laboratory in the Tropical Countries

Similar to other regions of the world, the quality system is necessary for all laboratories in the tropical countries. Since quality is universal, therefore, it can be applied in any setting. Hematology has a key role in diagnosis and patient management by selecting tests for their clinical relevance and utility for the specific circumstances, and ensuring their technical reliability when used in health clinics and point-of-care testing [20]. Although they lack resources, quality management is necessary for the developing countries. WHO has proposed a basic menu of tests in three categories: (a) tests such as hemoglobin screen which can be performed by nurses, midwives, health-aides or community doctors, (b) tests such as hemoglobinometry, microhaematocrit and microscopic examination of stained preparations which can be performed by a technician or laboratory assistant in a health centre, (c) tests requiring greater technical expertise of a laboratory technician or trained doctor [20]. Concerning developing countries, Lewis said that the peripheral health clinics and district laboratories should be familiar with the guidelines on standardized methods for collecting and storing specimens and transporting them to a regional laboratory or a reference center [20]. Lewis also noted that a training syllabus should be provided at the health centres and district laboratories, and this should include on-site instruction from supervisors and access to training manuals and distance-learning material [20]. Of particular concern is the reliable diagnosis and management of anemia [20]. Lewis said that a periphery laboratory has an important potential role in the resource-limited environment where anemia screening presently usually depends on unreliable clinical examination [20]. Therefore, the quality management is necessary in any setting including the periphery laboratory. Concerning the quality system for the hematology laboratory in tropical countries, there are some previous reports on this topic. The details of some interesting publications are presented as the following.

1. Tropical Asia

Tatsumi and Lewis said that international standardization on hematology was focused on the developed system but not for the developing system [21]. Tatsumi and Lewis noted that established standardized documents therefore would not be unsuitable for Asian societies [21]. International Council for Standardization in Hematology (ICSH) for Asia has been found and is divided into 5 region sub-groups, including the three tropical regions: Southeast Asia, South Asia and West Asia [21]. In Southeast Asia, Bunyaratvej said that there were around 2,000 clinical laboratories in private and government hospitals in Thailand and by the end of the year 2004, all of these laboratories are required to use the same or comparable standards nationwide [22 - 23]. At this time, Thailand is very conscious of quality in every field, including hospitals, and internal and external quality controls are one of the recommendations of the quality standard [24]. To run the standard system of hematology laboratories in Thailand, Bunyaratvej proposed three main aspects: standardization in process, method selection and academic interpretation [22]. Because of the wide spectrum of anemic blood diseases in Thailand: thalassemia, iron deficiency anemia and G6PD deficiency hemolytic disease, Bunyaratvej said that the analysis and interpretation of laboratory results using different technology were of great importance [22 -23]. Veloso *et al.* reported the overview of the two National External Quality Assessment Schemes (NEQAS) in Hematology in [25]. The first survey was conducted in December 1999 and the second in August 2000, with 95 and 187 laboratories, using mostly automated analyzers, participating respectively [25]. According to the first survey, no outlier were detected in each peer group after analysis by the 'Peer Group Mean and SDI' method [25]. Using the clinical laboratory improvement act of 1988 proficiency testing criteria (CLIA'88), all results were satisfactory for hemoglobin [25]. For the second survey, about 23 (12.6%) participants showed an abnormality in at least one parameter after analysis by the 'Peer Group Mean and SDI' [25]. Using CLIA'88, 8 Hemoglobin (9.7%) and 15 hematocrit (19.0%) were unsatisfactory [25]. Veloso *et al.* mentioned that the second NEQAS study was marked by a much larger sample size and better results [25]. Timan *et al.* noted that the National Program on External Quality Assessment Scheme (NEQAS) in Indonesia was first started in 1979, organized by the Indonesian Ministry of Health collaborating with professional bodies [26]. The first trial was for clinical chemistry test with 2 cycles per year, followed by the hematology NEQAS in 1986 in collaboration with WHO-Royal Post Graduate Medical School London [26]. Timan *et al.* said that participation in this NEQAS was mandatory for obtaining the laboratory license, and the Ministry of Health uses these schemes as one of the means for monitoring and coordinating the performance of laboratories throughout Indonesia [26].

Concerning South Asia, Shukla noted that National External Quality Assessment Programme (NEQAP) was taken at the Annual conference at Bombay in December, 1989

[27]. Shukla said that its unique feature was that it was truly multiparametric including clinical chemistry, hematology, microbiology and cytology and it covers about 300 labs from all corners of India [27]. Sah *et al.* reported their experience of quality assurance in hematology laboratory at B.P. Koirala Institute of Health Sciences, Nepal. They said that variations related to errors in manual and autopipetting, calibration and inter-observer differences had been noted from time to time and rectified [28]. Concerning West Asia, Bilto performed interlaboratory surveys to assess the analytical quality of Jordanian haematology laboratories [29]. The study surveyed 50 laboratories constituting the majority of clinical laboratories in the central region of Jordan using 15 control specimens of whole fresh blood and eight freshly prepared blood smears [29]. Bilto said that more than 97% of Jordanian laboratories using cell counters achieved the medically useful criteria for analytical performance, this figure was reduced to 84% in laboratories using manual methods [29]. Bilto noted that Jordanian laboratories were far from achieving the analytical goals that have been proposed based on intraindividual biological variation, therefore, there was a need for a national EQA scheme in hematology, to reach a common level of standardization [29].

2. Africa

The concepts of quality management in the hematology laboratory is widely used in Africa as well [30]. Dhatt *et al.* reported performance of South African laboratories in an External Quality Assurance scheme for hemoglobin A1c in South Africa [31]. Dhatt *et al.* said that a number of laboratories and methods did not meet the required analytical standards [31]. Dhatt *et al.* concluded that South African laboratories should adopt measures similar to other regional and national initiatives to significantly improve laboratory performance and bring about harmonization of hemoglobin A1c assays [31]. Kassu and Aseffa performed a study to identify current problems in laboratory services and elicit suggestions from the technicians aimed at improving the services in health centres within Amhara region, north Ethiopia and found that there was a great shortage of manpower, equipment, chemicals and other supplies to provide adequate laboratory services in the health centers within the region [32]. They noted that the laboratories were functioning below capacity consequently [32]. Gray and Carter also said that the technology had to be imported in most African countries by economies barely able to sustain the basic requirements of human life [33]. They said that health care was under the same capricious rule as all other public services: investment in laboratories was poor and most had no access to a professional laboratory at all and more investment, not less; expansion of pathology services not restricting them, was needed throughout the continent [33].

3. Latin America

Similar to other tropical areas, quality becomes the goal of hematology laboratories in the Latin America. However, Fink *et al.* said that many laboratories in Latin American countries did not have appropriate systems in place to evaluate and control quality [34]. Fink *et al.*

noted that the Pan American Health Organization sponsored a course in quality control in hematology during the XI Latin American Congress of Clinical Biochemistry (Mexico, 1993), in which representatives from Argentina, Chile, Cuba, Mexico, Paraguay, Dominican Republic, and Uruguay participated [34]. According to the course, the specific tasks carried out were: (1) determination of values for hemoglobin, hematocrit, and red and white blood cell counts by the procedures normally used in each laboratory; (2) recording of the data on special reporting forms; and (3) transmittal of those forms to the coordinator in each country [34]. According to this course, comparative analysis of the results showed the coefficients of variation (CV) of the hematocrit (4.5%), red blood cell count (11.0%), and white blood cell count (22.2%) to be higher than those reported from the United States of America and Europe and the only statistically significant result when analysis of variance (ANOVA) was used on data broken down by country and by procedure, was for leukocyte count [34]. Fink *et al.* concluded that training in the preparation of quality control materials and the subsequent use of these materials in pilot surveys could provide a starting point for establishing continuous internal and external quality assessment systems in hematology [34].

References

[1]   Wiwanitkit V. Types and frequency of preanalytical mistakes in the first Thai ISO 9002:1994 certified clinical laboratory, a 6 - month monitoring. *BMC Clin Pathol* 2001;1:5.

[2]   Freedman DB. Clinical governance--bridging management and clinical approaches to quality in the UK. *Clin Chim Acta* 2002;319:133-41.

[3]   Hernandez JS. Cost-effectiveness of laboratory testing. *Arch Pathol Lab Med* 2003;127:440-5.

[4]   Plebani M. Appropriateness in programs for continuous quality improvement in clinical laboratories. *Clin Chim Acta* 2003;333:131-9.

[5]   Dybkaer R. Quality assurance, accreditation, and certification: needs and possibilities. *Clin Chem* 1994;40(7 Pt 2):1416-20.

[6]   Dati F. Quality management and standardization programs in hemostaseology. *J Int Fed Clin Chem* 1996; 8:110-6.

[7]   Tatsumi N, Takubo T, Tsuda I, Hino M. Current problems in quality control (QC) in hematology. *Rinsho Byori*. 1997;45:997-1002.

[8]   Gulati GL, Hyun BH. Quality control in hematology. *Clin Lab Med* 1986;6:675-88.

[9]   Wiwanitkit V. Rejection of specimens for prothrombin time and relating pre-analytical factors in blood collection. *Blood Coagul Fibrinolysis* 2002;13:371-2.

[10] Banfi G, Dolci A. Preanalytical phase of sport biochemistry and haematology. *J Sports Med Phys Fitness* 2003;43:223-30.

[11] Narayanan S. *The preanalytic phase. An important component of laboratory medicine. Am J Clin Pathol* 2000;113:429-52.

[12] Wiwanitkit V. Modern concepts for venipuncture clinic setting. *Chula Med J* 2001; 45: 465 – 71.

[13] Wiwanitkit V. Laboratory information management system. *Chula Med J* 2000; 44: 887 – 91.

[14] Wiwanitkit V. Analysis and evaluation of unit cost of the laboratory investigations. *Srinagarind Med J* 2001; 16: 139 – 44.

[15] Carmichael ST. New laboratory start-up in the 21st century. *Trends Neurosci* 2002;25:287-8.

[16] Campbell NR, Edwards AL, Brant R, Jones C, Mitchell D. Effect on lipid, complete blood count and blood proteins of a standardized preparation for drawing blood: a randomized controlled trial. *Clin Invest Med* 2000;23:350-4.

[17] Garrib A, Griffiths W, Eldridge P, Hatton R, Worsley A, Crook M. Artifactually low glycated haemoglobin in a patient with severe hypertriglyceridaemia. *J Clin Pathol* 2003;56:394-5.

[18] Wong SS, Schenkel OJ. Quantification of plasma hemoglobin in the presence of bilirubin with bilirubin oxidase. *Ann Clin Lab Sci* 1995;25:247-51.

[19] Du ZL, Hu ZQ, Yang H, Chen L, Chen Q, Liu XQ. The influence of abnormally higher WBC on hemoglobin determination and its redress. *Sichuan Da Xue Xue Bao Yi Xue Ban* 2004;35:549-51.

[20] Lewis SM. Laboratory practice at the periphery in developing countries. *Int J Hematol* 2002;76 Suppl 1:294-8.

[21] Tatsumi N, Lewis SM. Restructuring of international council for standardization in haematology (ICSH) in Asia. *Int J Hematol* 2002;76 Suppl 1:281-5.

[22] Bunyaratvej A. Plan and process for hematology laboratory standard in Thailand. *Southeast Asian J Trop Med Public Health* 1999;30 Suppl 3:173-6.

[23] Bunyaratvej A. Strategic plan and action plan for standardization and harmonization of hematology laboratories in Thailand. *Southeast Asian J Trop Med Public Health* 2002;33 Suppl 2:83-5.

[24] Opartkiattikul N, Bejrachandra S. The external quality assessment schemes in Thailand. *Rinsho Byori* 2002;50:121-5.

[25] Veloso DJ, Saavedra MA Jr, Mendoza RD, Mauhay SM, Tulio RP, Shirakami A, Fujimoto K, Maramba TP. Second national external quality assessment scheme in hematology: the Philippine experience. *Southeast Asian J Trop Med Public Health* 2002;33 Suppl 2:48-56.

[26] Timan IS, Aulia D, Santoso W. External quality assessment scheme and laboratory accreditation in Indonesia. *Rinsho Byori* 2002; 50:126-30.

[27] Shukla PK. Report of NEQAP--the ten years growth success. *Indian J Pathol Microbiol* 2000;43:493-506.

[28] Sah SP, Raj GA, Prakash MB. Quality assurance programme in haematology at a teaching hospital in the eastern region of Nepal. *Indian J Pathol Microbiol* 1999;42:145-9.

[29] Bilto YY. Consensus and accuracy in haematology laboratories of developing countries: the Jordanian experience. *Clin Lab Haematol* 1999;21:11-5.

[30] Lema RA. Quality control in haematology and blood transfusion in sub-Saharan region of Africa. *East Afr Med J* 1993;70(4 Suppl):21-2.

[31] Dhatt GS, Pum JK, Viljoen A, Jenner W. Evaluation of HbA1C results in an external quality assessment scheme in South Africa. *Clin Chim Acta* 2003;331:147-51.

[32] Kassu A, Aseffa A. Laboratory services in health centres within Amhara region, north Ethiopia. *East Afr Med J* 1999;76:239-42.

[33] Gray IP, Carter JY. An evaluation of clinical laboratory services in sub-Saharan Africa. Ex Africa semper aliquid novi? *Clin Chim Acta* 1997;267:103-28.

[34] Fink NE, Fernandez Alberti A, Mazziotta D. External assessment of analytic quality in hematology: a necessity in Latin America. *Rev Panam Salud Publica* 1997;2:181-8.

Index

B

C

J

K

N

S

U

V

W

X

Y